CNS RECEPTORS:
FROM MOLECULAR PHARMACOLOGY TO BEHAVIOR

Advances in Biochemical Psychopharmacology
Volume 37

Advances in Biochemical Psychopharmacology

Series Editors

E. Costa, M.D.

Chief, Laboratory of Preclinical Pharmacology
National Institute of Mental Health
Washington, D.C.

Paul Greengard, Ph.D.

Professor of Pharmacology
Yale University School of Medicine
New Haven, Connecticut

CNS Receptors:
From Molecular Pharmacology to Behavior

Advances in Biochemical Psychopharmacology
Volume 37

Volume Editors

Paul Mandel, M.D., Ph.D.
Professor of Biochemistry
Honorary Director, Centre de Neurochimie
du CNRS
Université Louis Pasteur
Faculté de Médecine
Strasbourg, France

Francis V. DeFeudis, Ph.D.
Professeur Conventionné
Université Louis Pasteur
Faculté de Médecine
Strasbourg, France

Raven Press ■ New York

Raven Press, 1140 Avenue of the Americas, New York, New York 10036

Made in the United States of America

Library of Congress Cataloging in Publication Data
Main entry under title:

CNS receptors.

    (Advances in biochemical psychopharmacology ; v. 37)
    Proceedings of an international symposium held in the
Couvent Ste.-Odile, France, Sept. 1–3, 1982, and sponsored
by the Centre national de la recherche scientifique.
    Includes bibliographical references and index.
    1. Neurotransmitter receptors—Congresses. 2. Drug
receptors—Congresses. 3. Neural receptors—Congresses.
4. Central nervous system—Congresses. I. Mandel, Paul,
1908– . II. DeFeudis, F. V. III. Centre national
de la recherche scientifique (France) IV. Title: C.N.S.
receptors. V. Series. [DNLM: 1. Receptors, Drug—
Congresses. 2. Receptors, Endogenous substances—Congresses. W1 AD437 v.37 / WK 102 C651 1982]
RM315.A4   vol.37   615′.78s   [615′.78]   83-11175
[QP364.7]
ISBN 0-89004-827-4

Preface

During the past ten years, there has occurred an exponential development of studies on CNS receptors. This activity has been stimulated by the introduction of radioligand-binding methods, as well as by improvements in other methodologies (e.g., electrophysiology, autoradiography, photoaffinity-labeling). However, it should be understood that the ligand-binding method is limited by the lack of linkage between ligand-receptor interaction and those molecular mechanisms that underlie the physiological response. Also, the significance of multiple ligand-binding sites, identified by either agonist or antagonist interaction, is not yet fully understood, although such heterogeneity could be related to the principal effect and to secondary effects of various ligands. Hence, it seems evident that further emphasis should be placed on isolating and characterizing the membrane receptors themselves. In any case, studies that have been conducted at the biochemical and physiological levels have led to the development of more sophisticated behavioral analyses, and thus to an expression of certain physiological mechanisms and certain behaviors in terms of changes in CNS receptor function.

It is for these reasons that we organized this volume. The latest research efforts of outstanding workers from various countries are presented. Receptor studies that are emphasized include those on inhibitory (e.g., GABA, glycine) and excitatory (e.g., glutamate, aspartate) amino acids, dopamine, acetylcholine, benzodiazepines, serotonin, and norepinephrine. Results obtained with a wide variety of techniques are described.

Taken together, the information provided herein should be of great value in further stimulating research on CNS receptor functions and should lead to advances in the therapeutic management of certain neurological-psychiatric disorders.

This volume will be of interest to neurobiologists, neuropharmacologists, and clinicians who wish to increase their knowledge of CNS receptors.

P. Mandel, M.D., Ph.D.
F. V. DeFeudis, Ph.D.

Acknowledgments

This volume presents the proceedings of an international symposium held in the Couvent Ste.-Odile, France, September 1–3, 1982. We wish to thank all the participants of the meeting, the members of the organizing committee, and Mme Caroline Charras, Mlle Simone Ott, and Mlle Nicole Salsmann, all of whom contributed significantly to the considerable success of the conference. We gratefully acknowledge the Centre National de la Recherche Scientifique for sponsoring the symposium.

Contents

Receptors for Excitatory Amino Acids

Contributors

T. Abe
Laboratory of Insect Toxicology
Institute of Physical and Chemical Research
Wako-City, Saitama 351, Japan

J. A. Apud
Institute of Pharmacology and Pharmacognosy
University of Milan
Via A. Del Sarto, 21
20129 Milan, Italy

M. S. Arenson
Department of Pharmacology
St. Bartholomew's Hospital Medical College
University of London
Charterhouse Square
London EC1M 6BQ, England

J. M. Arrang
Unité 109 de Neurobiologie
Centre Paul Broca de l'INSERM
2 ter, rue d'Alésia
75014 Paris, France

R. Ashkenazi
Rappaport Medical Research Center
Department of Pharmacology
Haifa, Israel

A. Barat
Centro de Biologia Molecular
CSIC-UAM
Canto Blanco
Madrid-34, Spain

A. Batuecas
Centro de Biologia Molecular
CSIC-UAM
Canto Blanco
Madrid-34, Spain

M. Baudry
Department of Psychobiology
University of California
Irvine, California 92717

J. Benavides
Centre de Recherche Delalande
10 rue des Carrières
92500 Rueil-Malmaison, France

D. Ben-Shachar
Rappaport Medical Research Center
Department of Pharmacology
Haifa, Israel

C. P. Berrie
Division of Molecular Pharmacology
National Institute for Medical Research
Mill Hill
London NW7 1AA, England

E. Berry-Kravis
Departments of Biochemistry and Pediatrics
Joseph P. Kennedy, Jr. Mental Retardation
Research Center
University of Chicago
H.M. Box 82; and
Wyler Children's Hospital
950 East 59th Street
Chicago, Illinois 60637

N. J. M. Birdsall
Division of Molecular Pharmacology
National Institute for Medical Research
Mill Hill
London NW7 1AA, England

J. J. Bourguignon
Centre de Neurochimie du CNRS
Université Louis Pasteur
5 Rue Blaise Pascal
67084 Strasbourg Cedex, France

R. C. Bourne
Division of Psychiatry
MRC Clinical Research Centre
Northwick Park Hospital
Harrow HA1 3UJ, England

C. Braestrup
A/S Ferrosan
Sydmarken 5
DK-2860 Soeborg, Denmark

C. L. Broekkamp
CNS Pharmacology Unit
Organon, Oss, The Netherlands

T. P. Burch
Division of Molecular Pharmacology
Department of Pharmacology
University of Texas Health Science Center
7703 Floyd Curl Drive
San Antonio, Texas 78284

A. S. V. Burgen
Division of Molecular Pharmacology
National Institute for Medical Research
Mill Hill
London NW7 1AA, England

I. C. Campbell
Department of Biochemistry
Institute of Psychiatry
De Crespigny Park
London SE5 8AF, England

C. Cash
Centre de Neurochimie du CNRS
Université Louis Pasteur
5 rue Blaise Pascal
67084 Strasbourg Cedex, France

B. Chan
Psychopharmacology Section
Clarke Institute of Psychiatry
250 College Street
Toronto, Ontario M5T 1R8, Canada

L. Ciesielski
Centre de Neurochimie du CNRS
Université Louis Pasteur
5 rue Blaise Pascal
67084 Strasbourg Cedex, France

D. Cocchi
Institute of Pharmacology
University of Milan
Via A. Del Sarto, 21
20129 Milan, Italy

J. Costentin
Laboratoire de Pharmacodynamie et de
    Physiologie
Université de Rouen
Avenue de l'Université, B.P. 97
76800 St. Etienne du Rouvray, France

C. W. Cotman
Department of Psychobiology
University of California
Irvine, California 92717

I. Creese
Department of Neurosciences
School of Medicine
University of California, San Diego
La Jolla, California 92093

A. J. Cross
Division of Psychiatry
MRC Clinical Research Centre
Northwick Park Hospital
Harrow HA1 3UJ, England

D. R. Curtis
Department of Pharmacology
The Australian National University
Canberra City, A.C.T. 2601, Australia

G. Dawson
Departments of Biochemistry and Pediatrics
Joseph P. Kennedy, Jr. Mental Retardation
    Research Center
University of Chicago
H.M. Box 82; and
Wyler Children's Hospital
950 East 59th Street
Chicago, Illinois 60637

F. V. DeFeudis
Faculté de Médecine
Université Louis Pasteur
67085 Strasbourg Cedex, France

B. A. Demeneix
Institut de Physiologie et de Chimie Biologique
Université Louis Pasteur
21 rue René Descartes
F-67084 Strasbourg, France

G. DeMontis
Second Department of Pharmacology
University of Cagliari
Cagliari, Italy

M. Désarménien
Institut de Physiologie et de Chimie Biologique
Université Louis Pasteur
21 rue René Descartes
F-67084 Strasbourg, France

E. Desaulles
INSERM U-243
Faculté de Pharmacie
Université Louis Pasteur
67-Illkirch-Graffenstaden, France

R. Di Carlo
Institute of Pharmacology (2nd Chair)
University of Turin
Corso Raffaello, 30
10125 Torino, Italy

J. Drejer
Department of Biochemistry A
The Panum Institute
University of Copenhagen
DK-2200 Copenhagen, Denmark

I. Dubuc
Laboratoire de Pharmacodynamie et
    Physiologie
Université de Rouen
Avenue de l'Université, B.P. 97
76800 St. Etienne de Rouvray, France

A. M. Duchemin
Unité 109 de Neurobiologie
Centre Paul Broca de l'INSERM
2 ter, rue d'Alésia
75014 Paris, France

G. E. Fagg
Friedrich Miescher Institut
P.O. Box 273
CH-4002 Basel, Switzerland

E. Falch
Department of Chemistry BC
The Royal Danish School of Pharmacy
2 Universitetsparken
DK-2100 Copenhagen, Denmark

P. Feltz
Institut de Physiologie et de Chimie Biologique
Université Louis Pasteur
21 rue René Descartes
F-67084 Strasbourg, France

G. A. Foster
Department of Physiology and Pharmacology
School of Biochemical and Physiological
    Sciences
University of Southampton
Southampton S09 3TU, England

P. A. Frankham
Department of Biochemistry
The Medical School
Queen's Medical Centre
Nottingham NG7 2UH, England

S. J. Gamble
Division of Psychiatry
MRC Clinical Research Centre
Northwick Park Hospital
Harrow HA1 3UJ, England

M. Garbarg
Unité 109 de Neurobiologie
Centre Paul Broca de l'INSERM
2 ter, rue d'Alésia
75014 Paris, France

M. A. Gillman
Department of Experimental and Clinical
    Pharmacology
University of Witwatersrand Medical School
Johannesburg, South Africa

C. Goetz
Groupe NB, INSERM U-114
Collège de France
F-75005 Paris, France

C. Gomeni
Centre de Recherche Delalande
10 rue des Carrières
92500 Rueil-Malmaison, France

J. Gómez-Barriocanal
Centro de Biologia Molecular
CSIC-UAM
Canto Blanco
Madrid-34, Spain

H. Gozlan
Groupe NB, INSERM U-114
Collège de France
F-75005 Paris, France

J. M. Hall
Department of Biochemistry
The Medical School
Queen's Medical Centre
Nottingham NG7 2UH, England

R. Hammer
Division of Molecular Pharmacology
National Institute for Medical Research
Mill Hill
London NW7 1AA, England

M. Hamon
Groupe NB, INSERM U-114
Collège de France
F-75005 Paris, France

J. A. Heltzel
Biosciences Research
3M Center
St. Paul, Minnesota 55144

T. Honoré
A/S Ferrosan
Sydmarken 5
DK-2860 Soeborg, Denmark

E. Hösli
Department of Physiology
University of Basel
CH-4051 Basel, Switzerland

L. Hösli
Department of Physiology
University of Basel
CH-4051 Basel, Switzerland

E. C. Hulme
Division of Molecular Pharmacology
National Institute for Medical Research
Mill Hill
London NW7 1AA, England

Y. Ito
Department of Pharmacology
Kyoto Prefectural University of Medicine
Kawaramachi-Hirokoji
Kamikyo-ku, Kyoto 602, Japan

E. Iuliano
Institute of Pharmacology and Pharmacognosy
University of Milan
Via A. Del Sarto, 21
20129 Milan, Italy

N. Kawai
Department of Neurobiology
Tokyo Metropolitan Institute for Neurosciences
Fuchu-City, Tokyo 183, Japan

E. Kempf
Centre de Neurochimie du CNRS
Université Louis Pasteur
5 rue Blaise Pascal
67084 Strasbourg Cedex, France

P. Kontro
Department of Biomedical Sciences
University of Tampere
Box 607
SF-33101 Tampere 10, Finland

G. W. Kreutzberg
Nerve Cell Biology Group
Max Planck Institute for Psychiatry
Kraepelinstrasse 2
8 Munich 40, Federal Republic of Germany

P. Krogsgaard-Larsen
Department of Chemistry BC
The Royal Danish School of Pharmacy
2 Universitetsparken
DK-2100 Copenhagen, Denmark

K. Kuriyama
Department of Pharmacology
Kyoto Prefectural University of Medicine
Kawaramachi-Hirokoji
Kamikyo-ku, Kyoto 602, Japan

J. D. Leah
Department of Pharmacology
The Australian National University
Canberra City, A.C.T. 2601, Australia

K. S. Lee
Nerve Cell Biology Group
Max Planck Institute for Psychiatry
Kraepelinstrasse 2
8 Munich 40, Federal Republic of Germany

S. Leff
Department of Neurosciences
School of Medicine
University of California, San Diego
La Jolla, California 92093

R. Lehmann
Department of Physiology
University of Basel
CH-4051 Basel, Switzerland

J. E. Leysen
Department of Biochemical Pharmacology
Janssen Pharmaceutica
B-2340 Beerse, Belgium

F. J. Lichtigfeld
Department of Experimental and Clinical
Pharmacology
University of Witwatersrand Medical School
Johannesburg, South Africa

K. G. Lloyd
CNS Pharmacology Unit
L.E.R.S.-Synthélabo
31 Avenue P.V. Couturier
F-92220 Bagneux, France

V. Locatelli
Institute of Pharmacology
University of Milan
Via A. Del Sarto, 21
20129 Milan, Italy

J. P. Loeffler
Institut de Physiologie et de Chimie Biologique
Université Louis Pasteur
21 rue René Descartes
F-67084 Strasbourg, France

T. W. Lutz
Department of Physiology
University of Basel
CH-4051 Basel, Switzerland

G. Lynch
Department of Psychobiology
University of California
Irvine, California 92717

G. Mack
Centre de Neurochimie du CNRS
Université Louis Pasteur
5 rue Blaise Pascal
67084 Strasbourg Cedex, France

B. K. Madras
Psychopharmacology Section
Clarke Institute of Psychiatry
250 College Street
Toronto, Ontario M5T 1R8, Canada

M. Maitre
Centre de Neurochimie du CNRS
Université Louis Pasteur
5 rue Blaise Pascal
67084 Strasbourg Cedex, France

P. Mandel
Centre de Neurochimie du CNRS
Université Louis Pasteur
5 rue Blaise Pascal
67084 Strasbourg Cedex, France

E. Manrique
Centro de Biologia Molecular
CSIC-UAM
Canto Blanco
Madrid-34, Spain

J. C. Marvizon
Centre de Recherche Delalande
10 rue des Carrières
92500 Rueil-Malmaison, France

R. M. McKernan
Department of Biochemistry
Institute of Psychiatry
De Crespigny Park
London SE5 8AF, England

E. Meier
Department of Biochemistry A
The Panum Institute
University of Copenhagen
DK-2200 Copenhagen, Denmark

E. E. Mena
Department of Psychobiology
University of California
Irvine, California 92717

K. N. Mewett
Department of Pharmacology
The Medical School
University Walk
Bristol BS8 1TD, England

A. Miwa
Department of Neurobiology
Tokyo Metropolitan Institute for Neurosciences
Fuchu-City, Tokyo 183, Japan

H. Möhler
Pharmaceutical Research Department
F. Hoffmann-La Roche & Co., Ltd.
CH-4002 Basel, Switzerland

G. Muccioli
Institute of Pharmacology (2nd Chair)
University of Turin
Corso Raffaello, 30
10125 Torino, Italy

E. E. Müller
Institute of Pharmacology
University of Milan
Via A. Del Sarto, 21
20129 Milan, Italy

D. L. Nelson
Department of Pharmacology and Toxicology
College of Pharmacy
University of Arizona
Tucson, Arizona 85721

M. Nielsen
Sct. Hans Mental Hospital
4000 Roskilde, Denmark

C. J. E. Niemegeers
Department of Pharmacology
Janssen Pharmaceutica
B-2340 Beerse, Belgium

A. Nistri
Department of Pharmacology
St. Bartholomew's Hospital Medical College
University of London
Charterhouse Square
London EC1M 6BQ, England

D. J. Oakes
Department of Physiology
The Medical School
University Walk
Bristol BS8 1TD, England

G. Occhipinti
Istituto Fisiologia Umana
95125 Catania, Italy

S. S. Oja
Department of Biomedical Sciences
University of Tampere
Box 607
SF-33101 Tampere 10, Finland

R. W. Olsen
Division of Biomedical Sciences
Department of Biochemistry
University of California
Riverside, California 92521

H. J. Olverman
Department of Pharmacology
The Medical School
University Walk
Bristol BS8 1TD, England

J. M. Palacios
Preclinical Research
Sandoz, Ltd.
CH-4002 Basel, Switzerland

M. J. Peet
Department of Pharmacology
The Australian National University
Canberra City
A.C.T. 2601, Australia

P. Protais
Laboratoire de Pharmacodynamie et
 Physiologie
Université de Rouen
Avenue de l'Université, B.P. 97
76800 St. Etienne du Rouvray, France

S. Puglisi
Centre de Neurochimie du CNRS
Université Louis Pasteur
5 rue Blaise Pascal
67084 Strasbourg Cedex, France

T. T. Quach
Unité 109 de Neurobiologie
Centre Paul Broca de l'INSERM
2 ter, rue d'Alésia
75014 Paris, France

G. Racagni
Institute of Pharmacology and Pharmacognosy
University of Milan
Via A. Del Sarto, 21
20129 Milan, Italy

R. Ramanjaneyulu
Division of Molecular Pharmacology
Department of Pharmacology
University of Texas Health Science Center
7703 Floyd Curl Drive
San Antonio, Texas 78284

G. Ramírez
Centro de Biologia Molecular
CSIC-UAM
Canto Blanco
Madrid-34, Spain

M. Recasens
Department of Psychobiology
University of California
Irvine, California 92717

M. Reddington
Nerve Cell Biology Group
Max Planck Institute for Psychiatry
Kraepelinstrasse 2
8 Munich 40, Federal Republic of Germany

P. J. Roberts
Department of Physiology and Pharmacology
School of Biochemical and Physiological
Sciences
University of Southampton
Southampton S09 3TU, England

W. R. Roeske
University of Arizona
Health Sciences Center
Tucson, Arizona 85724

C. Rose
Unité 109 de Neurobiologie
Centre Paul Broca de l'INSERM
2 ter, rue d'Alésia
75014 Paris, France

J. F. Rumigny
Centre de Recherche Delalande
10 rue des Carrières
92500 Rueil-Malmaison, France

F. Saadoun
Department of Psychobiology
University of California
Irvine, California 92717

F. Santangelo
Istituto de Fisiologia Umana
95125 Catania, Italy

R. Schlichter
Institut de Physiologie et de Chimie Biologique
Université Louis Pasteur
21 rue René Descartes
F-67084 Strasbourg, France

A. Schousboe
Department of Biochemistry A
The Panum Institute
University of Copenhagen
DK-2200 Copenhagen, Denmark

P. Schubert
Nerve Cell Biology Group
Max Planck Institute for Psychiatry
Kraepelinstrasse 2
8 Munich 40, Federal Republic of Germany

J. C. Schwartz
Unité 109 de Neurobiologie
Centre Paul Broca de l'INSERM
2 ter, rue d'Alésia
75014 Paris, France

D. R. Sibley
Department of Neurosciences
School of Medicine
University of California, San Diego
La Jolla, California 92093

S. Simler
Centre de Neurochimie du CNRS
Université Louis Pasteur
5 rue Blaise Pascal
67084 Strasbourg Cedex, France

D. A. S. Smith
Department of Pharmacology
The Medical School
University Walk
Bristol BS8 1TD, England

F. A. Stephenson
Department of Biochemistry
Imperial College of Science and Technology
London SW7 2AZ, England

J. Stockton
Division of Molecular Pharmacology
National Institute for Medical Research
Mill Hill
London NW7 1AA, England

P. G. Strange
Department of Biochemistry
The Medical School
Queen's Medical Centre
Nottingham NG7 2UH, England

M. Strolin Benedetti
Centre de Recherche Delalande
10 rue des Carrières
92500 Rueil-Malmaison, France

W. Taylor
Department of Pharmacology and Toxicology
College of Pharmacy
University of Arizona
Tucson, Arizona 85721

F. Thuret
CNS Pharmacology Unit
L.E.R.S.-Synthélabo
31 Avenue P.V. Couturier
F-92220 Bagneux, France

R. Thyagarajan
Division of Molecular Pharmacology
Department of Pharmacology
University of Texas Health Science Center
7703 Floyd Curl Drive
San Antonio, Texas 78284

M. K. Ticku
Division of Molecular Pharmacology
Department of Pharmacology
University of Texas Health Science Center
7703 Floyd Curl Drive
San Antonio, Texas 78284

P. Van Gompel
Department of Biochemical Pharmacology
Janssen Pharmaceutica
B-2340 Beerse, Belgium

M. Verwimp
Department of Biochemical Pharmacology
Janssen Pharmaceutica
B-2340 Beerse, Belgium

G. Vincendon
Centre de Neurochimie du CNRS
Université Louis Pasteur
5 rue Blaise Pascal
67084 Strasbourg Cedex, France

W. H. Vogel
Department of Pharmacology
Thomas Jefferson University
Philadelphia, Pennsylvania 19107

J. L. Waddington
Royal College of Surgeons in Ireland
St. Stephen's Green
Dublin 2, Ireland

J. J. Warsh
Clarke Institute of Psychiatry
250 College Street
Toronto, Ontario M5T 1R8, Canada

J. C. Watkins
Department of Physiology
The Medical School
University Walk
Bristol BS8 1TD, England

M. Watson
University of Arizona
Health Sciences Center
Tucson, Arizona 85724

B. Weck
Department of Pharmacology and Toxicology
College of Pharmacy
University of Arizona
Tucson, Arizona 85721

C. G. Wermuth
Centre de Neurochimie du CNRS
Université Louis Pasteur
5 rue Blaise Pascal
67084 Strasbourg Cedex, France

M. Wheatley
Department of Biochemistry
The Medical School
Queen's Medical Centre
Nottingham NG7 2UH, England

P. M. Whitaker
Clarke Institute of Psychiatry
250 College Street
Toronto, Ontario M5T 1R8, Canada

E. H. F. Wong
Division of Molecular Pharmacology
National Institute for Medical Research
Mill Hill
London NW7 1AA, England

P. Worms
CNS Pharmacology Unit
L.E.R.S.-Synthélabo
31 Avenue P.V. Couturier
F-92220 Bagneux, France

H. I. Yamamura
Department of Pharmacology
University of Arizona
Health Sciences Center
Tucson, Arizona 85724

S. Yehuda
Rappaport Medical Research Center
Department of Pharmacology
Haifa, Israel

M. B. H. Youdim
Rappaport Medical Research Center
Department of Pharmacology
Haifa, Israel

C. Zehntner
Department of Physiology
University of Basel
CH-4051 Basel, Switzerland

M. J. Zigmond
Division of Molecular Pharmacology
National Institute for Medical Research
Mill Hill
London NW1 1AA, England

CNS Receptors—From Molecular Pharmacology to Behavior, edited by P. Mandel and F. V. DeFeudis. Raven Press, New York © 1983.

Molecular Pharmacology of the GABA Receptors and GABA Agonists

*P. Krogsgaard-Larsen, *E. Falch, †M. J. Peet, †J. D. Leah, and †D. R. Curtis

Department of Chemistry BC, The Royal Danish School of Pharmacy, DK-2100 Copenhagen, Denmark; and †Department of Pharmacology, The Australian National University, A.C.T. 2601, Australia

The neutral amino acid γ-aminobutyric acid (GABA) is an inhibitory neurotransmitter in the mammalian central nervous system (CNS) (11,33,57). GABA is involved in the central regulation of a variety of physiological processes including cardiovascular functions (19,20), secretion of certain hormones (21,25), food intake (5), and the sensation of pain (28) and anxiety (26). Furthermore, GABA appears to play a role in the pathophysiology of epilepsy (52) and Huntington's chorea (9). In Parkinson's disease there is an imbalance between GABA and dopamine (29), and neurochemical studies on brain tissue from patients dying with schizophrenia suggest impairments of the GABA functions in certain brain regions in this disease (61,63). Although the degree of complicity of GABA in schizophrenia and in neurological diseases (50) is unknown, there is an increasing interest in the pharmacology of GABA (34,39). In this review some aspects of the molecular pharmacology of GABA agonists will be discussed.

MULTIPLICITY OF GABA RECEPTORS

GABA neurones are ubiquitous in the mammalian CNS and most, if not all, central neurones are sensitive to GABA, rendering treatment of diseases with regioselective degeneration of GABA neurones with GABA agonists difficult. There is, however, evidence for the existence of different types of GABA receptors, and there is an urgent need for the development of specific GABA agonists and antagonists for each subpopulation of receptors.

Based on electrophysiological studies using the GABA antagonists bicuculline (BIC) or bicuculline methochloride (BMC) (14, 31) GABA receptors can be divided into two heterogeneous groups:

1) BIC-sensitive GABA receptors and
2) BIC-insensitive GABA receptors.

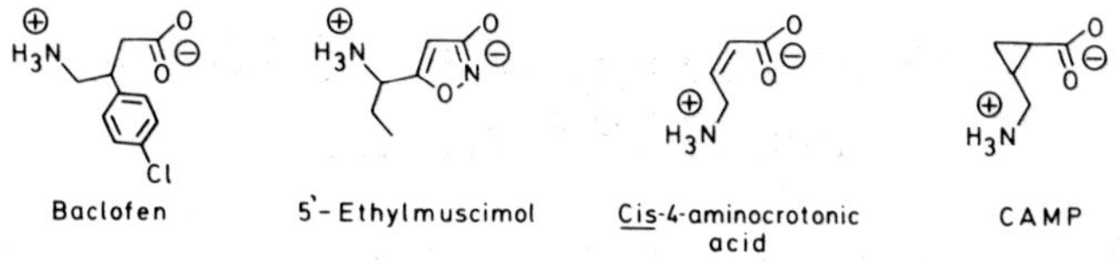

Baclofen   5'-Ethylmuscimol   Cis-4-aminocrotonic   CAMP
                                                  acid

FIG. 1. The structures of some BIC-insensitive GABA agonists.

Bicuculline-Sensitive GABA Receptors

The former class of receptors include *presynaptic* (axo-axonic) and *postsynaptic* (axo-somatic and axo-dendritic) receptors (10, 30). Studies on cat spinal neurones indicate that these receptors have very similar pharmacological characteristics (13). There is also evidence for *non-synaptic* GABA receptors (8,10). The physiological relevance of these receptors, which have agonist specificities different from those of synaptic GABA receptors (2), is unclear (1).

BIC-sensitive GABA receptors probably can be further subdivided. The relative potency of GABA and muscimol as BIC-sensitive neuronal depressants differs in the cat cerebral cortex and spinal cord (14,17). Furthermore, iso-THAZ (5,6,7,8-tetrahydro-4H-isoxazolo[3,4-d]azepin-3-ol) (Fig. 6) has antagonist properties at GABA receptors in the rat substantia nigra (4), whereas in the cat spinal cord iso-THAZ antagonizes glycine-induced neuronal depression without affecting the GABA receptors significantly (Fig. 7) (44). Finally, there is some evidence that BIC-sensitive GABA receptors in the neurohypophysis have characteristics different from those of the GABA receptors in cat spinal neurones (49).

Bicuculline-Insensitive GABA Receptors

The GABA analogue baclofen (Fig. 1) is a BIC-insensitive depressant of neuronal firing (15,18), and baclofen interacts with a population of binding sites, which bind GABA but not BIC or various BMC-sensitive GABA agonists (27). While these receptors seem to modulate the release of monoamines in the CNS (6) their relevance to the therapeutic effects of baclofen is unclear. Baclofen potently reduces monosynaptic excitation in the cat spinal cord, an effect which is unlikely to be mediated by GABA receptors (16).

Other groups of BIC-insensitive GABA receptors may exist in the mammalian CNS. While the depression of neuronal firing induced by 5'-ethylmuscimol (Fig. 1) is insensitive to BMC (46), this muscimol analogue does not interfere with the binding of baclofen (N. Bowery, unpublished). Furthermore, *cis*-4-aminocrotonic acid (32) and *cis*-2-(aminomethyl)cyclopropanecarboxylic acid

TABLE 1. Structure and activity *in vivo* and *in vitro* of GABA and some GABA analogues with known absolute configuration[a]

COMPOUND	REL. POTENCY OF BMC-SENSITIVE DEPRESSANT ACTION	INHIBITION OF THE RECEPTOR BINDING OF $IC_{50}(\mu M)$			ACTIVATION OF THE BINDING OF $EC_{50}(\mu M)$
		^3H-GABA	^3H-THIP	^3H-P4S	^3H-DIAZEPAM
GABA	— — —	0.033	0.014	0.021	3.8
(S)-(−)-5'-Methylmuscimol	— — (−)	0.64	0.74	5.8	230
(R)-(+)-5'-Methylmuscimol	— — (−)	19	9.5	8 3	2300
(S)-(−)-4-Methyl-trans-ACA	— — (−)	4.1	2.6	2 1	390
(R)-(+)-4-Methyl-trans-ACA	N.t.	1 4 8	8 8	6 7 0	>2000

[a]The binding studies using radioactive GABA, THIP, and P4S as ligands (23) and the studies on stimulation of diazepam binding (7) were performed as described earlier. The potency of the compounds *in vivo* was assessed relative to that of GABA (---) as described in detail in the legend for Fig. 2. N.t., not tested.

(CAMP) (3) (Fig. 1) are neuronal depressants insensitive to BMC or strychnine. More detailed studies of the mechanism underlying the effects of these GABA analogues must await the development of selective antagonists at BIC-insensitive GABA receptors.

The Postsynaptic GABA Receptor Complex

Electrophysiological methods, which offer the most direct approach to studies of receptor mechanisms, as well as receptor binding techniques have inherent limitations. The former method allows studies of alterations of neuronal membranes as a result of activation or blockade of the GABA receptors, but such experiments normally are not sufficiently precise to obtain quantitative data. The receptor sites studied in binding experiments (22), on the other hand, probably represent more or less disinte-

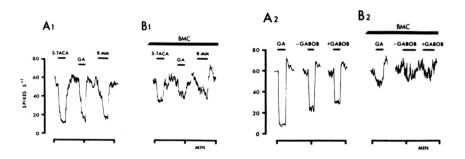

FIG. 2. A1–B1: Comparison of the effects of (S)-$(-)$-*trans*-4-me-
thyl-4-aminocrotonic acid (S-TACA; 0.1 M, pH 3.7, HCl, 45 nA),
GABA (GA; 0.2 M, pH 3, HCl, 25 nA), and (R)-$(+)$-5'-methylmuscimol
(R-MM; 0.1 M, pH 3.3, HCl, 50 nA) on a cat spinal Renshaw cell
(firing maintained with DL-homocysteic acid (DLH); 0.2 M, pH 7.5,
9 nA) before (A1), and just after (B1) the administration of BMC
(10 mM in 150 mM NaCl, 30 nA for 2.5 min). The effects of the
depressant amino acids recovered 5 min after B1. A2–B2: Comparison of the effects of GABA (GA; 0.1 M, pH 3, HCl, 20 nA) and
(S)-$(+)$- and (R)-$(-)$-3-hydroxy-GABA ($(+)$- and $(-)$-GABOB; 0.1 M,
pH 3.4, HCl, 20 nA) on the firing of a cat spinal Renshaw cell
(firing maintained by DLH: A2, 8 nA and B2 5.4 nA) before (A2)
and during (B2) the administration of BMC (10 mM in 150 mM NaCl,
20 nA for 3 min). The effects of the depressant amino acids recovered 2 min after B2.

grated forms of the physiological receptors, and interpretation
of binding data in terms of receptor mechanisms must be performed
with extreme care.
  As a result of an extensive amount of research using both
techniques a picture of the postsynaptic GABA receptor complex
begins to emerge. A chloride ionophore is controlled by a GABA
receptor, apparently consisting of three receptor sites (23,34)
and regulated by various additional units, which can be detected
as distinct binding sites for the benzodiazepines, the non-compe-

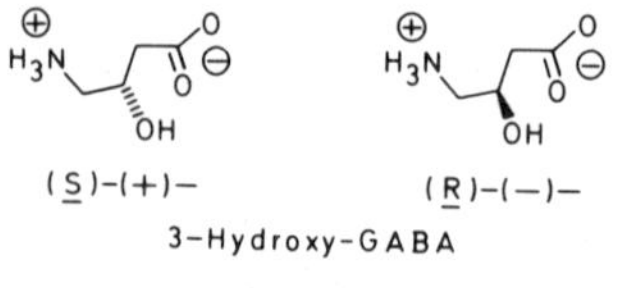

$$H_3\overset{\oplus}{N}\overset{}{\diagup}\underset{OH}{\overset{}{\diagdown}}\overset{O}{\underset{O_\ominus}{\diagup}}$$ $$H_3\overset{\oplus}{N}\overset{}{\diagup}\underset{OH}{\overset{}{\diagdown}}\overset{O}{\underset{O_\ominus}{\diagup}}$$

   $(\underline{S})$-$(+)$- $(\underline{R})$-$(-)$-

            3-Hydroxy-GABA

FIG. 3. The structures of (S)-$(+)$- and (R)-$(-)$-3-hydroxy-GABA.

titive GABA antagonist picrotoxinin, and the avermectins (30, 53). The physiological relevance of these additional sites in the GABA receptor complex, which have ligand specificities distinctly different from that of the receptor sites, is unknown.

BICUCULLINE-SENSITIVE GABA AGONISTS

Stereostructure-Activity Studies

There normally is a positive correlation between the potency of GABA agonists as inhibitors of GABA binding and as BIC-sensitive depressants of neuronal firing (36,45,55). Studies on some GABA analogues with known absolute configuration have, however, disclosed apparent discrepancies between *in vivo* and *in vitro* effects.

While (S)-(-)-5'-methylmuscimol is much more potent than the R-isomer as an inhibitor of the binding of radioactive GABA, THIP (4,5,6,7-tetrahydroisoxazolo[5,4-c]pyridin-3-ol), and P4S (piperidine-4-sulphonic acid) (23), these optical isomers were approximately equipotent, and slightly weaker than GABA, as BMC-sensitive neuronal depressants (Fig. 2, Table 1). Both optical enantiomers were tested on 17 cat spinal neurones. Similar relative and absolute potencies were observed for the S-(+)- and R-(-)-isomers of 3-hydroxy-GABA (Fig. 3) as BMC-sensitive depressants of cat spinal interneurones (14 interneurones tested) (D.R. Curtis, J.D. Leah, and M.J. Peet, unpublished) (Fig. 2), although the S-form (IC50 0.4 μM) is more potent than the R-form (IC50 2.0 μM) as an inhibitor of GABA binding. As reported earlier for (RS)-3-hydroxy-GABA (12) both isomers were slightly less potent than GABA.

Since neither (R)-(+)- nor (S)-(-)-5'-methylmuscimol interact with the GABA transport systems *in vitro* (34) it is unlikely that the rate of removal of these isomers from the synaptic environments after microelectrophoretic application is different. Consequently, these results seem to indicate that the degree of stereoselectivity of the GABA receptors and the GABA binding sites is different. The equipotency of the enantiomers of 3-hydroxy-GABA as depressants of neuronal firing compared with the difference in potency of these compounds as inhibitors of GABA binding may support this conclusion. The different relative potencies of these optical isomers *in vivo* and *in vitro* may, however, at least to some extent, be explained by the finding that the S-isomer is slightly more potent than the R-isomer in inhibiting glial and neuronal GABA uptake *in vitro* (58) and (A. Schousboe and P. Krogsgaard-Larsen, unpublished) suggesting that the S-form is being taken up more effectively than the R-isomer.

The difficulties in comparing the real effectiveness as GABA agonists of compounds with different affinities for the GABA uptake systems is exemplified in Fig. 2.A1. GABA is at least two orders of magnitude more potent than both (R)-(+)-5'-methylmuscimol and (S)-(-)-trans-4-methyl-4-aminocrotonic acid ((S)-(-)-4-methyl-trans-ACA) in inhibiting GABA binding (Table 1). Neverthe-

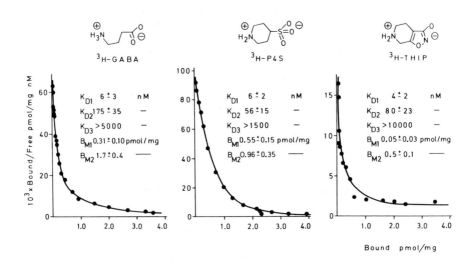

FIG. 4. Scatchard plots of the specific binding of radioactive
GABA, P4S, and THIP to rat brain synaptic membranes. The binding
parameters are derived from computer fitted non-linear regression
analysis of the data (23).

less, the apparent *in vivo* activity of GABA is only slightly
greater than those of the compounds concerned, none of which interact significantly with GABA uptake *in vitro* (34,59).

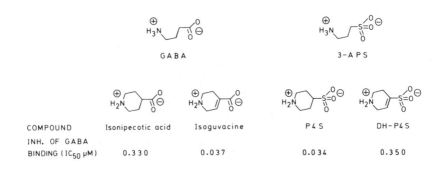

FIG. 5. The structures of GABA, 3-aminopropanesulphonic acid
(3-APS), and some cyclic analogues. The IC50 values of these
cyclic amino acids as inhibitors of GABA binding are from (43,45)
and (E. Falch and P. Krogsgaard-Larsen, unpublished).

P4S and Related GABA Agonists

Like isonipecotic acid and isoguvacine (41) the structurally
related amino sulphonic acid P4S is a very potent and specific
BMC-sensitive GABA agonist (43) indicating that these cyclic amino acids reflect the "receptor-active conformation" of GABA and
3-aminopropanesulphonic acid (3-APS), respectively (Fig. 5).
The very similar binding characteristics of GABA and P4S
(Fig. 4) (23,42) are in agreement with the conclusion from comparative microelectrophoretic studies that both compounds bind
to the same class of bicuculline-sensitive GABA receptors. This
is further supported by the same relative potency of a series of
optically active GABA analogues as inhibitors of the binding of
3H-GABA and 3H-P4S (Table 1) (23,34). If these compounds had to
compete with GABA and P4S for binding to different receptor sites
their *relative* potencies would have been different. On the other
hand, the *absolute* potencies of the inhibitors in these two series of experiments are different suggesting that the mechanism
of interaction of GABA and P4S with the GABA receptor sites is
somehow different. Accordingly, GABA and P4S affect the binding
of the benzodiazepines to the GABA receptor complex differently
in vitro (7,62). This difference is most pronounced at low temperatures and in the absence of chloride ions. Under these conditions GABA activates the binding of benzodiazepines, whereas
P4S is a deactivator. Under certain conditions the binding of
P4S has proved to be more sensitive to stimulation by barbiturates than the binding of GABA (54).
The effects of introduction of a double bond into the molecules of isonipecotic acid and P4S are different. While isoguvacine is an order of magnitude more potent than isonipecotic acid
as an inhibitor of GABA binding (43,45) and as a BMC-sensitive
neuronal depressant (41) the unsaturated analogue of P4S,
1,2,3,6-tetrahydropyridine-4-sulphonic acid (DH-P4S) is ten times
weaker than P4S as an inhibitor of GABA binding (Fig. 5) (E.
Falch and P. Krogsgaard-Larsen, unpublished). This observation
seems to support the conclusion that the replacement of the car-
boxylate group by a sulphonate group affects the mechanism of interaction of the compounds concerned with BIC-sensitive GABA receptors. The character of these changes is still unknown. It is
interesting to note that P4S is virtually inactive at receptors
in central neurones of the invertebrates *Periplaneta* and *Limulus*,
which otherwise have agonist specificities similar to that of
BIC-sensitive GABA receptors in the mammalian CNS (56).

Muscimol, THIP and Related Compounds

Muscimol and the structurally related compounds dihydromusci-
mol and thiomuscimol (Fig. 6) are more potent than GABA as BMC-
sensitive GABA agonists (45). Lack of specificity does, however,
limit the importance of these compounds as tools for studies of
GABA receptor mechanisms (45).
An extensive number of analogues of muscimol have been pre-

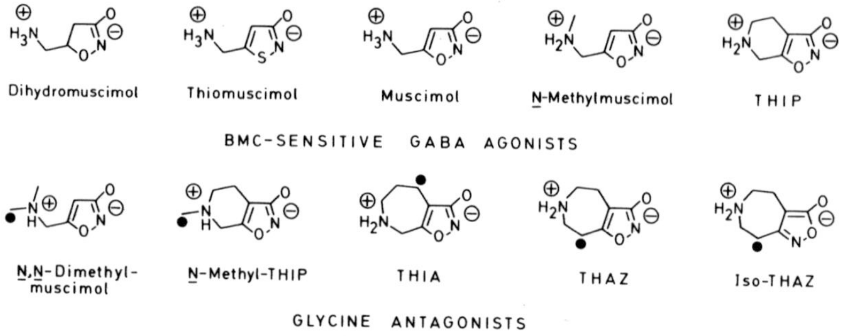

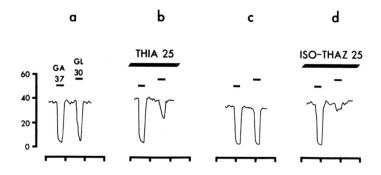

| Dihydromuscimol | Thiomuscimol | Muscimol | N-Methylmuscimol | THIP |

BMC-SENSITIVE GABA AGONISTS

| N,N-Dimethyl-muscimol | N-Methyl-THIP | THIA | THAZ | Iso-THAZ |

GLYCINE ANTAGONISTS

FIG. 6. The structures of some BMC-sensitive GABA agonists and some closely related glycine antagonists. The dots indicate the positions of the additional carbon atoms, which have converted GABA agonists into glycine antagonists.

pared in an attempt to develop specific agonists. With the exception of the S- and R-isomers of 5'-methylmuscimol (Table 1) and 5'-ethylmuscimol (Fig. 1), which depress the firing of central neurones in a manner sensitive and insensitive to BMC, respectively, most simple analogues of muscimol have little or no effect on GABA receptors *in vivo* or *in vitro* (36,37,46). These studies have demonstrated that at least two hydrogen atoms on the

FIG. 7. The effects of THIA and iso-THAZ on the inhibition of a cat spinal interneurone by glycine (GL) and GABA (GA) administered electrophoretically with the indicated currents (nA) and for the times indicated by the horizontal bars (one unit is 30 sec). (a) Before and (b) during the administration of THIA (25 nA); (c) 2 min after THIA; (d) during the administration of iso-THAZ (25 nA). Complete recovery of the effects of glycine occurred 6 min after the ejection of iso-THAZ was terminated. For details see (44).

TABLE 2. <u>GABA agonist activity and I/U-ratios of some GABA ana-
logues</u>[a]

STRUCTURE	GABA AGONIST ACTIVITY		pK$_A$ VALUES	I/U-RATIO	PENETRATION
	Receptor affinity in vitro (IC$_{50}$, µM)	Rel. potency in vivo			of the blood brain barrier
GABA	0.033	— — —	4.0 ; 10.7	—	No
P4S	0.034	— — — —	< 1 ; 10.3	> 1000000	No
Isoguvacine	0.037	— — — —	3.6 ; 9.8	200000	No
THIP	0.13	— — — (−)	4.4 ; 8.5	500	Yes
Thio-THIP	42	—	6.1 ; 8.5	16	N.t.

[a]The inhibition of GABA binding (23), the BMC-sensitive effects
on cat spinal neurones (41,43), and the I/U-ratios (40) were measured as described earlier.

charged amino group is a necessary, but not sufficient condition
for GABA agonist activity. Thus, both *N*-methylmuscimol and THIP
are BMC-sensitive GABA agonists (Fig. 6), THIP being the more potent compound (Table 2) (41,44). Neither *N*,*N*-dimethylmuscimol
nor *N*-methyl-THIP possesses GABA agonist activity, whereas both
compounds antagonize glycine-induced depression of the firing of
cat spinal neurones (Fig. 6) (44).
   The potency and specificity of THIP as a BMC-sensitive GABA a-
gonist (41,45) prompted labelling of THIP (38) and studies of the
binding of radioactive THIP to rat brain synaptic membranes (23).
Like GABA and P4S, THIP apparently binds to three sites of the
GABA receptors *in vitro*, but in comparison with the former GABA
agonists, THIP exhibits an apparent selectivity for the medium-
affinity binding site (Fig. 4). The physiological relevance of
this observation is unknown. However, while GABA is capable of
activating synaptic as well as extrasynaptic GABA receptors in
the rat hippocampus, THIP selectively activates synaptic receptors (1). Since the membranes used in binding studies probably
contain both synaptic and extrasynaptic receptor sites, it is
tempting to assume that the medium-affinity binding sites reflect
BIC-sensitive synaptic receptors and the high-affinity sites ex-

trasynaptic receptors. The relevance of low-affinity GABA agonist binding (Fig. 4) is unknown, but the binding data shown in
Table 1 supported by other *in vitro* studies (34,53,55) suggest
that the GABA receptor-benzodiazepine binding site coupling, assumed to exist, involves a low-affinity GABA site.

   In addition to the effects of *N*-methylation of *N*-methylmusci-
mol and THIP introduction of an additional carbon atom into certain positions of the piperidine ring of THIP results in glycine
antagonists (Fig. 6) (44). Thus, THIA (5,6,7,8-tetrahydro-4*H*-is-
oxazolo[5,4-*c*]azepin-3-ol), THAZ (5,6,7,8-tetrahydro-4*H*-isoxazo-
lo[4,5-*d*]azepin-3-ol), and iso-THAZ reduce the effectiveness of
glycine as a depressant of the firing of cat spinal neurones
without affecting the effect of GABA (Fig. 7). Within this new
class of glycine antagonists iso-THAZ is the most potent compound. As mentioned earlier iso-THAZ has GABA antagonistic properties after local application in the rat substantia nigra (4).

Pharmacology of THIP

   All specific BIC-sensitive GABA agonists, so far known, have
zwitterionic structures, and such compounds normally do not easily penetrate the blood-brain barrier (BBB). The ability of neutral amino acids to penetrate the BBB does, however, depend on
their protolytic properties (34). The ratio between the ionized
and the unionized forms of the compounds (I/U-ratio) is a function of the difference between the pKA-I and pKA-II values, a
great difference being tantamount with a high I/U ratio (40,47).
Since amino acids are likely to penetrate the BBB in the unionized forms it is of interest to develop analogues of GABA with
a smaller difference in the pKA values than in GABA, which does
not enter the brain after systemic administration.

   In agreement with the data shown in Table 2, THIP, but not isoguvacine and P4S, enters the brain very easily after systemic administration (47). Thio-THIP (4,5,6,7-tetrahydroisothiazolo-
[5,4-*c*]pyridin-3-ol) has a very low I/U-ratio, but this analogue
of THIP is a weak BMC-sensitive GABA agonist emphasizing the very
high degree of structural specificity of the GABA receptors (P.
Krogsgaard-Larsen and D.R. Curtis, unpublished).

   These favourable pharmacokinetic properties of THIP compared
with its stability *in vivo* and low toxicity (35,60) have made a-
nimal behavioural studies and studies in the human clinic possible. Among various pharmacological effects of THIP, its anticonvulsant properties in animals (48,51), its naloxone-insensitive
analgesic effects in animals and humans (28,35), the decreases in
blood pressure after injection of THIP into the brain ventricles
of cats (24), and the inhibition of food intake in the rat after
administration of THIP (5) may have particular therapeutic interest. However, more profound studies are required before the therapeutic value of THIP can be estimated.

ACKNOWLEDGEMENTS

P.K.-L. is a recipient of The Hede Nielsen Research Award. This work was supported by grants from The Danish Medical Research Council and The Australian National University. The secretarial assistance of Mrs. B. Hare and the technical assistance of Mrs. P. Searle and Mr. S. Stilling are gratefully acknowledged.

REFERENCES

1. Alger, B.E. and Nicoll, R.A. (1982): *J. Physiol.* (in press).
2. Allan, R.D., Evans, R.H., and Johnston, G.A.R. (1980): *Br.J. Pharmacol.*, 70: 609-615.
3. Allan, R.D., Curtis, D.R., Headley, P.M., Johnston, G.A.R., Lodge, D., and Twitchin, B. (1980): *J. Neurochem.*, 34: 652-654.
4. Arnt, J. and Krogsgaard-Larsen, P. (1979): *Brain Res.*, 177: 395-400.
5. Blavet, N., DeFeudis, F.V., and Clostre, F. (1982): *Psychopharmacology*, 76: 75-78.
6. Bowery, N.G., Hill, D.R., Hudson, A.L., Doble, A., Middlemiss, D.N., Shaw, J., and Turnbull, M. (1980): *Nature*, 283: 92-94.
7. Braestrup, C., Nielsen, M., Krogsgaard-Larsen, P., and Falch, E. (1979): *Nature*, 280: 331-333.
8. Brown, D.A. (1979): *Trends Neurosci.*, 2: 271-273.
9. Chase, T.N., Wexler, N.S., and Barbeau, A., editors (1979): *Huntington's Disease*. Raven Press, New York.
10. Curtis. D.R. (1978): In: *Amino Acids as Chemical Transmitters*, edited by F. Fonnum, pp. 55-86. Plenum Press, New York.
11. Curtis, D.R. and Johnston, G.A.R. (1974): *Ergeb. Physiol.*, 69: 97-188.
12. Curtis, D.R. and Watkins, J.C. (1960): *J. Neurochem.*, 6: 117-141.
13. Curtis, D.R., Lodge, D., Bornstein, J.C., Peet, M.J., and Leah, J.D. (1982): *Exp. Brain Res.* (in press).
14. Curtis, D.R., Duggan, A.W., Felix, D., and Johnston, G.A.R. (1971): *Brain Res.*, 32: 69-96.
15. Curtis, D.R., Game, C.J.A., Johnston, G.A.R., and McCulloch, R.M. (1974): *Brain Res.*, 70: 493-499.
16. Curtis, D.R., Lodge, D., Bornstein, J.C., and Peet, M.J. (1981): *Exp. Brain Res.*, 42: 158-170.
17. Curtis, D.R., Duggan, A.W., Felix, D., Johnston, G.A.R., and McLennan, H. (1971): *Brain Res.*, 33: 57-73.
18. Davies, J. and Watkins, J.C. (1974): *Brain Res.*, 70: 501-505.
19. DeFeudis, F.V. (1981): *Neurochem. Int.*, 3: 113-122.
20. DiMicco, J.A., Gale, K., Hamilton, B., and Gillis, R.A. (1979): *Science*, 204: 1106-1109.
21. Enna, S.J. (1981): *Biochem. Pharmacol.*, 30: 907-913.
22. Enna, S.J. and Snyder, S.H. (1975): *Brain Res.*, 100: 81-97.

23. Falch, E. and Krogsgaard-Larsen, P. (1982): *J. Neurochem.*, 38: 1123-1129.
24. Gillis, R.A., Williford, D.J., Souza, J.D., and Quest, J.A. (1982): *Neuropharmacology*, 21: 545-547.
25. Grandison, L. and Guidotti, A. (1979): *Endocrinology*, 105: 754-759.
26. Guidotti, A. (1980): In: *Receptors for Neurotransmitters and Peptide Hormones*, edited by G. Pepeu, M.J. Kuhar, and S.J. Enna, pp. 271-275. Raven Press, New York.
27. Hill, D.R. and Bowery, N.G. (1981): *Nature*, 290: 149-152.
28. Hill, R.C., Maurer, R., Buescher, H.-H., and Roemer, D. (1981): *Eur. J. Pharmacol.*, 69: 221-224.
29. Hornykiewicz, O., Lloyd, K.G., and Davidson, L. (1976): In: *GABA in Nervous System Function*, edited by E. Roberts, T.N. Chase, and D.B. Tower, pp. 479-485. Raven Press, New York.
30. Johnston, G.A.R., Allan, R.D., and Skerritt, J.H. (1982): In: *Handbook of Neurochemistry*, 2. ed., Vol. 6, edited by A. Lajtha, (in press). Plenum Press, New York.
31. Johnston, G.A.R., Beart, P.M., Curtis, D.R., Game, C.J.A., McCulloch, R.M., and Maclachlan, R.M. (1972): *Nature New Biology*, 240: 219-220.
32. Johnston, G.A.R., Curtis, D.R., Beart, P.M., Game, C.J.A., McCulloch, R.M., and Twitchin, B. (1975): *J. Neurochem.*, 24: 157-160.
33. Krnjević, K. (1974): *Physiol. Rev.*, 54: 418-540.
34. Krogsgaard-Larsen, P. (1981): *J. Med. Chem.*, 24: 1377-1383.
35. Krogsgaard-Larsen, P. and Christensen, A.V. (1980): *Annu. Rep. Med. Chem.*, 15: 41-50.
36. Krogsgaard-Larsen, P. and Falch, E. (1981): *Mol. Cell. Biochem.*, 38: 129-146.
37. Krogsgaard-Larsen, P. and Johnston, G.A.R. (1978): *J. Neurochem.*, 30: 1377-1382.
38. Krogsgaard-Larsen, P., Johansen, J.S., and Falch, E. (1982): *J. Label. Cpds.*, 19: 689-701.
39. Krogsgaard-Larsen, P., Scheel-Krüger, J., and Kofod, H., editors (1979): *GABA-Neurotransmitters. Pharmacochemical, Biochemical and Pharmacological Aspects*. Munksgaard, Copenhagen.
40. Krogsgaard-Larsen, P., Falch, E., Mikkelsen, H., and Jacobsen, P. (1982): In: *Optimization of Drug Delivery*, edited by H. Bundgaard, A.B. Hansen, and H. Kofod, pp. 225-235. Munksgaard, Copenhagen.
41. Krogsgaard-Larsen, P., Johnston, G.A.R., Lodge, D., and Curtis, D.R. (1977): *Nature*, 268: 53-55.
42. Krogsgaard-Larsen, P., Snowman, A., Lummis, S.C., and Olsen, R.W. (1981): *J. Neurochem.*, 37: 401-409.
43. Krogsgaard-Larsen, P., Falch, E., Schousboe, A., Curtis, D.R., and Lodge, D. (1980): *J. Neurochem.*, 34: 756-759.
44. Krogsgaard-Larsen, P., Hjeds, H., Curtis, D.R., Leah, J.D., and Peet, M.J. (1982): *J. Neurochem.*, 39 (in press).
45. Krogsgaard-Larsen, P., Hjeds, H., Curtis, D.R., Lodge, D., and Johnston, G.A.R. (1979): *J. Neurochem.*, 32: 1717-1724.

46. Krogsgaard-Larsen, P., Johnston, G.A.R., Curtis, D.R., Game, C.J.A., and McCulloch, R.M. (1975): *J. Neurochem.*, 25: 803-809.

47. Krogsgaard-Larsen, P., Schultz, B., Mikkelsen, H., Aaes-Jørgensen, T., and Bøgesø, K.P. (1981): In: *Amino Acid Neurotransmitters*, edited by F.V. DeFeudis and P. Mandel, pp. 69-76. Raven Press, New York.

48. Löscher, W., Frey, H.-H., Reiche, R., and Schultz, D. (1982): *Neuropharmacology*, (in press).

49. Mathison, R.D. and Dreifuss, J.J. (1980): *Brain Res.*, 187: 476-480.

50. Meldrum, B.S. (1982): *Clin. Neuropharmacol.*, 5: 293-316.

51. Meldrum, B.S. and Horton, R. (1980): *Eur. J. Pharmacol.*, 61: 231-237.

52. Morselli, P.L., Lloyd, K.G., Löscher, W., Meldrum, B., and Reynolds, E.H., editors (1981): *Neurotransmitters, Seizures, and Epilepsy*. Raven Press, New York.

53. Olsen, R.W. (1981): *J. Neurochem.*, 37: 1-13.

54. Olsen, R.W. and Snowman, A.M. (1982): *J. Neurosci.*, (in press).

55. Olsen, R.W., Bergman, M.O., Van Ness, P.C., Lummis, S.C., Watkins, A.E., Napias, C., and Greenlee, D.V. (1981): *Mol. Pharmacol.*, 19: 217-227.

56. Roberts, C.J., Krogsgaard-Larsen, P., and Walker, R.J. (1981): *Comp. Biochem. Physiol.*, 69C: 7-11.

57. Roberts, E., Chase, T.N., and Tower, D.B., editors (1976): *GABA in Nervous System Function*, Raven Press, New York.

58. Roberts, E., Krause, D.N., Wong, E., and Mori, A. (1981): *J. Neurosci.*, 1: 132-140.

59. Schousboe, A., Thorbek, P., Hertz, L., and Krogsgaard-Larsen, P. (1979): *J. Neurochem.*, 33: 181-189.

60. Schultz, B., Aaes-Jørgensen, T., Bøgesø, K.P., and Jørgensen, A. (1981): *Acta Pharmacol. Toxicol.*, 49: 116-124.

61. Stevens, J., Wilson, K., and Foote, W. (1974): *Psychopharmacologia*, 39: 105-119.

62. Supavilai, P. and Karobath, M. (1980): *Neurosci. Lett.*, 19: 337-341.

63. Van Kammen, D.P. (1977): *Am. J. Psychiatry*, 134: 138-143.

CNS Receptors—From Molecular
Pharmacology to Behavior, edited by
P. Mandel and F. V. DeFeudis.
Raven Press, New York © 1983.

Glycine Binding to Rat CNS Membranes: Possible Cooperative Interaction

J. C. Marvizon, J. F. Rumigny, M. Strolin Benedetti, C. Gomeni, and J. Benavides

Centre de Recherche Delalande, 92500 Rueil-Malmaison, France

The importance of glycine as an inhibitory neurotransmitter in specific areas of the CNS has recently been reviewed (2, 3, 4, 17). The convulsant drug strychnine potently antagonizes natural inhibitory synaptic transmission in the spinal cord in a similar fashion to its antagonism of the inhibitory effect of iontophoretically applied glycine (5, 8, 12). Young and Snyder (28) reported that [3H]-strychnine could bind to synaptic membrane fractions isolated from spinal cord and brainstem in a specific and glycine displaceable manner, which indicates an association with the synaptic glycine receptor. Specific strychnine binding to the glycine receptor was then defined as the amount of [3H]-strychnine bound which can be displaced by 1 mM glycine. Further studies by Young and Snyder (29) strongly suggest that these two compounds may bind to the same receptor complex but at distinct sites, therefore interacting with each other in an allosteric fashion, the strychnine binding site being associated with the ionic conductance mechanism for chloride.

Analysis of neurophysiological data for glycine and other neurotransmitter systems suggests that two or more transmitter molecules may be required to activate a receptor (6, 25, 26, 27). Hill plots of [3H]-strychnine displacement from its binding sites by varying concentrations of non-radioactive strychnine and glycine were linear, with an n for strychnine of 1.0, while the n for glycine was 1.7 (29). This n value suggests that two or more molecules of glycine interact in a cooperative fashion to displace [3H]-strychnine from its binding site. Protein reagents like diazonium tetrazole and acetic anhydride may interfere with this cooperative interaction between the glycine and strychnine binding sites (29).

In direct studies with [3H]-glycine as ligand, De Feudis et al. (9, 10) found that the binding mechanism involved positive cooperativity, and had K_d values similar for all regions of the CNS that ranged from 80 to 160 nM. However, in a further report,

Kishimoto et al. (15) described glycine binding in CNS as varying significantly between the different CNS areas studied. Two populations of binding sites were found in spinal cord and medulla oblongata, but only one in cerebral cortex, midbrain and cerebellum. These results were not discussed with regard to the possibility of the existence of positive cooperativity.

In this paper, we have studied some of the properties of glycine binding to rat medulla oblongata and spinal cord membranes. The possible existence of a cooperative phenomenon has been taken into account to explain the characteristics of the glycine binding to its synaptic receptor.

MATERIAL AND METHODS

$[2-^3H]$-Glycine (specific activity 50 Ci/mmol) was purchased from C.E.A. (France). Triton X-100, Lubrol WX, Lubrol PX, glycine, glycine analogs and ethyleneglycol-bis-(β-aminoethyl-ether)-N,N'-tetra acetic acid (EGTA) were obtained from Sigma. 3-[3-cholamidopropyl)-dimethylammonio]-1-propane sulfonate (CHAPS) was obtained from Calbiochem. Diazonium tetrazole was synthesized from 5-amino tetrazole (1, 7, 22) purchased from Aldrich.

Membrane preparation

Male Wistar rats were decapitated, and the medulla oblongata was dissected from the brain. The spine was cut in the lumbar region and the spinal cord removed by applying compressed air to the cavity.Medullae oblongatae and spinal cords from 20 rats were combined and then homogenised in 20 volumes of ice-cold 0.32 M sucrose in a glass homogeniser fitted with a Teflon pestle (8 strokes at 1500 rpm). Each homogenate was centrifuged for 10 min at 1000 x g, the pellet Pl discarded, and the supernatant centrifuged for 20 min at 20000 x g.

The crude mitochondrial pellet (P2) was resuspended in a minimum volume of ice-cold distilled water. An equal volume of 2 M sucrose was added to obtain a suspension in 1 M sucrose that was included in a three-layer gradient with 1.2 M sucrose (12 ml) and 0.8 M sucrose (12 ml). The gradients were centrifuged at 22000 rpm (g_{av} : 65000) for 120 min in a SW 28 Beckman ultra-centrifuge rotor. After the centrifugation, two layers of membranes were observed in the 1.2 M – 1 M and 1 M – 0.8 M interfaces of the gradient, together with the mitochondrial pellet and a dense, white coat floating over the gradient. The two intermedium layers were collected, diluted five-fold with ice-cold distilled water and centrifuged at 48000 x g for 20 min. The resulting pellets were stored at – 20°C for at least 12 hr. Frozen pellets were resuspended in 50 mM-Tris-citrate buffer (pH 7.1 at 4°C) to a protein concentration of 1 mg protein/ml, and homogenised with an Ultra-Turrax mechanical homogeniser set to 1/4 of maximum speed for 30 sec. In some experiments, the membranes were pre-incubated at 37°C with various detergents and reagents (see results for details).

The membrane suspension was then centrifuged at 48000 x g for 20 min. The resulting pellets were resuspended in the original volume of buffer, homogenised using a Dounce homogeniser (3 strokes, pestle B) and recentrifuged. This procedure was repeated and the pellets were resuspended in buffer, homogenised (Dounce pestle B, 6 strokes) and used for the binding assay.

^{3}H-GLYCINE BINDING ASSAY

0.2 ml aliquots of the membrane suspension (0.2 - 0.6 mg of protein) were placed in Beckman type 25 rotor tubes containing 0.2 ml of [^{3}H]-glycine at the required concentration and 0.2 ml of either 50 mM-Tris-citrate buffer (pH 7.1 at 4°C) or non-labelled glycine or dilutions of various test compounds in Tris-citrate buffer. After incubation at 0°C for 30 min, the tubes were then centrifuged at 20000 rpm for 25 min in a Beckman Ultra-centrifuge type 25 rotor. The supernatants were aspirated and the pellets were rapidly rinsed twice with 1 ml of ice-cold buffer. Pellets were resuspended in 0.5 ml of 1 M NaOH and incubated for 30 min at 40°C. Dimilume (Packard) was added and the radio-activity determined with an Intertechnique liquid scintillation counter. Specific binding was defined as the binding displaceable by 1 mM non-radioactive glycine. Protein concentrations were determined by the fluorimetric method of Resch et al. (18) using bovine serum albumin as a standard.

Mathematical treatment of the saturation data

We have chosen the Hill approximation (16, 20, 24) to characterize the possible cooperative interaction of glycine with its binding sites. This approach is based on the assumption that the cooperativity is very marked, so that the concentrations of all receptor-ligand complexes containing less than n molecules of ligand will be negligible. In this case the binding can be represented by the "all-or-none" reaction:

$$P + nF \rightleftharpoons (P-F)_n \qquad \text{with } K = \frac{[P] [F]^n}{[(P-F)_n]}$$

(where K is the apparent dissociation constant, P the unoccupied receptor, F the free ligand, $(P-F)_n$ the receptor-ligand complex).

Generalizing the above reaction to m-subclasses of receptors, the model defined by the following equation is obtained:

$$B = \sum_{i=1}^{m} (R_i \cdot F^n_i) / (K_i + F^n_i)$$

where B is the amount of $[^3H]$-glycine specifically bound, F the concentration of free $[^3H]$-glycine in the incubation medium, R_i the concentration of binding sites in the ith subclass (B max_i), K_i the apparent dissociation constant of the ith subclass, n_i the Hill coefficient for the ith subclass ($n_i = 1$ indicates no cooperativity, $n_i > 1$ indicates positive cooperativity and $n_i < 1$ indicates negative cooperativity).

When $F = F_{50} = \sqrt[n_i]{K_i}$ the ith subclass reaches its half maximum saturation.

This model therefore does not take into account those molecules of receptor with a partial occupancy of its binding sites. That is why the n_i values observed are not necessarily integer numbers, and can not be considered as representing the actual number of binding sites in each of the ith subclass of receptor. The saturation data were analysed with a Tektronix 4052 computer. Values for K_i, n_i, R_i which gave the best fitting were determined using the Gauss-Newton iterative procedure (13).

RESULTS

The effect of several membrane treatments and changes in the incubation medium composition on specific glycine binding was studied at 5 or 10 nM $[^3H]$-glycine concentrations.

Preincubations for 15 min with several detergents (0.05 %, w/v) such as Triton X-100, CHAPS, Lubrol PX and Lubrol WX, with further washing, failed to modify glycine binding. Ultrasonic treatment of the membranes was also ineffective. Preincubation of the membrane preparation with the protein modifying reagents diazonium tetrazole (0.5 mM) and acetic anhydride (10 mM) for 60 min did not have any significant effect on glycine binding. Specific glycine binding was not affected when a Tris-HCl buffer replaced the Tris-citrate buffer. The addition of $CaCl_2$ (5 mM or 0.1 mM) to Tris-HCl buffer did not modify the binding that was however reduced to 60 % of control values by EGTA (3 mM). Specific glycine binding is not modified over a range of pH values between 6.4 to 7.6.

Saturation data

Specific glycine binding to membrane preparations isolated from medulla oblongata + spinal cord was saturable with increasing concentrations of $[^3H]$-glycine, while nonspecific binding increased linearly over the concentration range used (Fig. 1). Under the standard assay conditions, specific binding represented 30 - 40 % of the total binding.

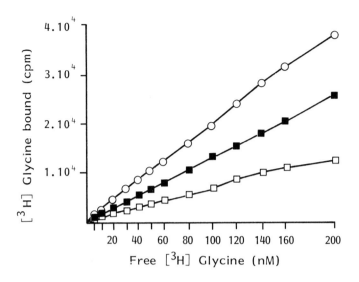

Fig. 1. Direct plot of total (O), non specific (■) and specific (□) glycine binding. Each point represents the mean of 4 determinations.

The Scatchard plot (Fig. 2) of the specific binding data is non-linear, and suggests the presence of two subclasses of receptors, at least one of them with positive cooperativity (curves convexing upward) (23). Using the Hill approximation with m = 2 (two subclasses), the system is characterized by the following parameters :

$(F_{50})_1$: 15 nM $(F_{50})_2$: 137 nM
R_1 : 151 $\pm$ 43 fmol/mg protein R_2 . 772 $\pm$ 47 fmol/mg protein
n_1 : 1.75 $\pm$ 0.83 n_2 : 2.34 $\pm$ 0.05

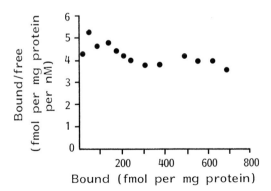

Fig. 2. Scatchard plot of specific glycine binding. This pattern could represent 2 subclasses of receptors, at least one of them with positive cooperativity (curve convexing upward).

The Gauss-Newton fitting of the saturation curve of the system is presented in Fig. 3.

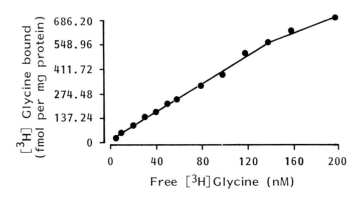

Fig. 3. Direct plot of specific glycine binding fitted with the Gauss-Newton itera-tive procedure using the Hill approximation. Two convexities are noted in the curve, corresponding to two subclasses of receptors.

Two classes of receptors and positive cooperativity were also found in an experiment with membranes obtained from spinal cord alone (data not shown).

Effect of glycine and glycine related compounds

Non-labelled glycine at 10 nM was found to slightly activate [^{3}H]-glycine binding. In a preliminary experiment an increase was also found with non — radioactive L-α-alanine, D-α-alanine, β-alanine and D-serine at concentrations between 10 and 100 nM.

DISCUSSION

With the membrane preparation method used in previous studies on ^{3}H-strychnine binding (28, 29) and [^{3}H]-glycine binding (15) we found that, while specific glycine binding in cerebral cortex represents more than 50 % of the total binding, in the spinal cord + medulla oblongata preparation the specific binding was between 20 and 10 % of the total binding. This may be due to the greater myelin content of the spinal cord and medulla oblongata ; in fact when the crude mitochondrial pellet (P2) was centrifuged in a density gradient to separate synaptic membranes from myelin and mitochondria, specific binding increased to more than 35 % of the total binding in the synaptic membrane fraction, while in the myelin (which accounts for more than 1/3 of the P2 protein content), it was less than 4 %.

Pretreatments of the membranes with detergents did not enhance specific glycine binding, as in the case of glutamate (21) and in

contrast with the findings for GABA (14, 18). Other conditions as
sonication, known to modify glutamate binding (21), were found
not to affect glycine binding. Young and Snyder (29) reported
that preincubation of synaptic membranes with the protein-
modifying reagents (1, 7, 22) diazonium tetrazole (0.25-0.75 mM)
and acetic anhydride (10 mM) strongly decreased the cooperativity
observed in the displacement of ^{3}H-strychnine by glycine.
Nevertheless, we did not find any effect on specific glycine
binding when our membrane preparations were treated with these
reagents.

Analysis of equilibrium binding at various glycine
concentrations indicates that specific glycine binding probably
involves more than one single population of receptor sites. Data
obtained from the Hill approximation, along with the enhancement
of [^{3}H]-glycine binding observed with low concentrations of
non-radioactive glycine or glycine-related amino-acids, are
compatible with the existence of positive cooperativity at least
for one subclass of receptors (see e.g. 11).

Our interpretation of glycine binding data in a positive
cooperative model is in agreement with the results reported by
Young and Snyder (29) for glycine displacement of ^{3}H-strychnine
binding and with the results for [^{3}H]-glycine binding of De
Feudis et al. (9, 10) who reported the possible existence of
positive cooperativity phenomena. Kishimoto et al. (14) did not
take into account the possibility of the existence of a positive
cooperativity, in spite of the fact that the Scatchard plot
obtained by them with spinal cord membranes is consistent with
such a model.

REFERENCES

1. Andres, S.F., and Atassi, M.Z. (1973): Biochemistry, 12:
   942-947.
2. Aprison, M.H. and Daly, E.C. (1978): In: Avances in Neurochemistry, vol. 3, edited by B.W. Agranoff, and M.H.
   Aprison, pp. 203-294, Plenum Publishing Corp., New York.
3. Aprison, M.H., and Nadi, N.S. (1978): In: Amino acids as
   Chemical Transmitters, edited by F. Fonnum. pp. 531-570,
   Plenum Publishing Corp., New York.
4. Borbe, H..O., Müllen, W.E., and Wollert, U. (1981): Brain
   Res., 205: 131-139.
5. Bradley, K., Easton, D.M., and Eides, J.C. (1953): J.Physiol.
   (London), 122: 474-488.
6. Brookes, N., and Werman, R. (1973): Mol. Pharmacol., 9:
   571-579.
7. Cuatrecasas, D.R. (1970):J. Biol. Chem., 245: 574-584.
8. Curtis, D.R., Duggan, A.W., and Johnston, G.A.R. (1971): Exp.
   Brain Res., 12: 547-565.

9. De Feudis, F.V., Fando, J., and Orensanz Munoz, L.M. (1977): Experientia, 33: 1068-1070.
10. De Feudis, F.V. (1979): J. Physiol. Paris, 75: 651-654.
11. De Lean, A., and Rodbard, D. (1979): In: The Receptors, a comprehensive Treatise, vol. 1, edited by R.D. O'Brien, pp. 143-192.
12. Dusser de Barenne, J.G. (1933): Physiol. Rev., 13: 325-335.
13. Harthley, H.O. (1961): Technometrics, 3: 269-280.
14. Hong, J.S., and Wong, D.T. (1978): J. Neurochem., 32: 1379-1386.
15. Kishimoto, H., Simon, J.R., and Aprison, M.H. (1981): J. Neurochem., 37: 1015-1024.
16. Molinoff, P.B., Wolfe, B.B., and Weiland, G.A. (1981): Life Sci., 29: 427-443.
17. Pycock, C.J., and Kerwin, R.W. (1981): Life Sci., 28: 2679-2686.
18. Redburn, D., and Mitchell, Ch.K. (1980): Life Sci., 28: 541-549.
19. Resch, K., Inm, W., Ferber, E., Wallach, D.M.F., and Fischer, M. (1971): Naturwissenschaften, 58: 200.
20. Segel, I.H. (1975): Enzyme Kinetics, pp. 346-385, Wiley Interscience Public. New York.
21. Sharif, N.A., and Roberts, P.J. (1980): J. Neurochem., 34: 779-784.
22. Sokolovsky, M., and Vallee, B.L. (1966): Biochemistry, 5: 3574-3581.
23. Thakur, A.K., Jaffe, M.L., and Rodbard, D. (1980): Analytical Biochemistry, 107: 279-295.
24. Weiland, G.A., and Molinoff, P.B. (1981): Life Sci., 29: 313-330.
25. Werman, R. (1969): Comp. Biochem. Physiol., 30: 997-1017.
26. Werman, R. (1972): Assoc. Res. Neur. Ment. Dis., 50: 147-180.
27. Werman, R. (1979): In: Advances Experimental Medicine and Biology, vol.123, edited by P. Mandel and F.V. De Feudis, pp. 287-301, Plenum Press, New York.
28. Young, A.B., and Snyder, S.H. (1973): Proc. Natl. Acad. Sci. USA, 70: 2832-2836.
29. Young, A.B., and Snyder, S.H. (1974): Mol. Pharmacol., 10: 790-809.

CNS Receptors—From Molecular
Pharmacology to Behavior, edited by
P. Mandel and F. V. DeFeudis.
Raven Press, New York © 1983.

Binding of Taurine to Brain Synaptic Membranes

Pirjo Kontro and S. S. Oja

Department of Biomedical Sciences, University of Tampere, SF-33101 Tampere 10, Finland

Taurine has been suggested to act, for example, as inhibitory neurotransmitter and -modulator, thermoregulator, endogenous antiepileptic agent or stabilizer of excitable membranes (see ref. 27). All these postulated functions presuppose interactions of taurine with neural membranes. A part of brain taurine is indeed sequestered into synaptic terminals, being particularly enriched in synaptic vesicles (15) and synaptic membrane fractions (24). So far, however, the nature of interactions of taurine with neural membranes has remained a matter of conjecture. In particular, no such binding which could represent association of taurine to its postulated postsynaptic receptor sites has been found with any certainty (13,21,22). In the present paper we describe our efforts to characterize taurine binding to isolated synaptic membranes and endeavours to disclose the specific sodium-independent binding considered characteristic of the attachment of ligands to postsynaptic receptor sites.

EXPERIMENTAL PROCEDURES

Materials

Animal brain samples were excised from adult (about 25 g) NMRI mice and Wistar (about 200 g) rats of both sexes. All mice and one group of rats received pelleted food and water ad libitum prior to the experiments, one group of rats were given 1 % (w/v) 2-guanidinoethanesulphonic acid solution instead of water in order to lower the brain taurine contents (12). Human brain samples were collected at autopsies from elderly (70-80 a) male and female subjects who had died of non-neurological diseases with no manifest brain pathology.

[1,2-^{3}H]Taurine (sp.act. 0.47 PBq/mol) and [2,3-^{3}H]GABA (sp. act. 2.37 PBq/mol) were purchased from the Radiochemical Centre, Amersham. Thiotaurine was synthesized by ourselves from hypotaurine (2). The anticonvulsant taurine derivatives MY-117

(2-phthalimidoethanesulphon-N-isopropylamide) (1) and 2-guanidino-
ethanesulphonic acid (GES) (12) were synthesized in the Research
Laboratories of Medica Pharmaceutical Company, Ltd., Helsinki.
Other reagents and drugs were obtained from commercial sources.

Preparation of synaptic membranes

In all procedures a crude mitochondrial pellet (P_2) was first
prepared from the brain samples (34). Synaptic membranes were
isolated and purified from the P_2 fraction according to Enna and
Snyder (4) and kept frozen for at least 2 days at 253 K. If not
otherwise stated, the membrane preparations were in the first
series of experiments subjected to the following standard treatment (procedure I) which was in the later series somewhat modified (procedure II). In procedure I the frozen membrane pellets
were thawed by suspending in water (1 g fresh tissue/10 ml),
maintained at 295 K for 20 min, centrifuged at 48 000 g for 20
min (4), and then suspended in incubation buffers for binding
assays. In procedure II the frozen membranes were thawed by incubating for 30 min at 310 K in 0.05 mol/l Tris-HCl buffer, pH
7.1, containing 0.05 % (v/v) Triton X-100, then sedimented during
10 min at 48 000 g, washed with water (6), and frozen again at
253 K. The Triton X-100 treatment was repeated 5 days later when
the final binding assays were carried out.

The protein content of the membrane preparations was determined
(23). It was about 2.8 % of the brain fresh weight. Taurine
contents were assayed by an automated amino acid analyzer (15).

Binding assays

The membrane preparations (0.8 or 1.6 g protein/l) were incubated generally for 1 or 10 min at 274 K in 0.5 ml of 0.05 mol/l
Tris-HCl buffer, pH 7.1 (sodium-independent binding) or in Krebs-
Ringer-HEPES medium, pH 7.4 (sodium-dependent binding) containing
varying amounts of [^{3}H]taurine with or without 1.0 mmol/l of
inactive taurine. Incubations were terminated by rapid filtration
through Millipore filters or by centrifugation for 5 min at
17 000 g with subsequent rinsing two or three times with cold
buffer. The binding of [^{3}H]GABA was assessed similarly.

Calculations

The filters with attached synaptic membranes, the sedimented
membrane pellets and samples from the incubation buffers were
measured for radioactivity (26). The counting efficiency (about
52 %) was determined with standard samples after correction for
quenching by the external-standard channels-ratio method.

The statistical significance of differences between two means
was assessed by Student's independent two-tailed t test. The
straight regression lines were fitted to the experimental data
and used for the estimation of binding parameters and their

confidence limits according to conventional statistical procedures (32).

RESULTS

Sodium-dependent binding

There occurred sodium-dependent binding of taurine to mouse
brain synaptic membranes frozen for two days according to procedure I. The binding was temperature-sensitive, being highest at
310 K (Fig. 1). The binding was somewhat higher to fresh than to
frozen and thawed membranes both at 310 K and 274 K (Table 1).
The sodium-dependent binding was readily displaceable by several
structural analogues, including hypotaurine, β-alanine and GABA
(Table 2). Furthermore, specific sodium-dependent binding could
be extracted from the total sodium-dependent binding. The former
was saturable in the concentration range of 0.06-1.0 μmol/l
(Fig. 2A). Only one class of binding sites was revealed by
Scatchard analysis (Fig. 3A). The parameters calculated for the
specific sodium-dependent binding are given in Table 6.

Sodium-independent binding

Procedure I
Sodium-independent taurine binding to mouse brain synaptic membranes frozen for two days could also be demonstrated. The binding was temperature-insensitive (Fig. 1) and remained constant
from 1 min up to 30 min of incubation. The binding was also
constant when measured with fresh or frozen and thawed membranes
both at 274 K and 310 K (Table 2). Furthermore, the total

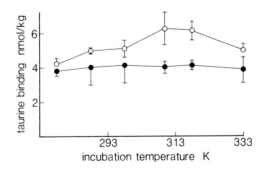

FIG. 1. Taurine binding to mouse brain synaptic membranes at
varying incubation temperatures. The membranes (procedure I)
were incubated for 1 min with [^{3}H]taurine (0.1 μmol/l, 30 MBq/l)
in Tris-HCl buffer, pH 7.1 (●-●, total sodium-independent binding) or in Krebs-Ringer-HEPES medium, pH 7.4 (o-o, total sodium-
dependent binding). The results are means (± S.E.M.) of five experiments.

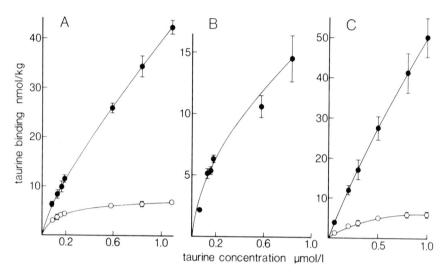

taurine concentration µmol/l

FIG. 2. Taurine binding to mouse brain synaptic membranes at
varying ligand concentrations. (A) The membranes (procedure I)
were incubated with varying concentrations of [3H]taurine (30
MBq/1) for 1 min at 274 K in Krebs-Ringer-HEPES medium, pH 7.4
(sodium-dependent binding). Specific binding (o-o) was determined
from the total binding (●-●) according to Enna and Snyder (4).
Means (± S.E.M.) of five experiments. (B) The membranes (procedure I) were similarly incubated in Tris-HCl buffer, pH 7.1
(sodium-independent binding). No specific binding could be extracted from the total binding (●-●). Means (± S.E.M.) of five
experiments. (C) The membranes (procedure II) were similarly incubated in Tris-HCl buffer. Specific sodium-independent binding
(o-o) was extracted from the total sodium-independent binding
(●-●) as above. Means (± S.E.M.) of 10 experiments.

TABLE 1. Effects of temperature on total taurine binding to
         mouse brain synaptic membranes[a]

Conditions of assays	Sodium-dependent binding	Sodium-independent binding
Fresh membranes, 274 K	100.0 ± 9.2	100.0 ± 9.0
Fresh membranes, 310 K	146.8 ± 4.6	98.2 ± 6.0
Frozen membranes, 274 K	59.0 ± 3.1	114.4 ± 9.4
Frozen membranes, 310 K	131.2 ± 6.1	103.1 ± 3.7

[a]Membranes, treated as indicated, were incubated with [3H]-
taurine as in Fig. 1. Results, means ± S.E.M. of 5 experiments,
are given in per cent of binding to fresh membranes at 274 K.

TABLE 2. Effects of structural analogues on total taurine binding to mouse brain synaptic membranes[a]

Effector[b] (mmol/1)		Sodium-independent binding[c] (% of control)		Sodium-dependent binding[c] (% of control)	
None (control)		100.0 ± 8.3	(16)	100.0 ± 2.0	(12)
GABA	1.0	110.6 ± 3.1	(3)	65.0 ± 4.1**	(8)
β-Alanine	1.0	77.6 ± 10.9	(4)	26.0 ± 0.8**	(4)
Hypotaurine	1.0	79.6 ± 7.4	(4)	25.4 ± 1.3**	(8)
Nipecotic acid	1.0	125.4 ± 15.3	(9)	102.0 ± 8.0	(8)
Muscimol	0.01	115.9 ± 6.6	(9)	87.5 ± 3.6**	(8)
L-DABA	1.0	124.1 ± 13.3	(4)	88.6 ± 7.6	(8)
Glycine	1.0	90.0 ± 3.1	(4)	96.1 ± 1.8	(8)
Cysteic acid	1.0	104.3 ± 2.7	(4)	97.2 ± 4.6	(8)
N-Methyltaurine	1.0	103.8 ± 5.3	(4)	109.1 ± 6.3	(8)
CSA	1.0	103.8 ± 5.0	(4)	148.1 ± 11.6**	(8)
Thiotaurine	1.0	150.1 ± 9.3**	(4)	67.8 ± 2.3**	(8)
GES	1.0	168.7 ± 9.3**	(4)	59.1 ± 2.9**	(8)

[a]The membranes prepared according to procedure I were incubated as in Fig. 1. [b]Abbreviations: L-DABA = L-2,4-diaminobutyric
acid, CSA = cysteinesulphinic acid, GES = 2-guanidinoethanesul-
phonic acid. [c]Means ± S.E.M. Number of experiments in parentheses. Significance of differences from controls: **P<0.01.

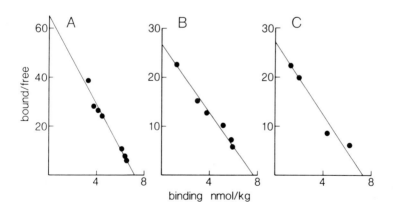

FIG. 3. Scatchard plots of the specific sodium-dependent taurine binding (A) and the specific sodium-independent binding (B
and C) to mouse brain synaptic membranes. The membranes were
subjected to procedure I and separated from medium by centrifugation in A, and in B and C procedure II was applied followed by
separation by filtration (B) or centrifugation (C).

sodium-independent binding was unaffected by the metabolic
poisons iodoacetate (1 mmol/1), 2,4-dinitrophenol (0.1 mmol/1)
and ouabain (0.1 mmol/1), and by structural analogues (Table 2)
with the exception of an enhancement by thiotaurine and GES. The
binding to synaptic membranes isolated from the human cerebral
and cerebellar cortices was similarly unaffected by GABA and
hypotaurine (data not shown). The total sodium-independent binding to mouse brain membranes was also unaffected by magnesium
ions and enhanced by 54 ± 6 % (mean ± S.E.M., n = 4) by 5 mmol/1
calcium ions, but no evident increment could be demonstrated with
human autopsy material (Table 3). Chlorpromazine and a number
of antiepileptic drugs (valproate, phenytoin, primidone, etho-
suximide, sultiame, clonazepam, carbamazepine, diazepam) failed
to influence significantly the total sodium-independent binding
in mouse brain preparations.

The binding of taurine in the absence of sodium ions was not
saturable in nature in the concentration range studied of 0.06-
1.0 μmol/1 (Fig. 2B). The specific binding displaceable by 1.0
mmol/1 inactive taurine could not be repeatedly and reproducibly
extracted from the total sodium-independent binding. When the
extraction was successful, the specific sodium-independent binding was 0.31 ± 0.03 nmol/kg (n = 8) of the total sodium-independent binding of 1.99 ± 0.27 nmol/kg fresh weight of membranes in
mouse brain preparations at a taurine concentration of 0.1 μmol/1.
In human brain preparations both total and specific sodium-independent binding were somewhat higher (Table 3). Correspondingly,
the specific sodium-independent binding was more frequently detectable in human autopsy samples. As a whole, procedure I did
not yield in our hands sufficiently reliable data on the specific
sodium-independent taurine binding. In contrast to taurine binding, the specific sodium-independent GABA binding, run in parallel

TABLE 3.   Effects of calcium on the sodium-independent binding
of taurine to human brain synaptic membranes[a]

Conditions of assay	Taurine binding (nmol/kg)[b]			
	Total		Specific	
Cerebral cortex, no Ca	3.42 ± 0.15	(16)	1.08 ± 0.05	(4)
+ 5 mmol/1 Ca	3.08 ± 0.16	(4)	0.70 ± 0.05	(4)**
Cerebellar cortex, no Ca	4.67 ± 0.41	(8)	1.36 ± 0.15	(4)
+ 5 mmol/1 Ca	3.82 ± 0.06	(4)	–	
Nucleus caudatus, no Ca	3.00 ± 0.25	(4)	1.52 ± 0.12	(4)
+ 5 mmol/1 Ca	3.59 ± 0.33	(4)	2.06 ± 0.09	(4)*

[a]The membranes were prepared and incubated with 0.1 μmol/1
[3H]taurine as in Fig. 1. [b]The results (means ± S.E.M.) are giv-
en per membrane wet weight. Number of experiments in parentheses. Significance of differences between samples with and without calcium: *P<0.05, **P<0.01.

experiments as a methodological control, could be invariably demonstrated.

Procedure II

The above inconsistency in the results on the specific sodium-independent taurine binding was the impetus for modifications of the standard treatment of the synaptic membrane preparations. In order to remove as much endogenous taurine or any other endogenous binding inhibitors as possible, the membranes were subjected to repeated freezing and thawing and thorough washings with Triton X-100 (Table 4). Such treatments seem to have exposed more sodium-independent taurine binding sites. Two freezing-thawing cycles combined with Triton X-100 treatments separated by 5 days gave the highest amount of specific sodium-independent binding and were therefore adopted as the second standard procedure (procedure II). The specific sodium-independent binding of taurine in procedure II was also uninfluenced by the metabolic inhibitors cyanide (1 mmol/l), 2,4-dinitrophenol (0.1 mmol/l) and p-hydroxymercuribenzoate (1.0 mmol/l). GABA may slightly enhance the binding, but homotaurine and some convulsants or anticonvulsants appeared strongly inhibitory (Table 5). The specific sodium-independent binding of GABA was also higher to mouse brain synaptic membranes subjected to procedure II than to procedure I. It was not modified by a concentration of 1 mmol/l of taurine.

The specific sodium-independent binding of taurine to the membranes treated twice with Triton X-100 and incubated for 10 min at 274 K was saturable in the concentration range of 0.06-1.0 μmol/l (Fig. 2C), exhibiting only one type of binding sites

TABLE 4. Effects of freezing and thawing and Triton X-100 on the specific sodium-independent taurine binding to mouse brain synaptic membranes[a]

Experimental conditions	Binding (pmol/kg)[b]	
Fresh membranes	n.d.	
I thawing, 2th day	222 ± 12	(4)
-Triton treated	n.d.	
II thawing, 4th day	–	
-Triton treated	780 ± 36	(4)
II thawing, 6th day	150 ± 24	(4)
-Triton treated	1350 ± 120	(8)
III thawing, 14th day	1284 ± 168	(4)
IV thawing, 28th day	516 ± 48	(4)

[a]The membranes treated as indicated were incubated with [3H]-taurine (0.09 μmol/l, 45 MBq/l) for 10 min at 274 K. [b]Results (means ± S.E.M.) are given in terms of membrane wet weight. Numbers of experiments in parentheses. n.d. = no specific binding detectable.

TABLE 5. Effects of structural analogues on the specific sodium-
          independent taurine binding to mouse brain synaptic
          membranes treated with Triton X-100[a]

Effector (mmol/1)		Binding[b] (% of control)	
None (control)		100.0 ± 6.5	(21)
Hypotaurine	1.0	111.2 ± 11.6	(7)
GABA	1.0	135.7 ± 4.3	(4)*
Muscimol	0.01	29.0 ± 12.1	(8)**
MY-117	0.1	35.0 ± 10.7	(18)**

[a]The membranes, prepared according to procedure II, were incubated as in Fig. 1. Taurine concentration: 60 nmol/1. [b]No binding was detected in the presence of strychnine, picrotoxin or
homotaurine (0.1 mmol/1). Means ± S.E.M. are given. Number of
experiments in parentheses. Significance of differences from
controls: *P<0.05, **P<0.01.

TABLE 6. Parameters for the specific taurine binding to
          synaptic membranes[a]

Preparation/ Conditions of assay	K_D (nmol/1)	B_{max} (nmol/kg)
Mouse brain		
Sodium-dependent binding, Procedure I	110 ± 10	7.2 ± 0.2
Sodium-independent binding, Procedure II, filtration	268 ± 43	7.3 ± 0.7
Sodium-independent binding, Procedure II, centrifugation	287 ± 21	7.7 ± 0.3
Rat brain		
Sodium-independent binding, Procedure II	549 ± 44	4.6 ± 0.2
+ GES for 2 weeks	102 ± 7	3.5 ± 0.1
+ GES for 4 weeks	122 ± 25	5.1 ± 0.4

[a]Constants with their 95 % confidence limits are given per
litre of incubation medium and per kg of membrane wet weight.

(Figs. 3B and 3C). The calculated binding parameters are given
in Table 6. Both separation methods, filtration and centrifugation, gave almost identical results. In rat brain membrane preparations the binding parameters could be similarly estimated for
the specific sodium-independent taurine binding. In the rat K_D

was greater and B_{max} smaller than in the mouse (Table 6). An attempt to reduce the rat brain taurine content in vivo by GES administration was also successful. After a 2 week GES adminis-tration the whole brain taurine content was reduced by 36.8 %. Both constants K_D and B_{max} were significantly (P<0.01) lowered, K_D more than B_{max}. After 4 weeks on GES there occurred a partial restoration of brain taurine levels to 85.0 % of the control values. Correspondingly, only K_D was still significantly (P<0.01) different from controls.

DISCUSSION

The receptors of the sodium-independent taurine binding described herein are obviously transport sites, because of the similarities in their properties to those of taurine uptake (14). Similar bind-ing has been demonstrated by a few earlier investigators with various membrane preparations (16,21,22,30); even the calculated binding parameters are of the same order of magnitude as those reported earlier for the rat brain (30). On the other hand, neither total nor specific sodium-independent binding could be regarded as interaction of taurine with transport sites, since they were unaffected by temperature, metabolic poisons and those structural analogues which interfere with the taurine uptake systems.

Earlier attempts to demonstrate sodium-independent taurine binding, which could represent attachment of taurine to the poss-ible postsynaptic receptor sites, have not been successful with membrane fractions isolated from the brain (13,22) or the retina (21). Our difficulties in consistent detection of the specific sodium-independent taurine binding with membranes subjected to procedure I, the original method of Enna and Snyder (4), are con-ceivable against the above background. The method was tailored for study of GABA binding and also now specific sodium-independ-ent GABA binding was invariably discernible.

The problems encountered in measurement of the sodium-independ-ent taurine binding may have several origins. Firstly, the number of binding sites can be very low, at the detection limit of our assay. The specific radioactivity of the available [3H]-taurine used as ligand is fairly low when compared to that of the [3H]GABA preparations. Secondly, the taurine binding sites may have been already saturated by high amounts of endogenous taurine in brain tissue. There are about 5 mmol/kg taurine in the mouse brain (28), and isolated membrane fractions still contain a considerable amount of taurine (24). Moreover, a part of taurine associated with membranes appears to be very tightly bound, unremovable even by various drastic measures, including washing with Triton X-100 (18). Thirdly, other endogenous inhibitor(s) besides taurine might also complicate the assay by masking specific binding. For instance, such factors have also hampered measurements of the postsynaptic GABA binding (8). Endogenous inhibitors of GABA binding have been removed and GABA binding

enhanced by freezing and thawing, several washes with buffer
(8,25) and Triton X-100 treatments (3,5,6,11,17,20,33) in various
membrane preparations. Detergents are thought to increase the
accessibility of receptor sites or to aid in washing out endogenous inhibitors by breaking open membrane pouches. On the other
hand, detergents can also destroy proteins responsible for binding, as has been observed with glutamate receptors (30). However,
multiple Triton X-100 extractions have not altered the parameters
of GABA binding (19).

In the present study at least a 5-fold increase in the specific binding of taurine occurred both after the fourth freezing-
thawing and washing cycle and after two Triton X-100 treatments.
As above, the increment may ensue from removal of endogenous
taurine and/or other binding inhibitors from the membrane preparations. In keeping, the taurine depletion by GES also improved
binding. To date, López-Colomé and Pasantes-Morales (22) have
observed no modification of the specific taurine binding to rat
brain membranes either after one Triton X-100 treatment with
various Triton concentrations, after four buffer washes or after
one sonication. Possibly more drastic washing and solublization
procedures than those currently used might be needed to reveal
all possible postsynaptic taurine receptors. Such attempts are
in progress in our laboratory.

The unmasked taurine binding was clearly saturable in nature
with a binding constant of the same order of magnitude as that of
glutamate binding (30) and that of the original low-affinity GABA
binding (29). However, the binding capacity for taurine was much
lower than that reported for GABA, for example (8,19,29). The
possibility that the specific sodium-independent taurine binding
represents binding to GABA receptors cannot yet be completely
ruled out, since taurine may be able to interact weakly with GABA
binding sites (9,10,35). However, in our frozen and thawed
membrane preparations even high amounts of taurine could not displace the specific sodium-independent GABA binding. The final
nature of the sodium-independent taurine binding could only be
ascertained using a specific postsynaptic taurine antagonist
which has not been available. Only during the course of this
work, the first communications proclaiming a selective taurine
(and β-alanine) antagonist have appeared (7,36).

SUMMARY

An account is given of our endeavours to demonstrate sodium-
independent and -dependent taurine binding to brain synaptic membranes. The total and specific sodium-dependent binding and the
total sodium-independent binding were fairly easily amenable to
characterization, but the disclosure of specific sodium-independent binding succeeded only after repeated freezing and thawing,
thorough buffer washes and two Triton X-100 treatments of the
membranes. The sodium-independent binding capacity for taurine

was rather small and only one type of relatively low-affinity binding site was revealed.

Acknowledgements: The financial support of the Medical Research Council of the Academy of Finland and the skilful technical assistance of Miss Riitta Mero are gratefully acknowledged.

REFERENCES

1. Andersén, L., Sundman, L.-O., Lindén, I.-B., Kontro, P., and Oja, S.S. (1982): J. Pharm. Sci., in press.
2. Cavallini, D., De Marco, C., and Mondovi, B. (1958): Bull. Soc. Chim. Biol., 40: 1711-1715.
3. Chiu, T.H., and Rosenberg, H.C. (1979): Eur. J. Pharmacol., 58: 335-338.
4. Enna, S.J., and Snyder, S.H. (1975): Brain Res., 100: 81-97.
5. Enna, S.J., and Snyder, S.H. (1977): J. Neurochem., 28: 857-860.
6. Enna, S.J., and Snyder, S.H. (1977): Mol. Pharmacol., 13: 442-453.
7. Girard, Y., Atkinson, J.G., Williams, M., Haubrich, D.R., and Yarbrough, G.G. (1981): J. Med. Chem., 25: 113-116.
8. Greenlee, D.V., Van Ness, P.C., and Olsen, R.W. (1978): Life Sci., 22: 1653-1662.
9. Greenlee, D.V., Van Ness, P.C., and Olsen, R.W. (1978): J. Neurochem., 31: 933-938.
10. Hitzeman, R.J., and Loh, H.H. (1978): J. Neurochem., 30: 471-477.
11. Horng, J.S., and Wong, D.T. (1979): J. Neurochem., 32: 1379-1386.
12. Huxtable, R.J., Laird, H.E., III, and Lippincott, S.E. (1979): J. Pharmacol. Exp. Ther., 211: 465-471.
13. Kontro, P. (1981): Abstracts, 8th Meeting of the International Society for Neurochemistry, Nottingham, p. 35.
14. Kontro, P., and Oja, S.S. (1981): Neurochem. Res., 6: 1179-1191.
15. Kontro, P., Marnela, K.-M., and Oja, S.S. (1980): Brain Res., 184: 129-141.
16. Kumpulainen, E., Jokisalo, V.J., and Lähdesmäki, P. (1978): Int. J. Neurosci., 8: 123-128.
17. Kurioka, S., Hayata, H., and Matsuda, M. (1981): J. Neurochem., 37: 283-288.
18. Lähdesmäki, P., Kumpulainen, E., Raasakka, O., and Kyrki, P. (1977): J. Neurochem., 29: 819-826.
19. Lester, B.R., Miller, A.L., and Peck, E.J., Jr. (1981): J. Neurochem., 36: 154-164.
20. Lloyd, K.G., and Dreksler, S. (1979): Brain Res., 163: 77-87.
21. López-Colomé, A.M., and Pasantes-Morales, H. (1980): J. Neurochem., 34: 1047-1052.
22. López-Colomé, A.M., and Pasantes-Morales, H. (1981): J. Neurosci. Res., 6: 475-485.

23. Lowry, O.H., Rosebrough, N.J., Farr, A.L., and Randall, R.S. (1951): J. Biol. Chem., 193: 265-275.
24. Marnela, K.-M., Kontro, P., Pitkänen, R.I., and Oja, S.S. (1980): Acta Univ. Oul. A 97, Biochem., 29: 11-16.
25. Napias, C., Bergman, M.O., Van Ness, P.C., Greenlee, D.V., and Olsen, R.W. (1980): Life Sci., 27: 1001-1011.
26. Oja, S.S., and Kontro, P. (1980): J. Neurochem., 35: 1303-1308.
27. Oja, S.S., and Kontro, P. (1982): In: Handbook of Neurochemistry, 2nd ed., vol. 3, edited by A. Lajtha, in press. Plenum Press, New York.
28. Oja, S.S., Lehtinen, I., and Lähdesmäki, P. (1976): Q. J. Exp. Physiol., 61: 133-143.
29. Olsen, R.W., Bergman, M.O., Van Ness, P.C., Lummis, S.C., Watkins, A.E., Napias, C., and Greenlee, D.V. (1981): Mol. Pharmacol., 19: 217-227.
30. Segawa, T., Inoue, A., Ochi, T., Nakata, Y., and Nomura, Y. (1982): In: Taurine in Nutrition and Neurology, edited by R.J. Huxtable, and H. Pasantes-Morales, pp. 311-324. Plenum Press, New York.
31. Sharif, N.A., and Roberts, P.J. (1980): J. Neurochem., 34: 779-784.
32. Snedecor, G.W. (1959): Statistical Methods, 5th ed.. Iowa State College Press, Ames.
33. Toffano, G., Guidotti, A., and Costa, E. (1978): Proc. Natl. Acad. Sci. USA, 75: 4024-4028.
34. Whittaker, V.P., and Barker, L.A. (1972): In: Methods of Neurochemistry, vol. 2, edited by R. Fried, pp. 1-52.
35. Williams, M., Risley, E.A., and Totaro, J.A. (1980): Life Sci., 26: 557-560.
36. Yarbrough, G.G., Singh, D.K., and Taylor, D.A. (1981): J. Pharmacol. Exp. Ther., 219: 604-613.

CNS Receptors—From Molecular
Pharmacology to Behavior, edited by
P. Mandel and F. V. DeFeudis.
Raven Press, New York © 1983.

Localization and Physiological Properties of Glycine and GABA Receptors in Cultures of Rat CNS

L. Hösli and Elisabeth Hösli

Department of Physiology, University of Basel, CH-4051 Basel, Switzerland

Biochemical and electrophysiological studies provide much evidence that GABA and glycine are inhibitory transmitter substances in the mammalian central nervous system (CNS) (3,4,16,23). Since nervous tissue cultures have proved to be an excellent tool to study the cellular localization of binding of various neurotransmitters by means of autoradiography, an attempt was made to visualize binding sites for glycine and GABA and their antagonists strychnine and bicuculline in cultures of rat CNS. The technique of tissue culture also provides a good model system to investigate electrophysiological properties of morphologically identified cells (neurones and glial cells) under direct visual control (13) and to study ionic mechanisms underlying the action of neurotransmitters by altering the ionic composition of the extracellular fluid (14).

MATERIAL AND METHODS

Explant cultures were prepared from spinal cord with or without attached dorsal root ganglia, from the lower brain stem and from the cerebellum of fetal or newborn rats (for details see 10, 15). The methods for the electrophysiological and the autoradiographic binding studies have been described previously (10,11,14,15).

RESULTS AND DISCUSSION

1. Autoradiographic localization of binding sites for GABA, glycine and their antagonists bicuculline and strychnine

A. Binding of ^{3}H-GABA and ^{3}H-bicuculline methiodide

a. Cerebellum. Binding sites for ^{3}H-GABA, the GABA-analogue ^{3}H-muscimol and the antagonist ^{3}H-bicuculline were observed on many cerebellar neurones. Figure 1 shows large neurones with long processes having the appearance of Purkinje cells. They are intensely labelled by ^{3}H-GABA (1A), ^{3}H-bicuculline (1B) and ^{3}H-flunitrazepam (1C), a potent benzodiazepine which is known to interact with neurotransmission mediated by GABA (7). Cerebellar interneurones such as stellate, basket and Golgi cells were also intensely labelled by these compounds (8,10). Similar results have been obtained by biochemical and autoradiographic binding studies in rat cerebellar slices (18,19,21,22,24).

The cell bodies of small neurones having the appearance of granule cells usually revealed no binding of the radio-ligands, but their dendrites and a great number of surrounding fibres showed an intense labelling (8,10). Autoradiographic studies on cerebellar slices have also demonstrated a high density of GABA binding in the granule cell layer, and it was suggested that these binding sites might be localized on granule cell dendrites which receive inhibitory inputs from Golgi cells (21,22).

b. Brain stem and spinal cord.   In cultures prepared from the lower brain stem, many large and medium-sized neurones were intensely labelled by ^{3}H-GABA (Fig. 2B), ^{3}H-bicuculline and ^{3}H-flunitrazepam over the soma and processes. In spinal cord cultures, however, mainly small to medium-sized neurones, probably interneurones, revealed binding of the radio-ligands (Fig. 3C,D) (10). Large unlabelled spinal neurones were often surrounded by labelled fibres which appeared to make contacts with these neurones (10). In cultures of dorsal root ganglia which remained attached to the spinal cord explant, many large neurones as well as the initial part of the bifurcated axons showed binding of ^{3}H-GABA (Fig. 2C).

Binding of all radio-ligands also occurred to nerve fibres, probably unmyelinated axons, which were growing out from the explants, suggesting the existence of non-synaptic GABA-receptors (1).

B. Binding of ^{3}H-glycine, ^{3}H-β-alanine and ^{3}H-strychnine

a. Cerebellum.   In contrast to the great number of binding sites for ^{3}H-GABA, ^{3}H-bicuculline and ^{3}H-flunitrazepam on cerebellar neurones, little or no binding was found for ^{3}H-glycine, ^{3}H-β-alanine and ^{3}H-strychnine.

b. Brain stem and spinal cord.   In brain stem cultures, many large and medium-sized neurones were labelled by ^{3}H-glycine (Fig. 2A), ^{3}H-β-alanine and ^{3}H-strychnine. Binding of ^{3}H-β-alanine was usually weaker than that of ^{3}H-glycine (9), which is consistent with biochemical studies on synaptosomal fractions from brain stem, demonstrating that the B_{max} for highest-affinity β-alanine binding is an order of magnitude lower than that for glycine (5).

In contrast to the findings with ^{3}H-GABA and ^{3}H-bicuculline which labelled mainly interneurones, binding of ^{3}H-glycine, ^{3}H-β-alanine and ^{3}H-strychnine was observed predominantly to large spi-

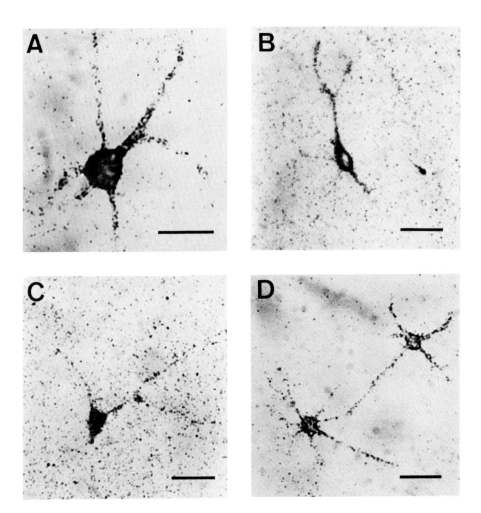

FIG. 1.   A: Purkinje cell showing binding sites for ³H-GABA
(10^{-8}M) over the cell body and dendrites. Culture 21 days <u>in vi-</u>
<u>tro</u> (incubation in Na⁺-containing medium). Bar: 20 μm (from <u>Hösli</u>
and Hösli, 8).   B: Purkinje cell which is heavily labelled by
the GABA antagonist ³H-bicuculline (10^{-8}M). Culture 16 days <u>in vi-</u>
<u>tro</u> (Na⁺-free incubation medium). Bar: 30 μm.   C: Large cerebel-
lar neurone having the appearance of a Purkinje cell which shows
binding of ³H-flunitrazepam (3×10^{-9}M). Culture 28 days <u>in vitro</u>.
Bar: 30 μm.   D: Two medium-sized cerebellar interneurones labelled by the GABA-analogue ³H-muscimol (10^{-8}M). Culture 20 days <u>in</u>
<u>vitro</u> (Na⁺-containing incubation medium). Bar: 30 μm.

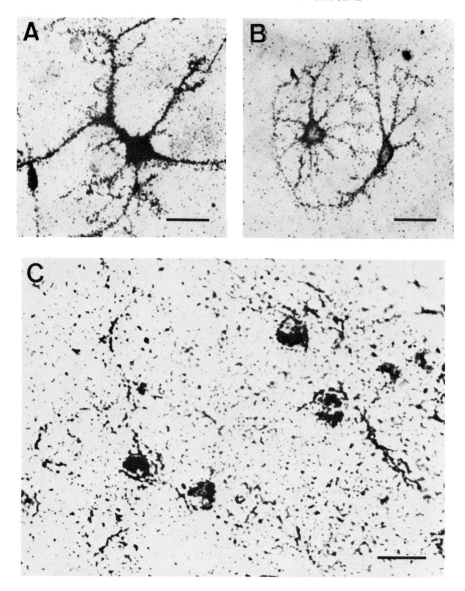

FIG. 2.   A: Large brain stem neurone which is intensely labelled
by ^{3}H-glycine (10^{-8}M) over the cell body and processes. Culture
14 days <u>in vitro</u> (Na$^+$-free incubation medium). Bar: 20 μm.
B: Two brain stem neurones showing binding of ^{3}H-GABA (10^{-8}M).
Culture 20 days <u>in vitro</u> (Na$^+$-free incubation medium). Bar: 20 μm.
C: Labelled dorsal root ganglion neurones after incubation with
^{3}H-GABA (10^{-8}M). Culture 10 days <u>in vitro</u> (Na$^+$-free incubation
medium). Bar: 50 μm (from Hösli et al., 10).

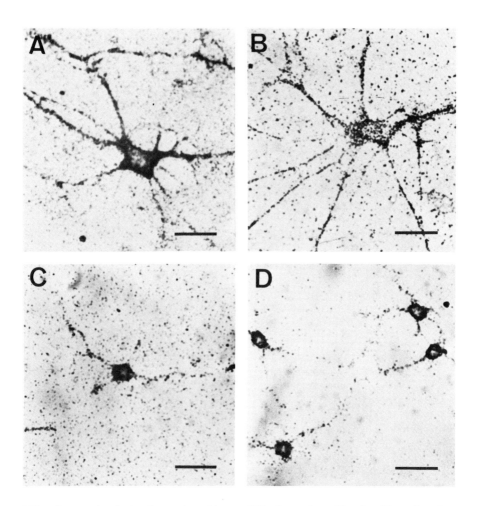

FIG. 3. A: Spinal cord culture (30 days in vitro) after incubation with ^{3}H-glycine (10^{-8}M, Na$^+$-containing medium). The cell
body and processes of the large neurone, probably a motoneurone,
are heavily labelled. B: Large spinal neurone showing binding
sites for ^{3}H-strychnine (10^{-8}M, Na$^+$-containing medium). Culture
21 days in vitro. C: Medium-sized spinal neurone, probably an
interneurone, showing binding sites for ^{3}H-GABA (10^{-8}M, Na$^+$-con-
taining medium). Culture 18 days in vitro. D: Medium-sized spinal neurones labelled by ^{3}H-flunitrazepam (3×10^{-9}M). Culture 20
days in vitro. Bars: 30 μm (A and B from Hösli and Hösli, 9;
C and D from Hösli et al., 10).

nal neurones, probably motoneurones (Fig. 3A,B). As was found in
brain stem cultures, the labelling by ^{3}H-β-alanine was weaker
than that by ^{3}H-glycine (9).

Binding of ^{3}H-GABA, ^{3}H-muscimol and ^{3}H-bicuculline was markedly reduced or inhibited by the addition of unlabelled GABA or bicuculline at high concentrations (10^{-3}M) (10). Addition of unlabelled glycine and strychnine (10^{-3}M) inhibited binding of ^{3}H-gly-
cine, ^{3}H-β-alanine and ^{3}H-strychnine (9). Binding of ^{3}H-flunitra-
zepam was inhibited by adding the pharmacologically potent benzodiazepine Ro-11-7800 (10).

C. Lack of binding sites for ^{3}H-GABA, ^{3}H-glycine and their
   antagonists on cultured glial cells

Although glial cells possess a high-affinity uptake mechanism
for amino acid transmitters (13), no binding of ^{3}H-GABA, ^{3}H-gly-
cine and their antagonists ^{3}H-bicuculline and ^{3}H-strychnine was
found to glial cells (8,9,10). Biochemical studies have also
shown that ^{3}H-GABA and ^{3}H-muscimol are not bound to subcellular
particles prepared from cultured astroblasts (20).

2. Electrophysiological studies of the action
   of glycine and GABA on cultured neurones

A. Action of glycine on neurones of brain stem and spinal cord

Glycine which was administered either microelectrophoretically
by means of multibarrel micropipettes (Fig. 4) or added to the bathing fluid at a concentration of 10^{-4}M (Fig. 5A) caused a hyperpolarization of the majority of cultured neurones tested (11,13,
14). This hyperpolarization was associated with a considerable increase in membrane conductance. As was observed in spinal motoneurones and brain stem neurones in situ (2,3,13,23), the effect of
glycine on neurones in tissue culture was reversibly blocked by
strychnine.

It has been suggested that the hyperpolarization by glycine is
due to an increase in the permeability of the neuronal membrane
for Cl$^-$ and K$^+$ (influx of Cl$^-$ and efflux of K$^+$) (2,3,23). This
suggestion is supported by the following observations which have
been made in our laboratory:
- Replacing Cl$^-$ in the extracellular fluid by acetate reversed the
  hyperpolarization by glycine to a depolarization (Fig. 5) (14),
  indicating that glycine alters the chloride permeability of cultured spinal neurones as it does in motoneurones in situ (2,3).
- Using ion-sensitive microelectrodes, we observed that the hyperpolarization of cultured spinal neurones by glycine is accompanied by an increase of the extracellular K$^+$-concentration $[K^+]_0$
  which is caused by an efflux of K$^+$ from the hyperpolarized cells
  (15).

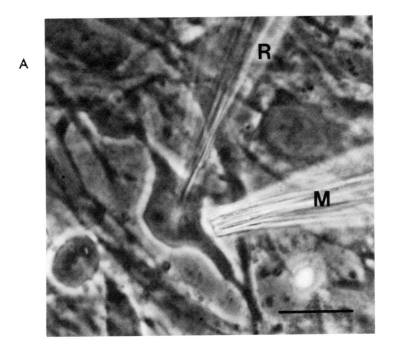

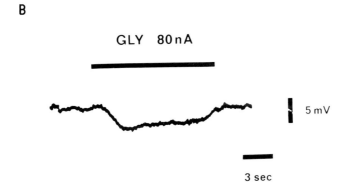

FIG. 4. A: Phase contrast picture of a cultured rat spinal neurone (20 days in vitro). R = microelectrode for intracellular recording. M = 4-barrel micropipette for microelectrophoretic administration of the amino acids. Bar: 20 μm. B: Hyperpolarization
of a cultured spinal neurone by microelectrophoretically-applied
glycine (80 nA) (culture 21 days in vitro; membrane potential
-42 mV) (from Hösli et al., 11).

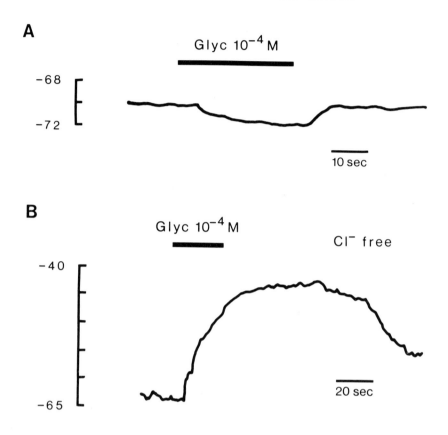

FIG. 5.   Action of glycine (Glyc 10⁻⁴M) on the membrane potential of two different spinal neurones in tissue culture.
A: in normal bathing fluid;   B: in Cl⁻-free bathing solution.
Duration of perfusion with glycine is indicated by horizontal bar
above tracings. Membrane potential in mV (from Hösli et al., 14).

B. Effects of GABA on neurones of the central and peripheral
   nervous system

GABA added to the bathing fluid at a concentration of 10⁻⁴M
caused a hyperpolarization of the majority of CNS neurones tested
(13). In contrast, GABA only had a depolarizing action on neurones
of cultured dorsal root ganglia (DRG, Fig. 7) (12). This depolarization of DRG neurones is consistent with the depolarizing action

of GABA on primary afferent terminals, suggesting that GABA is the transmitter mediating presynaptic inhibition (6). Both effects of GABA - hyperpolarization and depolarization - were associated with a marked increase in membrane conductance which appeared to be due to an increased permeability for Cl^- and K^+ (12,13). As was observed on dorsal root ganglion neurones in situ (6) and in the frog spinal cord (17), the action of GABA on cultured DRG and CNS neurones was accompanied by an increase of the $[K^+]_0$ (15). The effects of GABA were reversibly blocked by the convulsant bicuculline (12).

3. Indirect effects of GABA and glycine on cultured glial cells

In contrast to the hyperpolarizing action of GABA and glycine on cultured CNS neurones, both amino acids caused depolarizations of glial cells which were, however, not associated with a change in membrane resistance (12,15). Almost all glial cells which were depolarized by GABA and glycine were located in the vicinity of neurones; isolated glial cells in the outgrowth zone of the culture where no neurones are present were not affected by these amino acids. 4-Aminopyridine, a substance known to block K^+-conductance of excitable cells, reversibly abolished the depolarization by GABA and glycine of cultured astrocytes (12,15). From these observations it was suggested that the glial depolarization by the amino acids is an indirect effect which could be due to an efflux of K^+ from adjacent neurones. To further test this hypothesis, we have measured $[K^+]_0$ using ion-sensitive microelectrodes which were placed in close vicinity of neurones and glial cells during perfusion with GABA and glycine (15). Simultaneous intracellular recordings of the glial membrane potential revealed a good correlation in amplitude and time course between the depolarization and the increase in K^+-concentration (Fig. 6). From these electrophysiological investigations and the binding studies showing the absence of binding sites for glycine and GABA on glial cells it is suggested that unlike neurones, glial cells do not possess receptors for these amino acid transmitters, and that the glial depolarization by GABA and glycine is an indirect effect due to the efflux of K^+ from adjacent neurones.

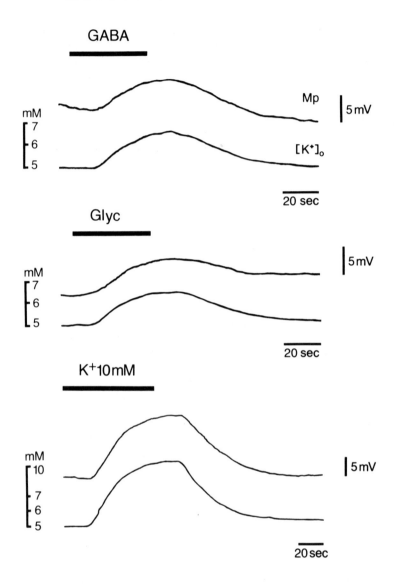

FIG. 6.   Simultaneous recordings of the effects of GABA, glycine
and K$^+$(10 mM)on the membrane potential (upper traces) of a cultured glial cell and on $[K^+]_0$ (lower traces) (spinal cord culture,
30 days in vitro). The resting potential of the glial cell was
-65 mV. Duration of perfusion with the amino acids (concentrations
10^{-4}M) and with K$^+$(10 mM) is indicated by horizontal bars above
tracings (from Hösli et al., 15).

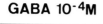

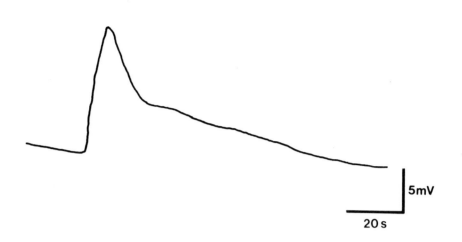

FIG. 7. Depolarization of a dorsal root ganglion neurone by GABA (10^{-4}M) (culture 18 days _in vitro_, membrane potential -60 mV).

SUMMARY AND CONCLUSIONS

Autoradiographic binding studies have shown that ^{3}H-GABA, ^{3}H-glycine, their antagonists ^{3}H-bicuculline and ^{3}H-strychnine were bound to many neurones of cultured rat CNS. In contrast, glial cells did not reveal binding sites for any of the compounds studied. The electrophysiological studies showed that GABA and glycine caused a hyperpolarization of cultured spinal neurones. This hyperpolarization was accompanied by a decrease in membrane resistance which is probably due to an increased membrane permeability to Cl$^-$ and K$^+$. On cultured glial cells, both GABA and glycine produced depolarizations which were, however, not associated with a change in membrane conductance. Measurements of the extracellular K$^+$-concentration using ion-sensitive microelectrodes indicated that the glial depolarization was caused by an efflux of K$^+$ from adjacent neurones. From our electrophysiological and autoradiographic studies it is suggested that unlike neurones, glial cells do not possess receptors for GABA and glycine.

REFERENCES

1. Brown, D.A. and Marsh, S. (1978): Brain Res., 156: 187-191.
2. Curtis, D.R., Hösli, L., Johnston, G.A.R. and Johnston, I.H. (1968): Exp. Brain Res., 5: 235-258.
3. Curtis, D.R. and Johnston, G.A.R. (1974): Rev. Physiol. Biochem. Pharmacol., 69: 79-188.
4. DeFeudis, F.V. (1979): Int. Rev. Neurobiol., 21: 129-216.
5. DeFeudis, F.V., Orensanz Muñoz, L.M., Moya, M.F., Latorre, A. and Fando, J.L. (1977): Gen. Pharmac., 8: 311-314.
6. Deschenes, M. and Feltz, P. (1976): Brain Res., 118: 494-499.
7. Haefely, W.E., Kulcsár, A., Möhler, H., Pieri, L., Polc, P. and Schaffner, R. (1975): In: Mechanisms of action of benzodiazepines, edited by E. Costa and P. Greengard, pp. 131-151. Raven Press, New York.
8. Hösli, E. and Hösli, L. (1980): Exp. Brain Res., 38: 241-243.
9. Hösli, E. and Hösli, L. (1981): Brain Res., 213: 242-245.
10. Hösli, E., Möhler, H., Richards, J.G. and Hösli, L. (1980): Neuroscience, 5: 1657-1665.
11. Hösli, L., Andrés, P.F. and Hösli, E. (1971): Brain Res., 34: 399-402.
12. Hösli, L., Andrés, P.F. and Hösli, E. (1978): Exp. Brain Res., 33: 425-434.
13. Hösli, L. and Hösli, E. (1978): Rev. Physiol. Biochem. Pharmacol., 81: 135-188.
14. Hösli, L., Hösli, E. and Andrés, P.F. (1973): Brain Res., 62: 597-602.
15. Hösli, L., Hösli, E., Andrés, P.F. and Landolt, H. (1981): Exp. Brain Res., 42: 43-48.
16. Krnjević, K. (1974): Physiol. Rev., 54: 418-540.
17. Kudo, Y. and Fukuda, H. (1976): Japan. J. Pharmacol., 26: 385-387.
18. Möhler, H. and Okada, T. (1977): Science, N.Y., 198: 849-851.
19. Möhler, H. and Okada, T. (1977): Nature (Lond.), 267: 65-67.
20. Ossola, L., DeFeudis, F.V. and Mandel, P. (1980): J. Neurochem., 34: 1026-1029.
21. Palacios, J.M., Young, W.S. III and Kuhar, M.J. (1980): Proc. Natl. Acad. Sci. USA, 77: 670-674.
22. Wamsley, J.K., Palacios, J.M., Young, W.S. III and Kuhar, M.J. (1981): J. Histochem. Cytochem., 29: 125-135.
23. Werman, R. (1972): In: Neurotransmitters. Res. Publ. A.R.N.M.D., 50: 147-180.
24. Young, W.S. III and Kuhar, M.J. (1979): Nature (Lond.), 280: 393-395.

CNS Receptors—From Molecular
Pharmacology to Behavior, edited by
P. Mandel and F. V. DeFeudis.
Raven Press, New York © 1983.

Trophic Actions of GABA on the Development of Physiologically Active GABA Receptors

E. Meier, J. Drejer, and A. Schousboe

*Department of Biochemistry A, The Panum Institute, University of Copenhagen,
DK-2200 Copenhagen, Denmark*

There is ample evidence that the interaction between GABA and
the synaptic membrane is mediated by pharmacologically distinctly
different classes of GABA receptors called A- and B-type receptors
(for references see DeFeudis & Mandel (5)). These are characterized by being bicuculline sensitive and insensitive, respectively
(16). Moreover, at least the A-type GABA receptor consists of a
complex of high and low affinity receptors since biphasic binding curves have repeatedly been reported in studies of GABA
binding to synaptic membranes prepared from different brain areas
(1, 11, 15, 21, 25, 26, 34, 39, 43). In addition, the total number
of $GABA_A$ receptor sites increases as a function of development
both in cerebrum and cerebellum (1, 21, 30, 34). In cerebellum
the period of the greatest increase in the number of receptor
sites coincides with the development of the granule cells (30)
in agreement with the repeated suggestion that a major fraction
of the $GABA_A$ receptors in cerebellum resides on this cell type
(17, 19, 21, 27, 29, 33, 41). On the contrary, $GABA_B$ sites
appear to be located primarily in the molecular layer in cerebellum with only a low density on the granule cells (41). In a
recent study of GABA binding to membranes prepared from cultured
cerebellar granule cells only high affinity $GABA_A$ receptors could
be detected. This may suggest that in vivo regulatory mechanisms
for $GABA_A$ receptors apparently were missing in the culture
system. Since it is known that certain neurotransmitters influence
the development of their respective receptors (for references see
Schousboe (32)) and that GABA may be important for synapse form-

ation (42) we decided to examine the effects of GABA in the culture media on the development of GABA receptors in cultured granule
cells. It was found that the presence of GABA during the culture
period led to the development of low affinity GABA receptors in
addition to the high affinity receptors which were always present
on the cells.

CELL CULTURES

Granule cells were cultured from cerebella of 7-day-old rats
essentially as described by Messer (23), Drejer et al. (7) and
Meier & Schousboe (21). Briefly, cells were isolated by mild tryp-
sinization followed by trituration in a DNAse solution containing
a trypsin inhibitor from soy beans. The cells were suspended at a
concentration of 3×10^7 cells/ml in Dulbecco's minimum essential
medium containing 10% fetal or newborn calf serum. This suspension was subsequently inoculated into poly-L-lysine-coated culture
flasks or Petri dishes. The culture medium contained in addition
to the usual constituents of Dulbecco's medium 24.5 mM KCl, 30 mM
glucose, 7 µM p-aminobenzoic acid and 100 mU/l insulin. After 2-3
days in culture 40 µM cytosine arabinoside was added and after 24
hours this medium was changed to an analogous medium without the
mitotic inhibitor. The cells were maintained in culture for
at least eight days.   Such cultures have been shown to consist
of 80 - 90 % granule cells and 5 - 10 % astrocytes (4). From a
distribution of the anodic and cathodic components of the D2 synaptic antigen in the cells (2) it may be concluded that they had

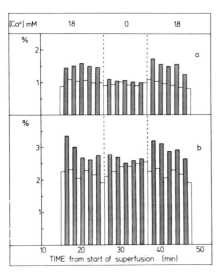

*FIG. 1. Fractional release (% in fraction of total radioactivity remaining in tissue prior to the fraction in question) of D-aspar-tate(a) or L-glutamate (b) from cultured cerebellar granule cells preloaded with ^{3}H-D-aspartate or ^{3}H-L-glutamate. Open bars repre-sent release into physiological (5.0 mM KCl) media and hatched bars represent release into high potassium (55 mM KCl) media. The Ca^{2+} concentration in the super-fusion media is indicated at the top of the figure.
From Drejer et al. (8).*

matured after 7 - 8 days in culture to a stage corresponding to that of cerebellum at the same postnatal age. Moreover, as can be seen from Fig. 1, such cells exhibit a pronounced potassium stimulated calcium dependent release of exogenously-supplied ^{3}H-L-glutamate or ^{3}H-D-aspartate which is in keeping with the presumed glutamatergic nature of cerebellar granule cells (e.g., 20, 45).

DEVELOPMENT IN VIVO

It is well established that the number of GABA binding sites increases in cerebellum as a function of postnatal development (1, 9, 21, 30, 34) and as can be seen from Table I this increase is reflected both in high and low affinity receptors. Moreover, from Fig. 2 it appears that the two receptor sites exhibit separate developmental patterns, the high affinity site reaching its maximum level at a much earlier developmental stage than the low affinity receptor. This might be interpreted as a differential   effect of endogenous regulators on the two receptor sites. It should be noted that the low affinity site (and only the low affinity site) may change also its affinity during development (Table I). Since a large fraction of the cerebellar GABA receptors are located on granule cells (cf. above) the developmental and functional properties of these receptors were studied in cultured granule cells.

Table I. *Kinetic constants (K_D and B_{max}) for GABA binding to membranes prepared from cerebella from rats of different postnatal ages.*

Age	K_D (nM)		B_{max} (pmol $\times$ mg^{-1})	
(days)	high affinity	low affinity	high affinity	low affinity
7	8.3 ± 0.3	158 ± 30	0.035 ± 0.002	0.123 ± 0.047
15	9.0 ± 0.5	163 ± 21	0.302 ± 0.021	0.561 ± 0.003
60	7.3 ± 0.3	753 ± 64	0.300 ± 0.010	1.262 ± 0.048

Kinetic constants were estimated from original binding data by computer analysis according to Olsen et al. (26). B_{max} values are expressed on the basis of total protein, i.e. the protein content in the cerebellar homogenates from which membranes were isolated as described by Meier & Schousboe (21). Values are averages ± S.E.M. of 3 individual experiments. From Meier and Schousboe (21).

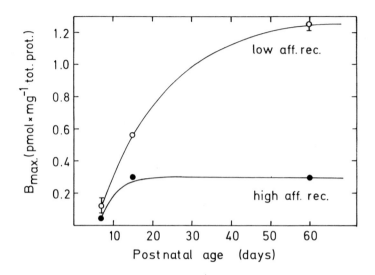

FIG. 2. B_{max} *for high and low affinity GABA receptors in cere-*
bellum as a function of the postnatal age of the rats. Values
have been taken from Table I. For further details, see legend
to Table I.

DEVELOPMENT IN VITRO

As can be seen from Fig. 3a and 3c,membranes prepared from
cultured cerebellar granule cells exhibited only the high affinity
GABA receptor regardless of the age of the cultures (culture period
8 - 21 days). This strongly indicated that an important endogenous
regulatory factor was missing in the culture system,and the transmitter itself might represent a strong candidate for such an endogenous regulator (14, 32). Since the granule cell culture lacks
the ability to release endogenous GABA (12) the granule cells were
cultured in the presence of 50 μM GABA. As shown in Fig. 3b this
treatment of the cultures led to the appearance of a low affinity
GABA receptor on the cultured cells. The kinetic properties of
this receptor were found to be almost identical to those of the low
affinity receptor found in cerebellar membranes prepared from cerebel·
la of the same ontogenetic age (cf. Table I and Fig. 3). The presence
of both high and low affinity GABA receptors on the GABA-treated
cultures is in agreement with results obtained for GABA binding to

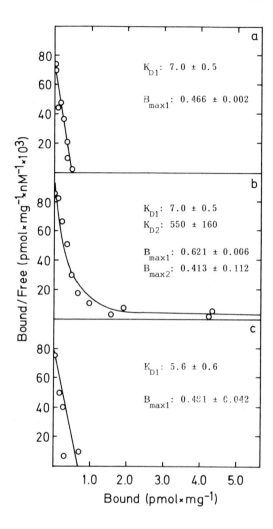

FIG. 3. Scatchard plots of ^{3}*H-GABA binding to membranes from cerebellar granule cells grown for 8 days in vitro in the absence (a) or presence (b) of 50 μM GABA or for 21 days without GABA (c). Binding conditions and membrane preparation were as described by Meier and Schousboe (21). Kinetic constants were obtained by computer analysis as described by Olsen et al. (26). Values are averages of 3 experiments ± S.E.M. and expressed as nM (K$_D$) and pmol bound × mg^{-1} membrane protein (B$_{max}$). From Meier et al. (22).*

membranes from cultures of cerebral cortical neurons maintained in culture for 3 weeks (38). The presence of only the high affinity site in cultures grown under standard conditions (i.e., without GABA) agrees, however, with analogous studies on cortical neurons cultured for only 3 days (6). This difference in the expression of high and low affinity GABA receptors on 3-day-old and 21-day-old cultures of cerebral cortical neurons, respectively might be explained by the absence of extracellular GABA in the younger cultures and presence of GABA in the older ones. In cultured cortical neurons the ability to synthesize and release GABA does not develop until the second and the third week in culture (35) consistent with the appearance of low affinity receptors in cultures of this age. These observations accordingly strongly indicate that GABA might play an important role in vivo as a regulatory substance for the development of GABA receptors. In support of this, it has been observed that injections of nipecotic acid, a compound known to increase synaptic levels of GABA (44), into rat retina lead to an increased number of retinal GABA receptors (D.A. Redburn, personal communication).

FUNCTIONAL CORRELATIONS OF GABA RECEPTORS

In order to obtain information about the physiological properties of the GABA receptors on cultured granule cells the effect of GABA on evoked release of L-glutamate or D-aspartate, a non-metabolizable analogue of glutamate, was studied. As seen in Fig. 4, GABA inhibited the potassium-stimulated D-aspartate (or L-glutamate, results not shown) release only when the granule cells had been grown in the presence of GABA. Moreover, relatively high concentrations of external GABA (> 500 nM) were needed for the inhibition of evoked D-aspartate release. Hence, it is likely that the inhibitory effect of GABA on glutamate release is brought about either by the low affinity GABA receptor alone or by a concerted effect of GABA on high and low affinity receptors. The observation (Table I) that it is primarily the number of low affinity receptor sites which increases as a function of maturation indicates that also in the in vivo situation low affinity GABA-receptors are essential for the GABA induced activation/deactivation of the GABA-receptor ionophore complex.

In addition to the effect of GABA on the induction of low affinity receptors, GABA in the culture media also affected other

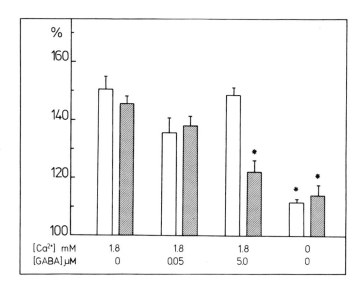

FIG. 4. Effect of external GABA on K^+-induced stimulation of ^3H-D-aspartate release from granule cells grown for 8 days in vitro in the absence (□) or in the presence (▨) of 50 μM GABA. Conditions were as described in Fig. 1. The columns represent the radioactivity (means ± S.E.M.) released in 5 successive stimulation (55 mM K^+) periods as percentage of the average release in the low potassium (5.0 mM K^+) medium. Asterisks indicate statistically significant differences from the stimulation exerted by 55 mM K^+ in the presence of Ca^{2+} (P < 0.025). From Meier et al. (22).

functional properties of the cells. It was found (Table II) that the presence of GABA in the culture media greatly enhanced neurite formation in the cultured cells. It is seen that the number of neurite-extending cells per mm^2 was increased by 50%. This finding is in perfect agreement with recent reports by Wolff et al. (42) and Spoerri & Wolff (36) of morphological changes at the electron microscope level of neurons exposed to extracellular GABA in vivo and of neuroblastoma cells cultured in the presence of GABA. These authors observed an increase in presynaptic thickenings and specialized synaptic contacts after exposure of the tissue to extracellular GABA which suggested a dual role of GABA in neurotransmission and in synaptogenesis.

Table II. *Effect of GABA on formation of neurites and neuronal colonies in granule cell cultures.*

Culture conditions	Neurite ext. cells/mm^2	Colonies/mm^2
- GABA (control)	629 ± 33	19 ± 4
+ GABA (50 µM)	931 ± 82*	43 ± 7*

Cells were cultured for 8 days in the absence or presence of 50 µM GABA and photomicrographs were taken and scored blindly for neurite-extending cells and colonies of cells. Non-neuronal flat cells (astroblasts) were not scored. Results are averages ± S.E.M. of 12 micrographs taken randomly of 3 cultures of each group. The asterisks indicate significant difference from control (P < 0.01). From Meier et al. (22).

The effects of GABA on the expression of receptor sites and on neurite growth might be anticipated to be reflected in the protein synthesis of the cells. As shown in Fig. 5,the addition of GABA to the culture medium led to changes in the protein composition of the cells. It is seen that extracts of granule cells cultured in the presence of GABA exhibited a distinct protein band at a molecular weight of approximately 70,000 whereas cells grown in the absence of GABA exhibited only a weak protein band at this position. The functional implication of this is as yet unclear but the finding demonstrates that the treatment with GABA leads to changes in the pattern of the protein synthesis in the cells.

The present results indicate that GABA is important for the development of at least part of the system required for GABA-mediated neurotransmission. In this context it seemed logical also to investigate benzodiazepine binding to cultured granule cells since an association between GABA and benzodiazepine binding sites has been repeatedly suggested (13, 18, 24, 31, 37, 40). As shown in Table III,very little binding of flunitrazepam could be demonstrated in membranes from cultured granule cells regardless of whether or not the cells had been cultured in the presence of GABA. This indicates that at least in cerebellar granule cells there does not appear to be an association between GABA and benzodiazepine receptors which is in line with autoradiographic studies of cerebellar slices by Palacios and Kuhar (28). The finding, however, also poses the question of an endogenous 'anxiety-ligand' which could have trophic actions on the benzodiazepine receptors and which may be missing in the culture system. The existence of such an endogenous benzodiazepine related ligand has been reported (10).

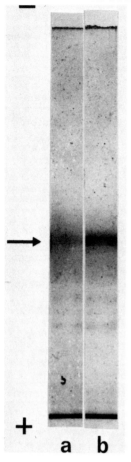

FIG. 5. SDS-polyacrylamide gel electrophoresis of granule cells cultured for
2 days in the absence (panel a) or presence of 50 μM GABA - during the last
24 hours - (panel b). Cells were harvested and solubilized by boiling for
3 min in 0.125 M Tris-HCl (pH 6.8) containing 0.2 mM EDTA, 1.25% SDS, 12.5%
glycerol, 0.5% mercaptoethanol and
0.0075% bromphenol blue. Samples (∿ 15
μg protein) were run in a discontinuous
Lammelli gel system for 3 hours at 50 mA.
Gels were subsequently fixed and stained
with coomassie brilliant blue. The arrow
indicates the position of proteins having a molecular weight of approximately
70,000.
E. Meier, unpublished.

Table III. Brain specific benzodiazepine receptor binding to membranes from rat cerebellum and from cerebellar granule
cells cultured in the presence or absence of 50 μM GABA.

	Specific binding (fmol × mg^{-1})	Relative dens. (cerebellum 100)	P
Cerebellum (60 days)	99 ± 3	100	< 0.001
Cult.gran.cells (8 DIV)	4.0 ± 0.7	4	0.01
Cult.gran.cells (8 DIV) + 50 μM GABA	7.3 ± 0.4	7	< 0.001
Cult.gran.cells (21 DIV)	19 ± 7	19	0.06

Benzodiazepine binding was determined using ^{3}H-flunitrazepam as
the radio-ligand and clonazepam to correct for unspecific binding
as described by Braestrup and Squires (3).Results are averages ±
S.E.M. of 3 experiments, and P-values < 0.05 indicate that specific binding is significantly different from zero.
From Meier et al. (22).

ACKNOWLEDGEMENTS

The technical assistance by Miss B. Marcussen and Mrs. G.M. Rossing is gratefully acknowledged. The work has been supported financially by grants from The Danish Medical Research Council (12-2309; 12-3229) to E. Meier and the Danish Natural Science Research Council (511-20817; 81-3256) and the NOVO Foundation to A. Schousboe.

REFERENCES

1. Aldinio, C., Balzano, M.A., and Toffano, G. (1980): Pharmacol. Res. Commun., 12: 495-500.
2. Balazs, R., Regan, C., Meier, E., Woodhams, G.L., Wilkin, G. P., Patel, L.J., and Gordon, R.D. (1980): In: Tissue Culture in Neurobiology, edited by E. Giacobini, A. Vernadakis, and A. Shahar, pp. 155-168. Raven Press, New York.
3. Braestrup, S., and Squires, R.F. (1977): Proc. Natl. Acad. Sci. U.S.A., 74: 3805-3809.
4. Currie, D.N. (1980): In: Tissue Culture in Neurobiology, edited by E. Giacobini, A. Vernadakis, and A. Shahar, pp. 75-87, Raven Press, New York.
5. DeFeudis, F.V., and Mandel, P., editors (1981): Amino Acid Neurotransmitters. Adv. Biochem. Psychopharmacol., 29: 1-572.
6. DeFeudis, F.V., Ossola, L., Schmitt, G., and Mandel, P. (1979): Neurosci. Lett., 14: 195-199.
7. Drejer, J., Larsson, O.M., and Schousboe, A. (1982): Exp. Brain Res., 47: 259-269.
8. Drejer, J., Larsson, O.M., and Schousboe, A. (1982): Neurochem. Res., submitted.
9. East, S.M., and Dutton, G.R. (1981): Febs Lett., 23: 307-311.
10. Ebstein, B., Guidotti, A., and Costa, E. (1982): In: Problems in GABA Research From Brain to Bacteria, edited by Y. Okada, and E. Roberts, pp. 348-354. Excerpta Medica, Amsterdam.
11. Falch, E., and Krogsgaard-Larsen, P. (1982): J. Neurochem., 38: 1123-1129.
12. Gallo, V., Ciotti, M.T., Coletti, A., Aloisi, F., and Levi, G. (1982): Proc. Natl. Acad. Sci. U.S.A., in press.
13. Gavish, M., and Snyder, S.H. (1981): Proc. Natl. Acad. Sci. U.S.A., 78: 1939-1942.
14. Giacobini, G., Filogamo, G., Weber, M., Boquet, P., and Changeux, J.-P. (1973): Proc. Natl. Acad. Sci. U.S.A., 70: 1708-1712.
15. Guidotti, A., Gale, K., Suria, A., and Toffano, G. (1979): Brain Res., 172: 566-571.
16. Hill, D.R., and Bowery, N.G. (1981): Nature (Lond.), 290: 149-152.
17. Hösli, E., Möhler, H., Richards, J.G., and Hösli, L. (1980): Neuroscience, 5: 1657-1665.

18. Huang, A., Barker, J.L., Steven, M.P., Moncada, V., and Skolnick, P. (1980): Brain Res., 190: 485-491.
19. Kingsbury, A.E., Wilkin, G.D., Patel, A.J., and Balazs, R. (1980): J. Neurochem., 35: 739-742.
20. McBride, W.J., Nadi, N.S., Altman, J., and Aprison, M. (1976): Neurochem. Res., 1: 141-152.
21. Meier, E., and Schousboe, A. (1982): Dev. Neurosci., 5: in press.
22. Meier, E., Schousboe, A., and Drejer, J. (1982): Nature (Lond.). Submitted.
23. Messer, A. (1977): Brain Res., 130: 1-12.
24. Möhler, H., Richards, J.G., and Wu, J.-Y. (1981): Proc. Natl. Acad. Sci. U.S.A., 78: 1935-1938.
25. Napias, C., Bergman, M.O., Van Ness, P.C., Greenlee, D.V., and Olsen, R.W. (1980): Life Sci., 27: 1001-1011.
26. Olsen, R.W., Bergman, M.O., Van Ness, P.C., Lummis, S.C., Watkins, A.E., Napias, C., and Greenlee, D.V. (1981): Mol. Pharmacol., 19: 217-227.
27. Olsen, R.W., and Mikoshiba, K. (1978): J. Neurochem., 30: 1633-1636.
28. Palacios, S.M., and Kuhar, M.S. (1980): In: GABA Neurotransmission. Brain Res. Bull., Vol. 5, Suppl. 2, edited by H. Lal, pp. 145-148. Ankho Internat. Inc. New York.
29. Palacios, J.M., Young, W.S., and Kuhar, J. (1980): Proc. Natl. Acad. Sci. U.S.A., 77: 670-674.
30. Patel, A.J., Smith, R.M., Kingsbury, A.E., Hunt, A., and Balazs, R. (1980): Brain Res., 198: 389-402.
31. Reisine, T.D., Overstreet, D., Gale, K., Rossor, M., Iversen, L., and Yamamura, H.I. (1980): Brain Res., 199: 79-88.
32. Schousboe, A. (1982): In: Neuroscience Approached Through Cell Culture, Vol. 1, edited by S.E. Pfeiffer, pp. in press. CRC Press, Boca Raton, Fl.
33. Simantov, R., Oster-Granite, M.L., Herndon, R.N., and Snyder, S.H. (1976): Brain Res., 105: 365-371.
34. Skerritt, J.H., and Johnston, G.A.R. (1982): Dev. Neurosci., 5: 189-197.
35. Snodgrass, S.R., White, W.F., Biales, B., and Dichter, M. (1980): Brain Res., 190: 123-138.
36. Spoerri, P.E., and Wolff, S.R. (1981): Cell Tissue Res., 218: 567-579.
37. Supavilai, P., and Karobath, M. (1981): Eur. J. Pharmacol., 70: 183-193.
38. Ticku, M.K., Huang, A., and Barker, S.L. (1980): Mol. Pharmacol., 17: 285-289.
39. Wang, Y.-S., Salvaterra, P., and Roberts, E. (1979): Biochem. Pharmacol., 28: 1123-1128.
40. White, W.F., Snodgrass, S.R., and Dichter, M. (1981): Brain Res., 215: 162-176.
41. Wilkin, G.P., Hudson, A.L., Hill, D.R., and Bowery, N.G. (1981): Nature (Lond.), 294: 584-587.

42. Wolff, S.R., Rickmann, M., and Chronwall, B.M. (1979): Cell
     Tissue Res., 201: 239-248.
43. Wong, D.T., Horng, J.S. (1977): Life Sci., 20: 445-451.
44. Wood, J.D., Schousboe, A., and Krogsgaard-Larsen, P. (1980):
     Neuropharmacology, 19: 1149-1152.
45. Young, A.B., Oster-Granite, M.L., Herndon, R.M., and Snyder,
     S.H. (1974): Brain Res., 73: 1-13.

CNS Receptors—From Molecular
Pharmacology to Behavior, edited by
P. Mandel and F. V. Defeudis.
Raven Press, New York © 1983.

Some Characteristics of Solubilized and Partially Purified Cerebral GABA and Benzodiazepine Receptors

Kinya Kuriyama and Yoshihisa Ito

Department of Pharmacology, Kyoto Prefectural University of Medicine, Kawaramachi-Hirokoji, Kamikyo-Ku, Kyoto 602, Japan

γ-Aminobutyric acid (GABA) has been established as a major inhibitory neurotransmitter in the mammalian central nervous system (11,15,20,34). Recently, Na-independent binding of [³H]GABA to synaptic membrane fractions obtained from the rat brain has been demonstrated (37), and this binding is considered to be representative of the association of GABA with its physiologically relevant GABA receptor. It has also been reported that muscimol has a potent agonistic action on GABA receptors (12,14), and [³H]muscimol has been used as a specific radioligand for the synaptic GABA receptor (2,9,10,24).

In various pharmacological (8) and neurophysiological (5,18) experiments, benzodiazepines have been found to facilitate GABAergic synaptic transmission. In addition, the existence of a specific and high affinity benzodiazepine receptor in the rat brain (21,31) has been demonstrated. Recent biochemical studies also provided evidence that benzodiazepines stimulate [³H]GABA receptor binding (9), while GABA agonists facilitate the benzodiazepine receptor binding (3,17,28,31). Furthermore, it has been demonstrated that barbiturates can influence the functional state of certain complexes associated with GABA receptors (22,33). These results suggest that the GABA receptor may be coupled with benzodiazepine and barbiturate recognition sites in cerebral synaptic membranes.

In order to facilitate the further characterization of cerebral GABA receptor, solubilization and purification of the receptor molecule must be achieved. In the present study, we have attempted to solubilize GABA receptor from synaptic membranes of the rat brain using Nonidet P-40, and to purify partially GABA and benzodiazepine receptors from these solubilized fractions.

SOLUBILIZATION OF GABA RECEPTOR FROM SYNAPTIC MEMBRANES

For the solubilization of GABA receptor from synaptic membranes, various detergents were used at solubilizing concentrations (1,4,6). As shown in Table 1, all detergents tested partially solubilized

TABLE 1. [³H]Muscimol binding to solubilized cerebral
          synaptic membranes

	Protein (mg)	[³H]Muscimol bound (fmol)	Specific binding (fmol/mg prot.)
P₂-membrane	28.3	386.9	13.6
Triton X-100(1.0%)			
Supernatant	15.9	629.6	39.6
Pellet	8.4	580.4	69.1
Deoxycholate(0.2%) + 1M KCL			
Supernatant	20.3	791.7	39.0
Pellet	5.7	200.0	35.1
Lysolecithin(0.25%)			
Supernatant	19.2	1244.2	64.8
Pellet	5.6	665.2	111.8
Nonidet P-40(1.0%)			
Supernatant	18.5	1087.8	58.8
Pellet	7.7	440.4	57.2
Digitonin(1.0%)			
Supernatant	14.7	130.8	8.9
Pellet	9.9	680.3	68.7

The frozen and thawed synaptic membrane fractions were washed 3
times with 50 ml of Tris-citrate buffer (pH 7.1) before use, and
this fraction was called P₂-membrane. The P₂-membranes were treated
with various detergents at 2°C for 20 min, and centrifuged at
105,000 g for 1 h. The resultant pellet was suspended in 50 mM
Tris-citrate buffer and this suspension was incubated with 1 nM
[³H]muscimol. The supernatant was dialyzed against 50 mM Tris-
citrate (pH 7.1) buffer containing 0.1% Triton X-100 at 2°C for
2 h. Finally, each fraction was incubated with 1 nM [³H]muscimol.
Each value represents the mean from 3 separate experiments done in
triplicate.   From Ito and Kuriyama (9).

---

the binding sites for [³H]muscimol from synaptic membrane. It has
been found that ammonium sulfate precipitation (ASP) induces a
significant increase in [³H]muscimol binding. A possible explanation for this increase in [³H]muscimol binding may be that the
endogenous inhibitory factor is solubilized with GABA receptor and
that this factor is removed by ammonium sulfate precipitation.
A similar type of increase in [³H]muscimol binding was noted following Triton X-100 treatment of crude synaptic membranes (16,30,
35,36). When the supernatant obtained following ammonium sulfate
precipitation was added to the assay mixture for [³H]muscimol
binding to solubilized (ASP) fraction, a marked inhibition of
[³H]muscimol binding was also demonstrated (9). Scatchard plot
analysis of the data from experiments on the supernatant-induced

inhibition of the specific [³H]muscimol binding revealed that the
apparent affinity of [³H]muscimol for the solubilized (ASP) fraction was decreased, whereas the maximal binding capacity was not
affected.

It is noteworthy that the solubilized (ASP) fraction obtained
by deoxycholate (DOC) + KCl is fairly unstable and showed a tendency to aggregate proteins. These results suggest that DOC + KCl
may not be a suitable detergent when the solubilized protein is
subjected to further purification. Among all detergents tested
(Table 1), Nonidet P-40 (1%) was found to possess good characteristics for solubilizing GABA receptor from synaptic membranes, such
as causing no interference with [³H]muscimol binding, yielding a high
specific activity of [³H]muscimol in the supernatant, rendering no
aggregation of the solubilized protein, maintaining a good stability of the solubilized GABA receptor. Although lysolecithin
(0.25%) was as potent a solubilizer as Nonidet P-40, the protein
solubilized by this agent showed a tendency for instability as
well as aggregation. Considering these experimental results, we
have decided that Nonidet P-40 is the best detergent for the solubilization of GABA receptor from cerebral synaptic membranes.

BIOCHEMICAL CHARACTERISTICS OF SOLUBILIZED GABA RECEPTOR

The binding capacity of solubilized GABA receptor after treatment with Nonidet P-40 was stable for 4 days at 4°C and for 2
weeks at -20°C. Pronase and trypsin treatments or exposure to
50°C for 15 min significantly inhibited the binding of [³H]musci-
mol, whereas treatment with phospholipase-C, α-glycosidase and
β-galactosidase had no effect. These results indicate that the
function of GABA receptor is dependent upon the integrity of the
protein.

A Hill plot showed that the Hill coefficients were 1.1 and 1.0
for synaptic (P_2) membrane and soluble (ASP) fractions, respectively
(Fig. 1). These results clearly indicate that cooperativity does not
change following solubilization and ammonium sulfate precipitation.
It has been reported that the conductance change induced by exo-
genously-applied GABA in arthropod tissues exhibits a typical
sigmoid curve, with slope close to 2 for Hill plots of the dose
vs response (26,27) or of Cl⁻ uptake (29). Considering these
results coupled with the present findings, it is conceivable that
the mechanism of cooperativity found in electrophysiological
studies may be present at the level of activation of ionophore, but
not at the level of GABA receptor binding.

The Scatchard plot of [³H]muscimol binding to the solubilized
(ASP) fraction revealed the presence of at least two different
types of binding site, as shown in the case of synaptic (P_2) and
Triton X-100-treated membranes (Fig. 2). The B max values for high
affinity binding sites in the solubilized (ASP) fraction and in
0.05% Triton X-100-treated membranes were greater than those found
in synaptic (P_2) membranes, whereas the Kd value for the low

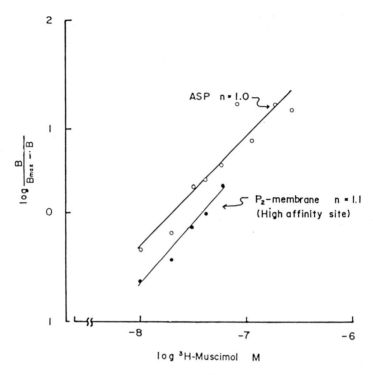

Fig. 1. Hill plots of binding of [³H]muscimol to the synaptic
(P₂) membrane and solubilized (ASP) fractions.
From Ito and Kuriyama (9).

---

affinity site in the solubilized (ASP) fraction was lower than
that found in synaptic (P₂) membranes. In addition, it was found
that relative proportions of the high affinity component in solubilized (ASP) fractions were larger than those in synaptic membranes. These results clearly indicate that solubilization and
ammonium sulfate precipitation of GABA receptor induce the increase
in the B max value of the high affinity component, as well as the
increase in the affinity of low affinity sites, possibly due to the
removal of the inhibitor for GABA receptor binding. Although it
has been found that this inhibitory substance is dialyzable and
heat-stable and induces a reduction in the affinity of [³H]muscimol
for GABA receptor sites without altering the B max value, exact
properties of the inhibitor remain to be determined by further
studies.

FUNCTIONAL ASSOCIATION OF GABA AND BENZODIAZEPINE RECEPTORS:
COEXISTENCE OF BOTH RECEPTOR SITES IN SOLUBILIZED
MACROMOLECULAR PROTEIN

The addition of 10^{-5} M diazepam slightly but significantly
increased the binding of $[^3H]$muscimol, not only to synaptic (P_2)
and Triton X-100-treated membranes, but also to the solubilized

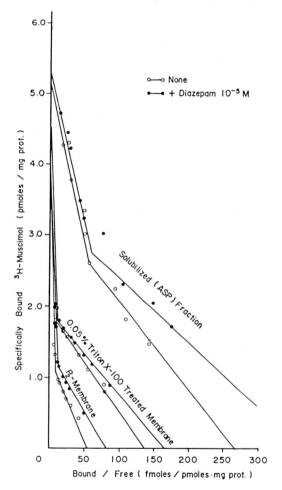

Fig. 2. Scatchard plot analysis of $[^3H]$muscimol binding to various fractions and effect of diazepam on the binding. Each fraction was incubated with 10 pmol $[^3H]$muscimol in the presence of
varying concentrations of non-radioactive muscimol up to 230 pmol.
Triton X-100 (0.05%)-treated membrane was prepared as follows:
The frozen synaptic membrane was treated with 0.05% Triton X-100
at 25°C for 20 min. Following the centrifugation at 48,000 g for
20 min, each sample was used for the determination of $[^3H]$muscimol
binding.   From Ito and Kuriyama (9)

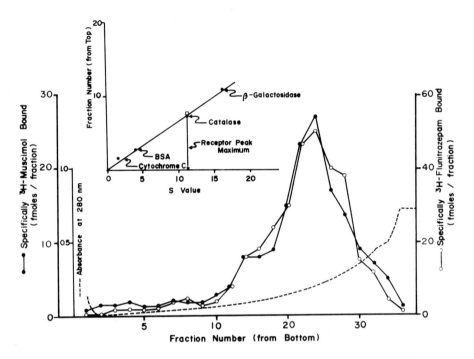

Fig. 3. Sucrose density gradient centrifugation of solubilized receptor protein fraction. One ml of the residue obtained following
Amicon XM 100-A filtration (approximately 5 mg protein) was subjected to 23 ml of a linear sucrose (5 - 25%) density gradient
(containing 50 mM Tris-citrate (pH 7.1), 150 mM NaCl and 0.1%
Nonidet P-40) centrifugation. Centrifugation was carried out for
20 hrs at 24,000 RPM in the Hitachi RPS-25 rotor (6°C). One-ml
fractions were collected, and 300-μl aliquots of each fraction were
used to determine the specific binding of [³H]muscimol and [³H]-
flunitrazepam and protein.

(ASP) fraction. Furthermore, these increases in [³H]muscimol binding by diazepam were always due to a change in the Kd value, but
not in the B max value, of the high affinity site (Fig. 2).
Several reports are available which indicate that a single macromolecular receptor protein complex possesses the ability to bind
GABA as well as benzodiazepines (7,9,25). In the present study we
have also found that benzodiazepine binding site is co-chromato-
graphed with GABA receptor, having a molecular weight of
260,000 - 270,000 daltons on gel filtration by Sephadex G-200 (9).
Similarly, the peak of [³H]flunitrazepam binding site also appeared
in the identical fraction with that of [³H]muscimol binding site
when the solubilized fraction was subjected to a linear sucrose
density gradient centrifugation (Fig. 3). The molecular weight
estimated by the latter method was found to be approximately

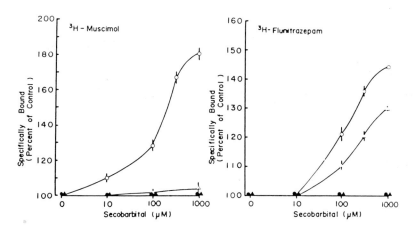

Fig. 4. Effect of secobarbital on [³H]muscimol and [³H]Flu binding to synaptic membrane and solubilized fraction. Binding to synaptic membrane in the absence (△) or presence (o) of 120 mM NaCl. Binding to solubilized fraction in the absence (▲) or presence (●) of 120 mM NaCl.

240,000. These values are essentially in agreement with those reported previously (1,9,23). In addition, it has been found that the apparent molecular weight of benzodiazepine binding site is estimated to be 51,000 daltons when solubilized GABA receptor fraction (ASP fraction) was photolabelled using [³H]flunitrazepam in the presence of UV light (9,10). These results strongly suggest that GABA receptor may be coupled to benzodiazepine receptor and may constitute a GABA/benzodiazepine molecular complex.

GABA AND BARBITURATE RECEPTORS:
DISAPPEARANCE OF STIMULATORY EFFECT OF BARBITURATE ON
[³H]MUSCIMOL BINDING DURING SOLUBILIZATION

It has been reported that barbiturates can influence the functional state of certain complexes associated with GABA receptors, leading to a decreased rate of dissociation of GABA (32,33). Secobarbital, pentobarbital and thiopental stimulated both [³H]-muscimol and [³H]flunitrazepam binding to synaptic membranes in the presence of NaCl (Fig. 4). These stimulatory effects were dose-dependent and were antagonized by picrotoxin. Kinetic analysis of secobarbital-stimulated [³H]muscimol and [³H]flunitrazepam binding to synaptic (P₂) membranes revealed that secobarbital induced an increase in B max value of high affinity [³H]muscimol binding site as well as an increase in affinity (decrease in Kd value) at [³H]flunitrazepam binding site (Table 2). In contrast, no stimulatory effect of secobarbital on either [³H]muscimol or [³H]flunitrazepam binding was detected in solubilized receptor fraction. In addition, it was found that the pretreatment of

TABLE 2. Kinetic analysis of secobarbital-stimulated[^{3}H]muscimol
and [^{3}H]flunitrazepam binding to cerebral synaptic
membrane in the presence of 120 mM NaCl

A) [^{3}H]Muscimol binding site

Treatment	High affinity site		Low affinity site	
	Kd(nM)	Bmax(pmoles/ mg prot.)	Kd(nM)	Bmax(pmoles/ mg prot.)
None	47.0	0.7	350	2.1
Secobarbital (3 × 10^{-4}M)	50.0	1.1	330	2.1

B) [^{3}H]Flunitrazepam binding site

Treatment	Kd(nM)	Bmax(pmoles/mg prot.)
None	1.48	1.05
Secobarbital (3 × 10^{-4}M)	0.89	1.06

synaptic (P$_2$) membranes with 0.1 - 1%   Nonidet P-40 completely
eliminated the stimulatory effect of secobarbital on the binding.
These results strongly suggest that the stimulatory effects of
barbiturates on [^{3}H]muscimol and [^{3}H]flunitrazepam binding are different in nature, and barbiturate recognition sites coupled with
GABA/benzodiazepine receptor complexes may be easily dissociated
or inactivated during solubilization procedures. It has been
postulated that barbiturate receptor has phospholipid components
(13). Synaptic membrane phospholipids were also found to play
multiple modulating roles on cerebral GABA/benzodiazepine receptor
complex: modulating roles on GABA receptor binding, benzodiazepine
receptor binding, and the coupling of GABA and benzodiazepine receptors, respectively (17,31). Considering the fact that the
treatment of synaptic membranes with various detergents removes
some phospholipids, it is likely that barbiturate receptor, which
is in part lipid in nature, may be removed and/or destroyed by
Nonidet P-40 treatment.

PARTIAL PURIFICATION OF SOLUBILIZED GABA
AND BENZODIAZEPINE RECEPTORS

To evaluate the relationship of [^{3}H]muscimol and [^{3}H]flunitra-
zepam binding sites, the binding of the two radioligands after
various purification procedures was examined. Application of the
solubilized receptor proteins to DEAE-Sepharose CL-6B and hydroxylapatite column chromatography provided some degree of purification
of both [^{3}H]muscimol and [^{3}H]flunitrazepam binding sites ([^{3}H]-

TABLE 3. Purification of solubilized GABA and benzodiazepine receptors on DEAE-Sepharose CL-6B and Hydroxylapatite column chromatography

	Volume (ml)	Protein (mg)	[³H]Muscimol Bound (at 5 nM)		[³H]Flunitrazepam Bound (at 1 nM)	
			Specific (fmoles/mg)	Total (fmoles)	Specific (fmoles/mg)	Total (fmoles)
Solubilized fraction	100	88.1	253.3	22290	190.0	16720
DEAE Sepharose CL-6B	28	40.1	561.1	20644	242.5	9700
Hydroxylapatite	13	10.2	637.8	9495	267.5	2728

TABLE 4. Purification of Solubilized GABA and Benzodiazepine Receptors by Affinity Column Chromatography using Nitrazepam-acetoamide-AH-Sepharose 4B

	Volume (ml)	Protein conc. (mg/ml)	Total prot. (mg)	[³H]Muscimol Bound (at 5 nM)		[³H]Flunitrazepam Bound (at 1 nM)	
				Specific (fmoles/mg)	Total (fmoles)	Specific (fmoles/mg)	Total (fmoles)
Solubilized fraction	110	1.31	145	165.3	21489	142.8	20706
PEG treated *	28	4.42	124	316.7	39270	124.5	15438
Column run-through	40	2.80	112	50.9	5700	18.3	2049
NaCl (1M) eluent	6	0.043	0.26	14337.0	3727	5525.6	1436
NaSCN (1M) eluent	12	0.068	0.81	21050.0	17050	8288.4	6713

* Polyethyleneglycol treated.

muscimol binding: 2.2 and 2.5-fold; [³H]flunitrazepam: 1.3 and
1.4-fold; Table 3), but extent of the enrichments was minimal.
In contrast, the application of solubilized GABA and benzodiazepine
receptors to affinity column chromatography using nitrazepam-
acetoamide-AH-Sepharose followed by elution with 1 M NaSCN resulted in a considerable degree of purification (Table 4). The specific activities of [³H]muscimol and [³H]flunitrazepam binding in
the NaSCN eluate were 128 and 58 times higher, respectively, than
those found in the original solubilized fraction.
    It is noteworthy that both [³H]muscimol and [³H]flunitrazepam
binding sites are not separable from each other and are co-purified
under the experimental conditions employed in this study, although
somewhat lower purification is noticed in the case of the [³H]-
flunitrazepam binding site than for the [³H]muscimol binding site.
These results are essentially in agreement with several reports
published previously (7,19,25), and indicate that GABA and benzodiazepine receptors might be part of a macromolecular complex.
It is becoming increasingly apparent, however, that there is a
multiplicity of GABA and benzodiazepine receptor complexes, and
that some GABA receptors are not linked to benzodiazepine receptors
and/or barbiturate recognition sites (13). The fact that the puri-
fications of GABA receptor and benzodiazepine receptor do not pro-
ceed to the same extent (Tables 3 and 4) may suggest the presence
of such a benzodiazepine receptor-independent GABA receptor protein
in the solubilized fraction. The suitability of such a concept,
however, should be clarified after obtaining a reasonable purification of both receptor proteins.

CONCLUSION

    γ-Aminobutyric acid (GABA) receptor was solubilized from synap-
tic membranes of the rat brain by various detergents. Nonidet P-40,
a non-ionic detergent, was found to be an effective solubilizing
agent. Ammonium sulfate precipitation of the solubilized supernatant significantly increased the binding of [³H]muscimol to GABA
receptor, possibly by removing heat-stable, low molecular weight
inhibitory substances. The specific [³H]muscimol binding to the
soluble fraction obtained by Nonidet P-40 treatment and subsequent
ammonium sulfate precipitation was saturable and consisted of high
and low affinity components. The enhancement of the [³H]muscimol
binding by diazepam, as found in synaptic membrane, was also detected
in the soluble fraction. The molecular weight of these solubilized re
ceptor sites was estimated to be 260,000 - 270,000 by Sephadex G-200
gel filtration or 240,000 by sucrose density gradient centrifugation.
The application of photoaffinity labelling with [³H]flunitrazepam
([³H]Flu) to the solubilized fraction and its subsequent analysis by
SDS-polyacrylamide gel electrophoresis indicated that the photolabelled component had a molecular weight of 51,500. It had also been foun
that barbiturates such as secobarbital and pentobarbital enhance [³H]
muscimol and [³H]Flu binding in the presence of chloride anion.

The Nonidet P-40 (1%) treatment of synaptic membranes, however, induced a complete loss of the stimulatory effect of barbiturates on the binding of both ligands to both solubilized supernatant and insoluble pellet fractions. Furthermore, solubilized GABA and benzodiazepine receptors were co-purified approximately 6٦ 130-fold by affinity chromatography using nitrazepam-acetoamide-AH-sepharose 4B. These results indicate that cerebral GABA and benzodiazepine receptors are co-solubilized as well as co-purified without altering the function and interaction of GABA/benzodiazepine receptors, while the barbiturate recognition site may inactivate and/or dissociate during solubilization.

ACKNOWLEDGMENT

This work was supported,in part, by Grant-in-Aid for Scientific Research (Nos 56480104 and 57870019, 1982) from the Ministry of Education, Science and Culture, Japan).

REFERENCES

1. Asano, T., and Ogasawara, N., (1980):Life Sci.,26: 1131-1137.
2. Beaumont K., Chilton, W., Yamamura, H.I., and Enna, S.J.(1978): Brain Research, 148: 153-162.
3. Briley, M.S., and Langer, S.Z., (1978): Eur. J. Pharmac., 52: 129-132.
4. Chude, O., (1979): J. Neurochem., 33: 621-629.
5. Choi, D.W., Farb, D.H., and Fischbach,G.D., (1977): Nature (Lond), 269: 342- 344.
6. Gavish, M., Chang, R.S.L., and Snyder, S.H. (1979): Life Sci., 25:783-790.
7. Gavish, M., and Snyder, S.H. (1981): Proc. nat. Acad. Sci. U.S.A.,78:1939-1942.
8. Guidotti, A., Toffano, G., and Costa, E., (1978): Nature (Lond), 275:553-555.
9. Ito, Y., and Kuriyama, K.,(1982): Brain Research, 236:351-363.
10. Ito, Y., Kuriyama, K., Ueno, E., Nishimura, C.,and Yoneda,Y., (1982): In: Problems in GABA Research from brain to bacteria, edited by Y. Okada, and Roberts, E., pp. 316-327. Excerpta Medica, Amsterdam.
11. Iversen, L.L., and Bloom, F.E. (1972): Brain Research, 41:131-143.
12. Johnston, G.A.R., (1976): In: GABA in Nervous System Function, edited by E. Roberts, T.N. Chase, and D.B. Tower, pp.395-411. Raven Press, New York.
13. Johnston, G.A.R., and Willow, M., (1982): Trends Pharmacol. Sci., 3:328-330.
14. Krogsgaard-Larsen P., Johnston, G.A.R., Curtis, D.R., Game, C.J.A., and McCulloch, R.H. (1975): J. Neurochem., 25:803-809.
15. Kuriyama, K., Haber, B., Sisken, B., and Roberts, E. (1966): Proc. nat. Acad. Sci. U.S.A., 55:846-852.
16. Kuriyama, K., Kurihara, E., Ito, Y., and Yoneda, Y. (1980):

J. Neurochem., 35:343-348.
17. Kuriyama, K., and Yoneda, Y., (1983): In: Neural Membrane, edited by G.Y. Sun, A.Y. Sun and J-Y. Wu, Humana Press, New Jersey, In Press.
18. MacDonald, R., and Barker, J. L., (1977): Nature (Lond), 271: 563- 564.
19. Martini, C., Lucacchini, A., Ronca, G., Hrelia, S., and Rossi, C.A., (1982): J. Neurochem., 38:15-19.
20. Miyata, M.Y., and Otsuka, M. (1972): J. Neurochem., 19:1833-1834.
21. Möhler, H., and Okada, T., (1977): Sci. 198:849-851.
22. Nicoll, R.A.(1980) In: Handbook of Psychopharmacology, edited by L.L. Iversen, S.D. Iversen, and S.H. Snyder, pp.187-234, Plenum Press, New York.
23. Sherman-Gold, R., and Dudai, Y., (1980): Brain Research 198: 485-490.
24. Snodgrass, S.R., (1978): Nature (Lond), 273:392-394.
25. Stephenson, F.A., Watkins, A.E., and Olsen, R.W. (1982): Eur. J. Biochem., 123:291-298.
26. Takeuchi, A., and Takeuchi, N.,(1969): J. Physiol. (Lond), 212: 337-351.
27. Takeuchi, A., and Takeuchi, N., (1975): Neuropharmacology, 14: 627-634.
28. Tallman, J.F., Thomas, J.W., and Gallager, D.W., (1978): Nature (Lond), 274:383-385.
29. Ticku, M.K., and Olsen, R.W., (1977): Biochim. Biophys. Acta, 464:519-529.
30. Toffano, G., Guidotti,A., and Costa, E., (1978): Proc. nat. Acad. Sci., U.S.A., 75:4024-4028.
31. Ueno, E., and Kuriyama, K., (1981): Neuropharmacology, 20: 1169-1176.
32. Willow, M., and Johnston, G.A.R. (1981 a):Neurosci. Lett., 23: 71-74.
33. Willow, M., and Johnston, G.A.R., (1981 b): J.Neurosci. 1:364-367
34. Yoneda, Y., and Kuriyama, K.,(1978): J. Neurochem., 30:821-825.
35. Yoneda, Y., and Kuriyama, K.,(1980 a): Nature (Lond), 285:670-673.
36. Yoneda, Y., Kuriyama, K., (1980 b): Brain Research, 197:554-560.
37. Zukin, S.R., Young, A.B., and Snyder, S.H., (1974): Proc. nat. Acad. Sci. U.S.A., 71:4802-4807.

CNS Receptors—From Molecular
Pharmacology to Behavior, edited by
P. Mandel and F. V. Defeudis.
Raven Press, New York © 1983.

Biochemical Pharmacology of the GABA Receptor-Ionophore Protein Complex

[1]F. Anne Stephenson and Richard W. Olsen

Division of Biomedical Sciences, Department of Biochemistry, University of California, Riverside, California 92521

Biochemical evidence now exists for direct interactions in vitro between distinct receptor binding sites for the inhibitory neurotransmitter γ-aminobutyric acid (GABA) and receptors for two classes of drugs whose actions on the nervous system appear to be at least partly due to modulation of GABAergic synaptic transmission, namely (a) the benzodiazepines, and (b) the barbiturates and related depressant agents and picrotoxinin and related excitatory agents (6,15,34). These three receptor classes show reciprocal chloride-dependent allosteric interactions in both membrane fractions of brain homogenates and in a partially-purified detergent-solubilized protein complex of discrete molecular properties, thus demonstrating the existence of a three receptor-chloride ion channel complex mediating the postsynaptic membrane function of GABA in the nervous system (25,27,37).

PHYSICAL PROPERTIES OF THE GABA/BENZODIAZEPINE RECEPTOR COMPLEX FROM MAMMALIAN BRAIN

Receptor-specific binding sites for [^{3}H] GABA and the potent and specific agonist [^{3}H] muscimol were found to be rather difficult to solubilize with retention of binding activity, consistent with the integral membrane nature of the GABA receptor protein. Numerous mild detergents and salt treatments yielded little solubilization, but a reasonable yield (33% of membrane sites and 50% of recovered sites) was solubilized from rat brain with 2% (w/v) sodium deoxycholate (14). The soluble binding activity was shown to have unequivocal receptor-specific properties (13): K_D values for muscimol and GABA of about 50 nM, with inhibition by other GABA agonists and bicuculline, but no inhibition by 2,4-diaminobutyrate. The receptor protein migrated on gel filtration columns as a discrete protein peak with apparent molecular weight of

---

[1]Present address: Department of Biochemistry, Imperial College of Science and Technology, London SW7 2AZ, England.

900,000 compared to globular standards (14). The binding activity was unstable in deoxycholate solution, declining significantly in 24 hr at 0°C. This problem was alleviated by immediate switching of the deoxycholate extract into the detergent Triton X-100 by means of Sephadex G-50 column chromatography, which simultaneously provides the removal of endogenous GABA solubilized from even well-washed membranes (12,14,24,33). The binding activity was stable in 0.5% Triton X-100 for days at 0-4°C and indefinitely at -20°C. In addition, a lower concentration of deoxycholate (0.5%, w/v) was found equally suitable for solubilization and better for stability (33).

It had been reported that pharmacologically relevant receptor sites in brain for the benzodiazepine drugs (5,22), whose action had been shown to involve an enhancement of GABA-mediated inhibitory synaptic transmission (6,15,34), were allostericaly enhanced in vitro by GABA receptor agonists (37). Furthermore, GABA receptor ligands were reported to protect benzodiazepine receptor binding activity from heat inactivation (30), and benzodiazepine receptor ligands showed a reciprocal protection of GABA binding sites (10). Therefore we examined the soluble GABA receptor preparation for benzodiazepine receptors.

Deoxycholate extracts of bovine cortex were found to contain GABA-enhanced benzodiazepine receptor binding activity in roughly equivalent quantities to GABA receptor binding (generally 2-4 GABA sites per benzodiazepine site solubilized). $[^3H]$ Muscimol binding showed a K_D of 12 nM and B_{max} of 1.56 pmol/mg protein; $[^3H]$ GABA binding gave a K_D of 50 nM and B_{max} of 1.55 pmol/mg; $[^3H]$ flunitrazepam had a K_D of 8 nM and a B_{max} of 0.8 pmol/mg. Soluble $[^3H]$ flunitrazepam binding was inhibited by nanomolar concentrations of flunitrazepam, diazepam, and the "brain-specific" analogue, clonazepam, but not by micromolar concentrations of the "peripheral" benzodiazepine RO5-4864. Soluble benzodiazepine receptor binding had a low affinity for ethyl β-carboline-3-carboxylate ($IC_{50} \simeq 50$ nM) and for the anxiolytic triazolopyradazine CL 218,872 ($IC_{50} \simeq 1$ μM). The yield of $[^3H]$ muscimol binding sites was 31% (58% of recoverable activity), with another 25% remaining active in the detergent-treated membranes. By contrast, 63% of the total $[^3H]$ flunitrazepam binding sites were solubilized, representing 90% of the recoverable sites. Protease inhibitors could improve these yields (33).

Soluble $[^3H]$ flunitrazepam binding was enhanced about 2-fold by muscimol ($EC_{50} \simeq 0.6$ μM) and GABA ($EC_{50} \simeq 2$ μM), even following protein separation procedures (33), suggesting that the two receptors could still interact in solution. Indeed, the two binding activities were found to co-migrate on several columns and sucrose gradients (33), a result also observed by other groups (1,11). We found the deoxycholate-solubilized $[^3H]$ muscimol and $[^3H]$ flunitrazepam binding activities to co-migrate as a single peak on Sepharose 6B gel filtration columns in Triton X-100, with a Stokes radius of 6.8 nm (33). Sucrose gradient centrifugation in H_2O and D_2O also showed co-migration of the two activities and estimation of a sedimentation coefficient of 12.5 S, a partial specific volume $\bar{v}$ of 0.73 ml/g, and a calculated molecular weight of 355,000. It is possible that some of this mass reflects bound detergent, but the anomalous molecular seiving/sedimentation properties could also reflect a nonglobular shape, and a frictional coefficient f/fo of 1.46 was calculated. Both binding activities appear to reside on a single protein complex (33). This complex was found to contain the 50,000 molecular weight subunit on SDS gels following photoaffinity labeling of the column-purified material with [^{3}H] flunitrazepam, as previously described by others (23). It is not yet known whether these or other subunits carry the binding sites for GABA/muscimol.

A similar Sepharose 6B profile with GABA and benzodiazepine receptor activity co-migrating at a position at or slightly prior to the elution of the marker <u>E. coli</u> β-galactosidase (Stokes radius 6.8 nm, molecular weight 550,000) and significantly ahead of catalase (Stokes

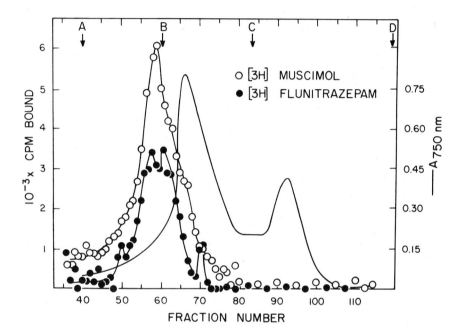

FIG. 1. Gel Filtration of GABA/Benzodiazepine Receptor Complex from Bovine Cerebellum.

Crude P_2 + P_3 membranes from 5g of frozen and thawed bovine cerebellum were solubilized in 10 ml of 0.5% (w/v) deoxycholate in 50 mM Tris-HCl, 50 mM KCl, pH 8.0 plus protease inhibitors (32,33), for 30 min at 0°C, followed by centrifugation (100,000 x g-hr). The supernatant fraction was applied to a column (3 x 47 cm) of Sepharose 6B and eluted with the same buffer substituting 0.5% (v/v) Triton X-100. Fractions (2 ml) were assayed for protein (A_{750}) and for binding of [^{3}H] flunitrazepam and [^{3}H]muscimol by centrifugation with bovine globulin and polyethylene glycol. The letters A, B, C, and D signify the positions of molecular weight markers, blue dextran, β-galactosidase, catalase, and cytochrome <u>c</u>.

radius 5.2 nm, molecular weight 240,000) was observed for several preparations. These included bovine cortex membranes solubilized with the detergent CHAPS (32) or Triton X-100, whole rat brain solubilized with 0.5% deoxycholate, or bovine cerebellum solubilized with 0.5% deoxycholate (Fig. 1), all chromatographed in 0.5% (v/v) Triton X-100. The soluble cerebellum binding activity had similar pharmacological properties, and bound [^{3}H] flunitrazepam with a K_D of 13 nM, B_{max} of 0.25 pmol/mg protein, and [^{3}H] muscimol with a K_D of 30 nM, B_{max} of 0.9 pmol/mg. Approximately 85% of the recoverable benzodiazepine receptor sites were solubilized, but over 40% of the GABA receptor sites remained in the detergent-treated membrane, a similar or even greater percentage than that observed with cortex. The other detergents such as Triton X-100 or CHAPS solubilized even less of both benzodiazepine and GABA receptors. The residual membrane-bound GABA binding was best described by two affinities as generally observed in untreated membranes (12,24,26), but the soluble activity could be described by a single affinity, although the possibility of heterogeneity was not eliminated. Similar observations were made with cortex.
Some [^{3}H] flunitrazepam "binding" was observed at smaller molecular weight regions of the Sepharose 6B column chromatogram such as that shown in Fig. 1, but this was almost completely nonspecific since it was not displaceable by nonradioactive 10 μ M flunitrazepam. In some cases a small amount of displaceable binding was observed at fractions corresponding to molecular weights smaller than the major peak seen in Fig. 1; however, this was never the case with extracts solubilized and chromatographed in the presence of protease inhibitors, when only the one peak of activity was observed. Thus any smaller species would appear to be artifactually produced by proteolysis. We have never observed any significant amount of a second size species of benzodiazepine binding protein, nor any separation from the GABA binding activity, using several detergents, brain regions and species. As far as we can tell, all of the benzodiazepine receptor activity seems to be associated with GABA receptor activity. Likewise the bulk of the solubilized GABA receptor activity seems to be associated with benzodiazepine receptor activity. On the other hand, the residual GABA receptor activity not solubilized by deoxycholate would appear to lack this association with the benzodiazepine receptor (and also with the picrotoxinin/barbiturate receptor sites and chloride channels as discussed below).
The soluble GABA and benzodiazepine receptor binding activities were also observed to co-migrate on ion-exchange columns (1,11), on lectin-agarose (11), and on a benzodiazepine affinity column which afforded a partial purification (11). We have achieved a partial purification of some 30-fold on a Sepharose 6B column plus chromatography on insolubilized lectin-agarose (Lens culinaris), plus several hundreds-fold by affinity chromatography. A total purification factor of about 5000 appears to be required. Current studies are aimed at a reproducible purification to homogeneity, determination of the subunit structure with identification of the various drug binding sites, reconstitution of GABA-regulated chloride ion channels into a membrane, and production of antibodies against the receptor.

ASSOCIATION OF BARBITURATE/PICROTOXININ RECEPTOR SITES AND CHLORIDE ION CHANNELS WITH THE GABA/BENZODIAZEPINE RECEPTOR COMPLEX.

Picrotoxinin is a small molecular weight compound of plant origin which contains no nitrogen atom. It has convulsant activity, primarily due to a universal antagonism of GABA-mediated inhibitory synaptic transmission (25,27). Picrotoxinin blocks the GABA receptor-activated membrane chloride channels involved in inhibitory postsynaptic responses without interfering with the binding of GABA to its recognition site, the receptor (38). In order to probe the site of action of picrotoxinin further, we synthesized a radioactive biologically active analogue of picrotoxinin, [^{3}H] α-dihydropicrotoxinin (DHP). This ligand was shown to bind to specific sites in brain membranes related to the site of action of picrotoxinin by virtue of chemical and tissue specificity, density, and affinity (38).

[^{3}H] DHP binding is inhibited by biologically active picrotoxinin analogues (convulsants which block GABA synapses [38]), by "cage" compounds such as alkyl bicyclophosphates and tetramethylenedisulfotetramine (also convulsants which block GABA synapses [40]), by a convulsant benzodiazepine, RO5-3663 (19), and by excitatory and depressant barbiturates (39), drugs which also are known to modulate GABA postsynaptic responses (15,34). Despite this circumstantial relationship of [^{3}H] DHP sites to the GABA receptor-ionophore system, it has been difficult to study [^{3}H] DHP sites due to a relatively low affinity (K_D = 1 μM) for the only available radioactive ligand. Furthermore, initial studies revealed no reciprocal allosteric interactions in vitro between GABA receptor binding sites and [^{3}H] DHP sites (13,25,38). However, recent studies show interactions between these two populations of drug receptor sites which leave little doubt that there is indeed a picrotoxinin/barbiturate receptor site associated with the GABA receptor-ionophore complex.

A class of anxiolytic drugs, the pyrazolopyridines (e.g. etazolate = SQ20009), were observed to enhance, rather than inhibit, the binding of radioactive benzodiazepines to brain membrane receptors in vitro (3,42). This effect was augmented by chloride ions and blocked by picrotoxin (35). We observed that not only is the etazolate enhancement blocked by concentrations of picrotoxinin that bind to [^{3}H]DHP sites, but that the pyrazolopyridines, at concentrations that enhance benzodiazepine binding, also inhibit [^{3}H] DHP binding (20). Furthermore the enhancement by etazolate of benzodiazepine binding is inhibited by appropriate concentrations of other convulsant drugs which inhibit [$_3$H]DHP binding (17,20), while the depressant drugs which inhibit [^{3}H] DHP binding like barbiturates show an effect like that of etazolate and enhance benzodiazepine receptor binding (18).

The barbiturate enhancement of benzodiazepine receptor binding in brain membranes was shown to involve a two-fold increase in affinity without any change in the number of binding sites (18,29,41). The effect was stereospecific and chemically specific (18,21,29,41) in a manner correlating highly for a series of barbiturates as sedative-hypnotic

agents in vivo and as potentiators of GABA synaptic responses in tissues
(4). Furthermore the enhancement was dependent on the presence of
certain anions and only those anions demonstrated to permeate chloride
channels which mediate barbiturate-enhanced inhibitory postsynaptic
responses in the nervous system (8). The same anions were shown by
others to enhance baseline benzodiazepine receptor binding (7) and the
binding of the antagonist bicuculline to GABA receptor sites (9).

These interactions show that picrotoxinin/barbiturate/pyrazolo-
pyridine sites are coupled to benzodiazepine receptor sites and chloride
ion channels. The previously mentioned (37) allosteric enhancement of
benzodiazepine binding by GABA receptor ligands shows that GABA
receptors are also coupled to benzodiazepine receptors and therefore to
picrotoxinin/barbiturate receptors. Several other lines of evidence
support this hypothesis, including protection of benzodiazepine binding
sites against heat inactivation by both GABA receptor ligands (30) and by
picrotoxinin/barbiturate receptor ligands (31), the chloride- and
temperature-dependent enhancement of benzodiazepine binding by
picrotoxinin-like convulsants (17), the chloride- and temperature-
dependent allosteric inhibition of GABA receptor binding by
picrotoxinin-like convulsants (36), and the chloride-dependent,
picrotoxinin-sensitive allosteric enhancement of GABA receptor binding
by barbiturates (2,16,28,36) and pyrazolopyridines (36). Many of these
interactions appear to be most visible under more physiological
temperature and assay buffer conditions than are often employed in in
vitro binding studies. There have also been some reports of a small
enhancement of GABA binding by benzodiazepines, but this is
controversial.

We demonstrated that the same picrotoxinin/barbiturate receptor
sites were involved in enhancement of both benzodiazepine receptors and
GABA receptors, showing a specificity of barbiturates with DMBB >
secobarbital > pentobarbital > (+)hexobarbital = (-)mephobarbital =
amobarbital > (-)hexobarbital = phenobarbital > (+)mephobarbital =
metharbital = barbital (18,21,28). Enhancement was dependent on the
same anions mentioned above (chloride, bromide, iodide, perchlorate,
thiocyanate, nitrate or formate, but not fluoride, acetate, propionate,
azide, bicarbonate, phosphate, sulfite or sulfate [18,28]). Picrotoxinin
and related convulsants inhibited the enhancement (28,36). The
enhancement of GABA binding by barbiturates and pyrazolopyridines
involves an apparent increase in the number of sites (28,36); we have
provided evidence that this is probably due to an enhanced affinity of
low affinity sites which are normally detected with difficulty (28).

The existence of the three-receptor, chloride channel complex has
now been demonstrated in solution. We observed pentobarbital
enhancement of deoxycholate-solubilized GABA/benzodiazepine receptor
binding activity as described above, but the effect was irreproducible
and/or unstable (33). Use of the unique zwitterionic bile salt detergent
3- [(3-cholamido-propyl)-dimethylammonio]propanesulfonate (CHAPS)
allowed us to achieve a reproducible two-fold enhancement of both
GABA and benzodiazepine receptor binding in solution by barbiturates,
and this interaction was maintained following protein separation
procedures (32).

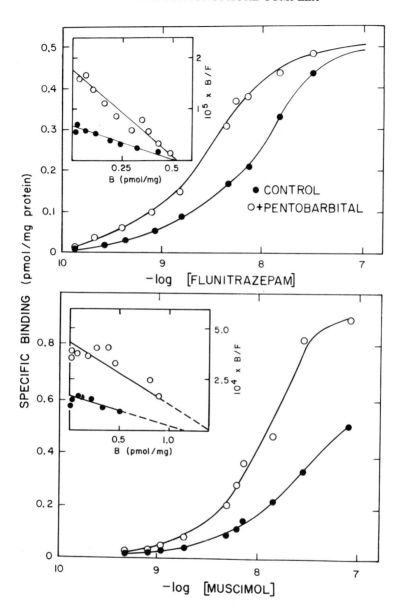

FIG. 2.   Enhancement   by   Pentobarbital   of   CHAPS-Solubilized
Benzodiazepine and GABA Receptor Binding in Bovine Cortex.
    Membranes were prepared and solubilized as in Fig. 1 except for the
substitution of 20 mM CHAPS for the deoxycholate.   Binding of
[³H] flunitrazepam (upper) and [³H] muscimol (lower) were measured
at varying concentrations of ligand, in the absence and presence of
pentobarbital (1 mM). The insets show Scatchard plots of the data shown
in the larger figures.

Solubilization of bovine cortex with CHAPS detergent resulted in a GABA/benzodiazepine receptor complex which migrated on Sepharose 6B column chromatography in 0.5% (v/v) Triton X-100 in a manner similar to deoxycholate extracts, eluting around the position of the marker β - galactosidase (32). The maximum yield of [^{3}H] flunitrazepam sites (25-40%) was obtained at 20 mM CHAPS, with a lower yield at higher detergent concentrations. Pentobarbital enhancement was 50-70% in 5, 10, or 20 mM CHAPS extracts and lower in a 30 mM CHAPS extract. The [^{3}H] flunitrazepam binding in solution (Fig. 2, upper) showed a K_D of 8 nM and B_{max} of 0.53 pmol/mg protein, while this was improved in affinity (K_D = 3 nM) in the presence of pentobarbital (1 mM), with no change in B_{max} (0.51 pmol/mg) (32). Pentobarbital gave a maximum effect of about 80% enhancement with an EC_{50} of 300 μM. The CHAPS-extracted membranes retained 60-75% of the [^{3}H] flunitrazepam binding activity (B_{max} = 1.59 pmol/mg), but showed no enhancement by pentobarbital (K_D = 4 nM without and 3 nM with pentobarbital). Barbiturate enhancement of the soluble [^{3}H] flunitrazepam binding was reversibly decreased by lowering the chloride concentration in the assays, and showed the same chemical specificity for barbiturates seen in membranes (18,32). The enhancement was diminished but still present (35%) following Sepharose 6B column chromatography, ruling out the possible role of GABA in mediating the barbiturate-benzodiazepine interaction (32).

[^{3}H] Muscimol binding activity solubilized by CHAPS (Fig. 2, bottom) showed receptor-like specificity and a K_D of about 40 nM with B_{max} of 1.2 pmol/mg (yield 30-40%). Pentobarbital enhanced the binding about 150% over control (250% of control) at maximal concentrations, with an EC_{50} of 300 μM. The binding curve showed a small increase in affinity (K_D = 30 nM in Fig. 2) as well as in B_{max} (1.4 pmol/mg). In three experiments there was always an apparent increase in B_{max}, as observed with membranes (28). This observation leads to the inescapable conclusion that the number of GABA receptor sites in the soluble complex is significantly higher (2-4 times) than the number of benzodiazepine receptor sites. Our results suggest that the soluble [^{3}H] muscimol binding, like in membranes, appears to show some low affinity (K_D = 0.1-1 μM) sites which are difficult to detect in the absence of barbiturates. An increase in affinity for these low affinity sites can account for the apparent increase in binding sites seen in the presence of barbiturates. The existence of low affinity GABA receptor sites would also be consistent with the high (micromolar) concentrations of muscimol and GABA needed to enhance [^{3}H] flunitrazepam binding.

Barbiturate enhancement of [^{3}H] muscimol binding, like the enhancement of [^{3}H] flunitrazepam binding, persists partially following various column separation procedures, indicating that this chloride- and picrotoxinin-sensitive barbiturate receptor site is a part of the GABA/benzodiazepine receptor complex which can be solubilized and isolated from brain. Biochemical studies on this complex should prove valuable in understanding the pharmacological actions of neurotransmitters and drugs at the molecular level.

ACKNOWLEDGEMENTS

This work was supported by NIH grants NS-12422 and Research Career Development Award NS-00224 and NSF Grant BNS 80-19722. We thank L.M.F. Leeb-Lundberg, A.E. Watkins, E.H.F. Wong and A.M. Snowman for helpful discussions, and Nancy Price for typing the manuscript.

REFERENCES

1. Asano, T., and Ogasawara, N. (1981) Life Sci. 29:193-200.
2. Asano, T. and Ogasawara, N. (1981) Brain Res. 225:212-216.
3. Beer, B., Klepner, C.A., Lippa, A.S. and Squires, R.F. (1978) Pharmac. Biochem. Behav. 9:849-851.
4. Bowery, N.G and Dray, A. (1978) Br. J. Pharmac. 63:179-215.
5. Braestrup, C. and Squires, R.F. (1977) Proc. Natl. Acad. Sci. USA 74: 3805-3809.
6. Costa, E. and Guidotti, A. (1979) Ann. Rev. Pharmac. Tox. 19:531-545.
7. Costa, T., Rodbard, D. and Pert, C.B. (1979) Nature 277:315-317.
8. Eccles, J., Nicoll, R.A., Oshima, T. and Rubia, F.J. (1977) Proc. R. Soc. Lond. B. 198:345-361.
9. Enna, S.J., and Snyder S.H. (1977) Mol. Pharmac. 13:442-453.
10. Gavish, M. and Snyder, S.H. (1980) Nature 287:651-652.
11. Gavish, M. and Snyder, S.H. (1981) Proc. Natl. Acad. Sci. USA 78: 1939-1942.
12. Greenlee, D.V., Van Ness, P.C. and Olsen, R.W. (1978). Life Sci. 22: 1653-1662.
13. Greenlee, D.V., Van Ness, P.C. and Olsen, R.W. (1978). J. Neurochem. 31:933-938.
14. Greenlee, D.V. and Olsen, R.W. (1979) Biochem. Biophys. Res. Comm. 88:380-387.
15. Haefely, W., Polc, P., Schaffner, R., Keller, H.H., Pieri, L. and Möhler, H. (1979) In GABA-Neurotransmitters (Krogsgaard-Larsen, P., Scheel-Kruger, J. and Kofod, H., eds.) pp. 357-375, Munksgaard, Copenhagen.
16. Johnston, G.A.R. and Willow, M. (1981) Adv. Biochem. Psychopharmac. 26: pp. 191-198, Raven Press, New York.
17. Karobath, M., Drexler, G. and Supavilai, P. (1981) Life Sci. 28:307-313.
18. Leeb-Lundberg, F., Snowman, A. and Olsen, R.W. (1980) Proc. Natl. Acad. Sci. USA 77:7468-7472.
19. Leeb-Lundberg, F., Napias, C. and Olsen, R.W. (1981) Brain Res. 216: 399-408.
20. Leeb-Lundberg, F., Snowman, A. and Olsen, R.W. (1981) J. Neurosci. 1:471-477.
21. Leeb-Lundberg, F. and Olsen, R.W. (1982) Mol. Pharmacol. 21:320-28.
22. Möhler, H. and Okada, T. (1977) Science 198:849-851.
23. Möhler, H., Battersby, M.K. and Richards, J.G. (1980) Proc. Natl. Acad. Sci. USA 77:1666-1670.

24. Napias, C., Bergman, M.O., Van Ness, P.C., Greenlee, D.V. and Olsen, R.W. (1980) Life Sci. 27:1001-1011.
25. Olsen, R.W. (1981) J. Neurochem. 37:1-13.
26. Olsen, R.W., Bergman, M.O., Van Ness P.C., Lummis, S.C., Watkins, A.E., Napias, C. and Greenlee, D.V. (1981). Mol. Pharmac. 19:217-227.
27. Olsen, R.W. (1982) Ann. Rev. Pharmac. Tox. 22:245-277.
28. Olsen, R.W., Snowman, A.M. (1982) J. Neurosci. in press.
29. Skolnick, P., Rice, K.C., Barker, J.L. and Paul, S.M. (1982) Brain Res. 233:143-156.
30. Squires, R.F., Klepner, C.A. and Benson, D.I. (1980) Adv. Biochem. Psychopharmac. 21:285-293.
31. Squires, R.F. and Saederup, E. (1982) In Pharmacology of Benzodiazepines, Paul et al., eds. Macmillan Press.
32. Stephenson, F.A. and Olsen, R.W. (1982) J. Neurochem. in press.
33. Stephenson, F.A., Watkins, A.E. and Olsen, R.W. (1982) Eur. J. Biochem. 123:291-298.
34. Study, R.E. and Barker, J.L. (1981) Proc. Natl. Acad. Sci. USA 78: 7180-7184.
35. Supavilai, P. and Karobath, M. (1979) Eur. J. Pharmac. 60:111-113.
36. Supavilai, P., Mannonen, A. and Karobath, M. (1982) Neurochem. Int. in press.
37. Tallman, J.F., Paul, S.M., Skolnick, P. and Gallager, D.W. (1980) Science 207:274-281.
38. Ticku, M.K. Ban, M. and Olsen, R.W. (1978) Mol. Pharmac. 14:391-402.
39. Ticku, M.K. and Olsen, R.W. (1978) Life Sci. 22:1643-1651.
40. Ticku, M.K. and Olsen, R.W. (1979) Neuropharmacology 18:315-318.
41. Ticku, M.K. (1981) Biochem. Pharmacol. 30:1573-1579.
42. Williams, M. and Risley, E.A. (1979) Life Sci. 24:833-841.

CNS Receptors—From Molecular
Pharmacology to Behavior, edited by
P. Mandel and F. V. DeFeudis.
Raven Press, New York © 1983.

Barbiturate Interactions with Benzodiazepine-GABA Receptor-Ionophore Complex

Maharaj K. Ticku, Troie P. Burch, Rajee Thyagarajan,
and R. Ramanjaneyulu

*Division of Molecular Pharmacology, Department of Pharmacology, The University of Texas
Health Science Center, San Antonio, Texas 78284*

The GABAergic synapse appears to be a site of action for a variety of centrally acting anxiolytic, depressant, convulsant and anticonvulsant drugs. The postsynaptic complex with which these drugs interact and affect GABAergic transmission is an oligomeric complex and appears to be composed of at least three interacting components: (a) GABA recognition (receptor) sites; (b) benzodiazepine binding sites; and (c) picrotoxinin binding sites. This complex represents the so-called benzodiazepine-GABA receptor-ionophore complex. The three components of this complex have been well characterized in vitro by radioligand binding assays (7,15,17,23,29,30). Recent in vitro studies have also demonstrated that drugs that modulate GABAergic transmission can bind to one of these components and, in turn, perturb or modulate the binding of ligands to other sites of this complex.

Neurophysiological studies suggest that depressant barbiturates like pentobarbital produce their therapeutic effects by facilitating GABAergic transmission (16,21). In this report, the interactions of barbiturates with the three components of the benzodiazepine-GABA receptor-ionophore complex will be discussed.

INTERACTION OF BARBITURATES WITH PICROTOXININ BINDING SITES

We have previously demonstrated that a biologically active radioactive analogue of picrotoxinin, [^{3}H]-α-dihydropicrotoxinin (DHP) binds to rat brain membranes in a specific and saturable manner (29). DHP binds to brain membranes with a K_D of 1-2 μM and a B_{max} of 5-10 pmol/mg protein. DHP binding also shows a similar but not identical subcellular and brain regional distribution and postnatal development as GABA and benzodiazepine binding sites (17,29-31).

The pharmacological specificity of DHP binding is demonstrated by the fact that its binding is inhibited by biologically active analogues of picrotoxin and not by inactive analogues. DHP binding is also inhibited by GABA antagonists and convulsant drugs like "cage" convulsants bicyclophosphate esters, a convulsant benzodiazepine RO5-3663, and pentylenetetrazole (17,29,32,33).

Besides convulsant drugs, DHP binding is also inhibited by depressant, convulsant and anticonvulsant barbiturates. Depres-- sant barbiturates like pentobarbital inhibit DHP binding competi- tively with an IC_{50} value of 50 μM. Convulsant barbiturates like CHEB (IC_{50} = 0.7 μM) and (+) MPPB (IC_{50} = 0.3 μM) were more potent and anticonvulsants like phenobarbital (IC_{50} = 400 μM) were less potent than pentobarbital. Besides racemic bar- biturates, the DHP binding is inhibited by stereoisomers of various barbiturates. Table 1 lists the IC_{50} values of various

TABLE 1. IC_{50} VALUES FOR INHIBITION OF DHP BINDING BY BARBITURATES

Barbiturate	IC_{50} (μM)
(±) DMBB	0.10
CHEB	0.70
(±) MPPB	1.00
(+) MPPB	0.30
(-) MPPB	3.00
(±) Mephobarbital	5.00
(+) Mephobarbital	2.00
(-) Mephobarbital	4.00
(±) Secobarbital	5.00
(+) Secobarbital	10.00
(-) Secobarbital	3.00
(±) Hexobarbital	12.00
(-) Hexobarbital	6.00
(+) Hexobarbital	2.00
(±) Pentobarbital	50.00
(+) Pentobarbital	82.00
(-) Pentobarbital	22.00
Phenobarbital	400.00

barbiturates for DHP binding. Figure 1 shows the displacement of DHP binding by racemic pentobarbital and its stereoisomers. (-) Pentobarbital was 4-fold more potent than (+) pentobarbital in inhibiting DHP binding. Stereoisomers of MPPB and DMBB which exhibit opposite pharmacological activities also inhibited DHP binding. The ability of stereoisomers of barbiturates to inhibit DHP binding is not surprising since both isomers are pharmacologically active (4,9). We have previously proposed that depressant and convulsant barbiturates may modulate GABAergic transmission via the DHP site (32). Recent biochemi- cal studies further support this notion (11,12,26,28,29; see below).

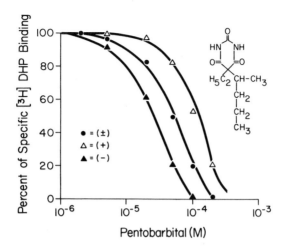

Pentobarbital (M)

FIG. 1. Displacement of specific [³H]DHP binding from rat brain membrane by racemic pentobarbital and its stereoisomers.

INTERACTION OF BARBITURATES WITH BENZODIAZEPINE BINDING SITE

Figure 2 shows that muscimol and pentobarbital produce a dose-dependent enhancement of [³H]diazepam binding to rat brain membranes. The pentobarbital enhancement of diazepam binding was due to an increase in the affinity of diazepam for its binding sites (28). Thus, 10^{-4}M (±) pentobarbital changed the K_D of diazepam from a control value of 9.23 ± 0.17 nM to 4.11 ± 0.22 nM (P<0.02) without altering the B_{max} (28). Although a variety of depressant barbiturates enhanced the diazepam binding, all barbiturates do not give the same maximal enhancement (28). Thus, pentobarbital and secobarbital give similar maximal enhancing effects (110% over basal values), while hexobarbital gave a maximal enhancement of 40 ± 6%.

Table 2 shows that (a) pentobarbital enhancement of diazepam binding was additive with that of muscimol, and (b) that pentobarbital potentiated the ability of muscimol to enhance diazepam binding. Similar results have been reported by others (11,17,22). Table 3 shows the effect of stereoisomers of MPPB on diazepam binding. [³H]Diazepam binding was enhanced by (-) MPPB (depressant) but not by (+) MPPB (convulsant). Furthermore, the effect of (-) MPPB was additive with that of muscimol, whereas (+) MPPB antagonized the muscimol enhancing effect. Thus, barbiturates exhibit stereoselectivity in inhibiting DHP binding (Table 1; 27) and in enhancing diazepam binding (Table 3; 17;28). Pentobarbital enhancement of [³H]diazepam binding is inhibited by convulsant drugs like picrotoxinin, bicyclophosphate esters and RO5-3663, which act at the picrotoxinin-sensitive site of the benzodiazepine-GABA receptor-ionophore complex (17,28).

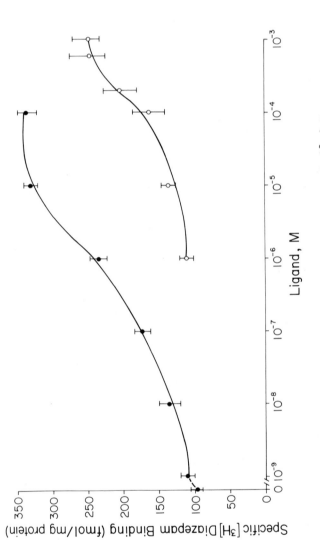

FIG. 2. Concentration-dependent enhancement of [³H]diazepam binding by muscimol (●-●) and (±) pentobarbital (o-o). Various concentrations of muscimol or pentobarbital were incubated with 1 nM [³H]diazepam and membranes, as described. The curves describe enhancement over the basal diazepam binding, which was approximately 100 fmoles/mg protein. Each value is the mean ± S.D. of three experiments, each done in triplicate. (Reprinted with permission from Ticku, Biochem. Pharmacol. 32:1573-1579, 1981, Pergamon Press, Ltd.;28.)

However, bicuculline, which acts at the GABA receptor level, also partially inhibits the pentobarbital-enhancing effect (17,28). These studies provide further evidence that various components of the GABA receptor complex interact in vitro.

In a manner similar to pentobarbital, pyrazolopyridines (like etazolate) also inhibit DHP binding (11) and enhance benzodiazepine binding in a picrotoxinin-sensitive fashion (25).

TABLE 2. EFFECT OF (±) PENTOBARBITAL ON MUSCIMOL EN-
HANCEMENT OF [³H]DIAZEPAM BINDING*

Treatments	Specific [³H]Diazepam Binding (fmoles/mg protein)	% Enhancement
Control	119.3± 8.7	---
+10⁻⁷M Muscimol	182.4± 8.2	53
+10⁻⁵M Muscimol	330.9± 6.9	177
+10⁻⁴M (±) Pentobarbital	152.5± 7.1	28
+5x10⁻⁴M (±) Pentobarbital	252.1± 4.5	111
+10⁻⁷M Muscimol +		
10⁻⁴M (±) Pentobarbital	232.3± 9.1	95
5x10⁻⁴M (±) Pentobarbital	355.7± 5.8	198
+10⁻⁵M Muscimol +		
10⁻⁴M (±) Pentobarbital	374.2± 8.8	214
5x10⁻⁴M (±) pentobarbital	414.1±10.7	247

*[³H]Diazepam binding was studied using 1 nM [³H]diazepam. Muscimol or (±) pentobarbital alone or in combination were present during the incubation. Each value is the mean ± S. D. of three experiments, each done in triplicate. (Reproduced with permission from 28.)

TABLE 3. EFFECT OF STEREOISOMERS OF MPPB WITH OPPOS-
ING PHARMACOLOGICAL ACTIVITIES ON [³H]DIAZE-
PAM BINDING*

Treatments	Specific [³H]Diazepam Binding (fmoles/mg protein)	% Enhancement
Control	93.1± 4.2	---
+10⁻⁶M (-) MPPB	112.5±3.7	21
+10⁻⁶M (+) MPPB	98.6±4.5	6
+10⁻⁵M Muscimol	257.7±7.3	177
+10⁻⁵M Muscimol + 10⁻⁶M (-) MPPB	274.8±5.4	195
+10⁻⁵M Muscimol + 10⁻⁶M (+) MPPB	233.7±9.6	151

*Muscimol and the (-) and (+) isomers of MPPB were incubated alone or in combination with 1 nM [³H]diazepam. Each value is the mean ± S.D. of two experiments each done in triplicate. (Reproduced with permission from 28.)

TABLE 4.   BARBITURATE ENHANCEMENT OF [^{3}H]GABA BIND-
ING TO CORTEX

| | Percent Enhancement over Basal Binding | |
Barbiturate	10^{-4}M	2 x 10^{-4}M
(-) DMBB	87 ± 6	N.T.
(+) DMBB	56 ± 8	N.T.
(-) Secobarbital	45 ± 7	85 ± 10
(+) Secobarbital	17 ± 2	55 ± 10
(-) MPPB	26 ± 6	60 ± 5
(+) MPPB	2 ± 2	8 ± 2
(-) Pentobarbital	28 ± 4	57 ± 10
(+) Pentobarbital	6 ± 3	14 ± 4
(-) Mephobarbital	30 ± 6	40 ± 5
(+) Mephobarbital	2 ± 2	4 ± 3
Phenobarbital	0	0

[^{3}H]GABA binding to extensively washed and freeze-thawed
membranes was studied by a centrifugation assay. Membranes
were resuspended in 0.05 M TRIS HCl, 0.05 M KCl, pH 7.I, at
0-4°C and incubated for I0 min with 4 nM [^{3}H]GABA in the
absence and presence of various barbiturates. NT refers to
not tested.

INTERACTION OF BARBITURATES WITH GABA RECEPTOR SITES

Although previous studies failed to demonstrate an interaction
between barbiturates and GABA receptor sites (18,32), several
studies have recently demonstrated such an interaction. Willow
and Johnston (34) were the first to show that barbiturates enhance GABA binding in Tris-citrate buffer. Others have shown
that barbiturates enhance GABA binding in Cl$^-$-containing buffer (1,10,17,19). Furthermore, this enhancing effect is stereospecific and is blocked by picrotoxinin.

Pentobarbital produces a dose-related enhancement of specific
[^{3}H]GABA binding to cerebral cortex membranes (see below).
Table 4 shows the effect stereoisomers of various barbiturates
on GABA binding to cortex. Depressant barbiturates like (±)
pentobarbital, (±) secobarbital and their (-) isomers, (-) DMBB
and (-) MPPB were more potent than their (+) isomers. Furthermore, convulsant barbiturates like (+) MPPB and CHEB, and
anticonvulsant barbiturates like phenobarbital and eterobarb did
not enhance the binding. However, (+) DMBB, which apparently
is a convulsant, does enhance [^{3}H]GABA binding. Similar results have been reported by others (17,19). The pentobarbital
enhancement of GABA binding was blocked by picrotoxinin.
Etazolate has also been reported to increase GABA binding in a
chloride-dependent manner and this enhancing effect is blocked
by picrotoxin (20,25). These results support the notion that
pentobarbital and etazolate may interact with the GABA receptor
sites via the picrotoxinin site of the benzodiazepine-GABA
receptor-ionophore complex.

TABLE 5. EFFECT OF STEREOISOMERS OF ETOMIDATE AND
($\pm$) PENTOBARBITAL ON [^{3}H]GABA AND [^{3}H]DIA-
ZEPAM BINDING TO CORTEX AND CEREBELLUM

| | SPECIFIC BINDING (Percent of Control) | | | |
| | [^{3}H]GABA | | [^{3}H]Diazepam | |
Treatment	Cortex	Cerebellum	Cortex	Cerebellum
None (Control)	100	100	100	100
10^{-5}M (+) Eto-midate (4)	160 $\pm$ 6	113 $\pm$ 5	166 $\pm$ 18	123 $\pm$ 7
10^{-5}M (-) Eto-midate (3)	96 $\pm$ 5	92 $\pm$ 9	113 $\pm$ 11	104 $\pm$ 8
2x10^{-4}M Pen-tobarbital (5)	163 $\pm$ 9	118 $\pm$ 6	147 $\pm$ 6	124 $\pm$ 5
10^{-3}M Pheno-barbital (2)	101 $\pm$ 4	104 $\pm$ 6	109 $\pm$ 12	103 $\pm$ 7

GABA binding to extensively washed and freeze-thawed membranes was studied in 0.05 M TRIS-HCl, 0.05 M KCl, pH 7.1 buffer,
by a centrifugation assay. Diazepam binding to extensively
washed fresh membranes was studied in 0.2 M NaCl, 10 mM sodium phosphate buffer, pH 7.0, by a filtration assay, as described (28). The concentrations used were [^{3}H]GABA = 4 nM
and [^{3}H]diazepam = 1.0 nM. The values are the means $\pm$ S.D.;
numbers of experiments indicated in parentheses.

Comparison of Pentobarbital and Etomidate Interactions
With [^{3}H]GABA and [^{3}H]Diazepam Binding

Besides barbiturates, several other drugs like the anxiolytic
etazolate, avermectin and etomidate also enhance [^{3}H]GABA and
[^{3}H]benzodiazepine binding. Etomidate, a hypnotic and anticonvulsant drug which is not structurally related to barbiturates,
has been shown to mimic GABA responses (8) and to enhance
GABA (35) and diazepam binding (2) which was not blocked by
picrotoxin. We have compared the effects of pentobarbital and
etomidate on these two binding sites of the benzodiazepine-GABA
receptor-ionophore complex. Table 5 shows that (+) etomidate
and pentobarbital enhance both GABA and diazepam binding in
cortex. Furthermore, the etomidate enhancing effect was stereospecific since the (-) isomer (which is pharmacologically inactive)
does not enhance either GABA or diazepam binding. In agreement with the results of Ashton et al (2), we observed that (+)
etomidate enhanced diazepam binding in cortex but was very
weak in cerebellum. Similarily, pentobarbital produces much
greater increases in both diazepam and GABA binding in cortex
relative to cerebellum. The EC$_{50}$ values for pentobarbital were
1.5x10^{-4}M for GABA binding and 1.1x10^{-4}M for diazepam binding.
The EC$_{50}$ values for (+) etomidate were 10^{-5}M for GABA binding
and 8x10^{-6}M for diazepam binding. Both pentobarbital and (+)
etomidate increased the affinity of diazepam for the binding site
(data not shown). In contrast, they increase the number of
both high- and low-affinity sites of GABA to cerebral cortex

(unpublished observation).

(+)Etomidate enhancement of GABA binding was additive with pentobarbital and etazolate; however, it was blocked by picrotoxinin, isopropylbicyclophosphate and (+)bicuculline (unpublished observations). Willow (35) has reported that picrotoxin did not alter etomidate enhancing effect on GABA binding. (+)Etomidate's enhancing effect on diazepam binding was additive with GABA and was also blocked by picrotoxinin, isopropyl bicyclophosphates, and (+)bicuculline (unpublished observations). These results indicate that (+)etomidate interacts with the GABA and diazepam binding sites via the picrotoxinin site. All these observations support the notion that depressant and anxiolytic compounds (like pentobarbital and etazolate) and convulsants like picrotoxin and bicyclophosphate esters, perturb GABA and benzodiazepine binding components (at least in part) via the dihydropicrotoxinin component of the benzodiazepine-GABA receptor-ionophore complex. Recent studies by other investigators which showed that (a) picrotoxinin and cage convulsant drugs produce a chloride- and temperature-dependent enhancement of benzodiazepine binding (l0), and (b) convulsants that act at the dihydropicrotoxinin site prevent heat inactivation of benzodiazepine binding sites (23), also support this notion. It has also been demonstrated that barbiturates enhance benzodiazepine and GABA receptor functions in Lubrol- and CHAPS-solubilized fractions (6,l9).

Effect of Protein-Modifying Reagents on Muscimol and Pentobarbital Enhancement of Benzodiazepine Binding:

To further understand the molecular interactions of drugs that modulate GABAergic transmission, we have investigated the effects of two protein modifying reagents on basal and stimulated benzodiazepine binding and on GABA binding. Pretreatment of cerebral cortex, cerebellum or hippocampus membranes with di-ethylpyrocarbonate (DEP; pH 6.0, 20 min at 0-4°C) or diazotized sulfanilate (pH 7.0, 20 min at 37°C) results in a dose-dependent inactivation of [^{3}H]diazepam, [^{3}H]flunitrazepam and [^{3}H]propyl-β-carboline-3-carboxylate (PrCC) binding in all the three regions (5). Both DEP and sulfanilate pretreatment decreased the B_{max} of benzodiazepine radioligands without altering the K_D. Following partial inactivation of [^{3}H]diazepam binding with 1 mM DEP (which produces 40-50% inhibition), muscimol and pentobarbital were still able to enhance [^{3}H]diazepam binding. The EC_{50} values of muscimol and pentobarbital were similar in control and DEP-pretreated regions. However, following partial inactivation of cerebral cortex or hippocampus membranes with 1 mM sulfanilate (which produces 60-68% inhibition), muscimol and pentobarbital were unable to enhance [^{3}H]diazepam binding (5).

We have also investigated the effect of DEP and sulfanilate on GABA binding. Sulfanilate but not DEP produced a dose-related inhibition of GABA binding to both cortex and cerebellum (5). Table 6 summarizes the effects of DEP and sulfanilate on [^{3}H]benzodiazepine binding, [^{3}H]GABA binding and on pentobar-

TABLE 6.   EFFECT OF PROTEIN MODIFYING REAGENTS ON
BENZODIAZEPINE-GABA RECEPTOR-IONOPHORE COMPLEX

	Diethylpyrocarbonate (DEP)	Diazotized Sulfanilate
A. LIGAND BINDING		
[^{3}H]Diazepam[a]	Inhibited	Inhibited
[^{3}H]PrCC[a]	Inhibited	Inhibited
[^{3}H]GABA[b]	No Effect	Inhibited
B. DIAZEPAM ENHANCEMENT[c]		
Pentobarbital	No Effect	Inhibited
Muscimol	No Effect	Inhibited

[a]: [^{3}H]Diazepam and [^{3}H]propyl-β-carboline-3-carboxylate (Prcc) was inhibited by pretreating cortex, cerebellum or hippocampus membranes with DEP (0.25 - 10 mM; pH 6.0, 20 min, 0°C) and diazotized sulfanilate (0.25 - 10 mM, pH 7.0, 30 min, 37°C) in a dose-related manner.

[b]: DEP (up to 5 mM) had no effect on GABA binding to cortex or cerebellum.   Diazotized sulfanilate (1 mM) abolished the low affinity GABA receptor sites without altering the high affinity site.

[c]: Pentobarbital   and   muscimol   enhancement   of   [^{3}H]diazepam binding was abolished by 1 mM diazotized sulfanilate but not by DEP.

bital and muscimol enhancement of [^{3}H]diazepam binding.   Scat-chard analysis of the binding data indicated that 1 mM sulfani-late pretreatment eliminates the low-affinity GABA receptor site in both cortex (Fig. 3) and cerebellum (data not shown).   Eli-mination of the low-affinity GABA receptor sites by 1 mM sul-fanilate and the inability of muscimol to enhance diazepam binding following sulfanilate pretreatment strongly suggests that low-affinity GABA receptors are involved in the stimulation of benzo-diazepine binding (5).

These results are consistent with other observations which utilized thiocynate (3), sulfhydral reagents (14) and diazepam enhancement of low-affinity GABA receptor (13) and provided evidence which implies that the activation of low-affinity GABA receptors stimulates benzodiazepine binding.   Sulfanilate, but not DEP, abolishes the enhancing effect of both muscimol and pentobarbital and the low-affinity GABA receptors.   It is reason-able that sulfanilate modifies some other groups besides histidine (e.g. tyrosine), or that it simply interacts with different histidine residues.   It is also feasible that sulfanilate affects the coupling mechanism between GABA and barbiturate receptors and the ben-zodiazepine receptors.   Further studies with these group selective reagents should provide valuable information about the functional groups that may be critical for the function of the benzodiaze-pine-GABA receptor-ionophore complex and the possible coupling mechanisms involved.

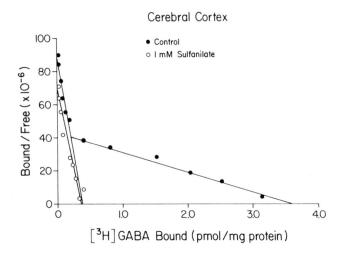

Cerebral Cortex

[^{3}H] GABA Bound (pmol/mg protein)

FIG. 3. [^{3}H]GABA Scatchard plot in control and 1 mM diazotized sulfanilate pretreated cortex.

ACKNOWLEDGEMENT

We thank Dr. Knabe (West Germany) for providing us with stereoisomers of MPPB, hexobarbital and mephobarbital; Dr. Downes (Oregon) for CHEB; and Dr. Leysen (Belgium) for the stereoisomers of etomidate, and Mrs. Marilyn Wilson for excellent secretarial assistance.

This work was supported, in part, by NIH Grant NS #15339.

REFERENCES

1. Asano, T. and Ogasawara, N. (1981): Brain Res., 225:212-216.
2. Ashton, D., Geerts, R., Waterkeyn, C. and Leysen, J.E. (1981): Life Science, 29:2631-2636.
3. Browner, M., Ferkany, J.W. and Enna, S.J. (1981): J. Neurosci., 1:514-518.
4. Büch, H.P., Schneider-Affeld, F., Rummel, W. and Knabe, J. (1973): Naunyn-Schmiedeberg's Arch. Pharmacol., 277:191-198.
5. Burch, T.P., Thyagarajan, R. and Ticku, M.K. (1983): Mol. Pharmacol., in press.
6. Davis, W.C. and Ticku, M.K. (1981): J. Neurosci., 1:1306-1042.
7. Enna, S.J. and Snyder, S.H. (1975): Brain Res., 100:81-97.
8. Evans, R.M. and Hill, R.E. (1978): Experientia, 34:1325-1326.

9. Grossman, W., Jurna, I. and Theres, C. (1974): Naunyn-Schmiedeberg's Arch Pharmacol., 282:367-377.
10. Karobath, M., Drexler, G. and Supavilai, P. (1981): Life Sci., 28:307-313.
11. Leeb-Lundberg, F., Snowman, A. and Olsen, R.W. (1980): Proc. Natl. Acad. Sci. U.S.A., 77:7468-7472.
12. Leeb-Lundberg, F., Snowman, A. and Olsen, R.W. (1981): J. Neurosci., 1:471-477.
13. Matsumoto, K. and Fukuda, H. (1982): Life Sci., 30:935-942.
14. Marangos, P.J. and Martino, A.M. (1981): Mol. Pharmac., 20:16-21.
15. Möhler, H. and Okada, T. (1977): Science, 198:849-851.
16. Nicoll, R.A., Eccles, J.C., Oshima, T.C. and Rubia, F. (1975): Nature, 258:625-627.
17. Olsen, R.W. (1981): J. Neurochem., 37:1-13.
18. Olsen, R.W., Greenlee, D., VanNess, P. and Ticku, M.K. (1978): In: Amino Acids as Chemical Transmitters, edited by F. Fonnum, pp. 467-486. Plenum Press, New York.
19. Olsen, R.W. and Snowman, A. (1982): J. Neurosci., in press.
20. Placheta, P. and Karobath, M. (1980): Eur. J. Pharmacol., 62:225-228.
21. Simmonds, M.A. (1981): Br. J. Pharmacol., 73:739-747.
22. Skolnick, P., Paul, S.M. and Barker, J.L. (1980). Eur. J. Pharmacol., 65:125-127.
23. Squires, R.F. and Braestrup, E. (1977): Nature, 266:732-734.
24. Squires, R.F. and Saederup, E. (1982): In: Pharmacology of Benzodiazepines, edited by S.M. Paul et al, in press, Macmillan Press, New York.
25. Supavilai, P. and Karobath, M. (1979): Eur. J. Pharmacol., 60:111-113.
26. Supavilai, P., Mannonen, A. and Karobath, M. (1982): Neurochem. Int., in press.
27. Ticku, M.K. (1980): Brain Res., 211:127-133.
28. Ticku, M.K. (1981): Biochem. Pharmacol., 30:1573-1579.
29. Ticku, M.K. (1982): Fed. Proc., in press.
30. Ticku, M.K., Ban, M. and Olsen, R.W. (1978): Mol. Pharmacol. 14:391-402.
31. Ticku, M.K., VanNess, P.C., Haycock, J.W., Levy, W.B. and Olsen, R.W. (1978): Brain Research, 150:642-647.
32. Ticku, M.K. and Olsen, R.W. (1978): Life Sci. 22:1643-1652.
33. Ticku, M.K. and Olsen, R.W. (1979): Neuropharmacology 18:315-318.
34. Willow, M. and Johnston, G.A.R. (1980): Neurosci. Lett. 18:323-327.
35. Willow, M. (1981): Brain Res. 220:427-431.

CNS Receptors—From Molecular
Pharmacology to Behavior, edited by
P. Mandel and F. V. DeFeudis.
Raven Press, New York © 1983.

Electrophysiological Study of GABA$_A$ Versus GABA$_B$ Receptors on Excitation-Secretion Coupling

*M. Désarménien, **F. Santangelo, **G. Occhipinti,
*R. Schlichter, *J. P. Loeffler, †E. Desaulles,
*B. A. Demeneix, and *P. Feltz

*Institut de Physiologie et de Chimie Biologique, Université Louis Pasteur,
F-67084 Strasbourg, France; **Istituto di Fisiologia Umana, 95125 Catania, Italy;
and †INSERM U-243, Department de Pharmacie, Université Louis Pasteur,
67-Illkirch-Graffenstaden, France

SUMMARY: Inwardly-directed Ca^{++}-currents are caused by numerous types of action potentials which would not otherwise cause secretion. This process is regulated electrically and by neurotransmitters. We have studied in vitro the ionic mechanisms of GABA-mediated presynaptic inhibition and thereby the distinctive characteristics of GABA$_A$ and GABA$_B$ receptors: i.e., the GABA$_A$ system, which produces such short-lasting changes that there is an instantaneous reduction of spike amplitudes, in particular by opening Cl$^-$-conductance, and the GABA$_B$ system, which results directly in inhibition of secretion due to a tonic depression of Ca^{++}-currents. The principal aim was to determine if GABA$_B$/Ca^{++} receptors could coexist on a membrane already possessing a large number of GABA$_A$/Cl$^-$ sites available for presynaptic inhibition. Intracellular recordings of Aδ and C dorsal root ganglion cell bodies were used as a model for the study of preterminal axonal membranes. Results were tentatively correlated with those obtained extracellularly by recording Ca^{++} and K$^+$ movements (Cl$^-$ being assessed indirectly) from a set of other cells which also secrete neuropeptides by exocytosis: e.g., endings of unmyelinated fibres in the neurohypophysis and clusters of innervated gland cells in the pars intermedia.

In recent years there has been a growing interest in receptors for neurotransmitters (e.g., monoamines, peptides, γ-aminobutyric acid) modulating Ca^{++}-dependent secretion in various biological systems (14-16,24,25,29,34). Modulation is possible either by changing the basic characteristics of the ionic currents during a standard action potential (Na$^+$/K$^+$ voltage transients being

markedly altered by repolarizing K^+ currents) or by any kind of
direct action on voltage-dependent Ca^{++}-channels: the latter will
allow Ca^{++} to enter the cell in graded amounts not only as parts
of well-defined Ca^{++}-spikes (16,14,39; see also 24,26,28) but
possibly also along complex sequences of tail-currents (for the
biophysics, see 28,29). Accordingly, it is essential to study
presynaptic actions of transmitters in systems where spikes can be
recorded, though presynaptic receptor activation can sometimes be
identified by other means than spiking patterns (e.g., membrane
effects in relation to other well-defined ionophores).

The study of cells which are in contact with synapses synthesizing and releasing γ-aminobutyric acid (GABA) has drawn much of the
attention given to these problems. The debate is not yet closed
as to whether GABA-receptor activation exerts an inhibitory action,
either by acting on Cl^--ionophores until diminishing spike amplitude and/or frequency (see 10,25,27), or by maintaining subsequent
Ca^{++}-currents in a depressed stage (15,16,21).

PHYSIOLOGICAL BASIS FOR MULTIPLE RECEPTORS
AT GABA-ergic SYNAPSES

In view of the multiple modes of action, two groups of workers
having used biochemical (3,8,23,38) and electrophysiological (6,9,
15,18) determinations of presynaptic inhibitory actions of
(-)β-p-chlorophenyl-GABA (baclofen),arrived at the conclusion that
GABA may have two different receptors. This notion has been pursued recently by Hill and Bowery so as to identify two independent
binding sites: $GABA_A$ versus $GABA_B$, with respective list headings
for agonist specificity being isoguvacine and (-)baclofen.
Additional criteria are the susceptibility of $GABA_A$ receptors to
antagonism by bicuculline and a typical relationship with Cl^--
ionophores. In contrast, the newly-discovered $GABA_B$ or baclofen-
receptor would cause direct inhibition of transmitter output by
restricting presynaptic Ca^{++} influx (3,8,15). However, the evidence
for this $GABA_B$ receptor being associated with voltage-dependent
Ca^{++}-channels is not as strong as that presented for $GABA_A$ linkage
with Cl^--ionophores.

One convenient way in which presynaptic receptors can be studied
by electrophysiological methods is to carry out experiments on
preparations which can be easily isolated, impaled with microelectrodes and superfused with a drug-containing medium or kept free
of Ca^{++}. Biochemical assays do not always allow sufficient pre-
cision to monitor the fine variations that result from modulation
of Ca^{++} entering secretory cells. Thus, the study of GABA-receptors
on the soma of primary afferent neurones has been essential for
predicting the modes of action of GABA as a major inhibitory transmitter at the presynaptic level (see reviews 9,27,and refs. in 20,
22,25,32). As discussed in many review articles (e.g., 9, 27,30),
the mammalian spinal cord has always been the subject of selected
physiological and/or pharmacological determinations of presynaptic
inhibition (recent reports in 10,17). However, the bulk of data
is on the distribution of only the first class of GABA-receptors,
those susceptible to antagonism by bicuculline. These $GABA_A$
receptors cause membrane depolarization, which argues not only
against inhibition but also against a possible reduction of Ca^{++}

entry. This apparent contradiction is generally ruled out by the consistent demonstrations of Na^+/K^+ spikes being electrically shunted by the GABA-mediated increase in Cl^- conductance (see 7,25,30). Moreover, the depolarizing actions of GABA may represent outwardly-directed Cl^--fluxes as nerve terminals of primary afferent cells would be heavily loaded with this anion (9,22,30). In turn, these Cl^--dependent depolarizations would diminish any Na/K voltage transient, thereby leaving less Ca^{++} to enter by means of voltage-dependent Ca^{++}-channels (less will open according to biophysical models: 29).

Our aim was first to use intracellular recordings of dorsal root ganglia (DRG) neurones tentatively identified with respect to their nerve endings; by this means we gained information on inherent cell membrane conductance and on Ca^{++}-currents as a result of the characteristics of action potentials (see 15,24,39). Ultimately, we studied the interrelated distribution of GABA-receptors by assuming that earlier studies on GABA-induced depolarizations of nerve trunks were predictive of GABA-receptors to be found on group C neurones (4,17,40). These cells have been of further interest to us because they may represent the source of neuropeptide secretion in the spinal cord (namely substance P and SRIF: 5,19). All experiments followed criteria accounting for the physiological classification of primary afferents (group 1_A, Aδ and C) and the precise pharmacological distinction between both types of presynaptic GABA-receptors, recently introduced by Bowery and colleagues (3,23). In the final part of the Results section we outline similar results obtained when studying modulatory effects of GABA on endocrine secretion, also known to be possibly under control of GABA-ergic synapses (31,34,37). We have consequently used as a model the neuro-intermediate lobe of the hypophysis in vitro, where voltage-dependent release of peptide hormones can easily be monitored (see 14,33,34), and,most interestingly,together with electrophysiological determinations of ionic fluxes (Fig. 6-8).

DISTRIBUTION ANALYSIS AT PRIMARY AFFERENT MEMBRANES OF GABA$_A$
AND GABA$_B$ RECEPTORS FOR PRESYNAPTIC INHIBITION

Sensory Ganglia as a Model

A depolarizing action of GABA has been demonstrated on the somatic membrane of virtually every dorsal root ganglion cell studied, whether in vivo (refs. in 12,13), in vitro (11,12,20,26), or in primary cell cultures (7,15,21,30). This effect on DRG cells is obtained with any defined GABA$_A$ agonist (see ref. 13 and Fig. 4), and corresponds to a primary increase in Cl^--conductance (7,11,22). As regards distribution studies of these responses, the most pertinent information from earlier studies is that metabolic conditions are critical (Cl^- gradients), and that great care must be taken to avoid receptor desensitization (10,20). This can be done by using the most rapid means of drug application (fast perfusion, micropressure, short pulse ionophoresis). Moreover, uptake of GABA into glial cells can easily be kept under control, by recording from single cells at the surface of superfused spinal ganglia (11,20).

As regards nerve terminals in the spinal cord, great advances have been made recently by the use of extracellular recordings of

identified single fibres, in particular for testing drug actions
at group 1$_A$ preterminal endings (9,10,27,32). These experiments
provided the best insight into the distribution patterns of the
first variety of known GABA-receptors causing membrane depolarization, precisely where neurally-supplied GABA is released. Notable
among such experiments based on measurements of single fibre excitability, mainly pursued by Curtis and his colleagues (see 10), is
the substantial demonstration that presynaptic GABA$_A$ receptors are
by themselves sufficiently potent in gating the excitation-secretion
process, independent of the GABA$_B$ system (but see 6,18). These
results are of interest in so far as they are related to physiological events at one particular group of primary afferents which
possibly release a transmitter related to glutamate or aspartate:
group 1$_A$ sensory cells with fast-conducting myelinated axons and
intense firing patterns of Na/K spikes.
     It is, however, important to realize that, with the exception
of some controversial studies on the release of either amino acids
or neuropeptides in the spinal grey and in other relay stations
of primary afferent terminals (16,18,35), most of the primary
afferent neurones are as yet unidentified in the context of the
newly discovered GABA$_B$ or baclofen receptor. Here we present
evidence that Aδ (slow-conducting myelinated fibres) and the bulk
of unmyelinated group C terminals are certainly the major target
for GABA$_B$ receptors in the adult rat. In contrast with a recent
report on chick sensory ganglia in culture (16), we could demonstrate that almost all groups of sensory neurones do show the
principal actions of GABA, typical of GABA$_A$ receptor activation,
although in the adult rat some cells may exhibit noticeable differences in sensitivity. This latter aspect of receptor distribution appears more relevant to developmental patterns and will be
examined in detail elsewhere.
     Irrespective of the precise patterns of receptor densities,
which may change from the somatic membrane up to the central preterminal axons (possible addition of regulatory sub-units), a
consistent finding is that the whole of the cell membrane of sensory
cells can display depolarizing currents in response to GABA$_A$ receptor activation. Any significant change in Cl$^-$ distribution would
either suppress or invert these GABA-induced currents (7,11,22),
but would not noticeably change the closely related extrasynaptic
response seen on some cells with 5-HT (also causing depolarization
on spinal and visceral C cells: 22).

GABA and Slow-Conducting Primary Afferents

     There are many reasons to believe that neurally-released GABA
would affect a whole series of nerve endings originating from
sensory ganglia. Anatomically, high densities of GABA terminals
are indeed located in all layers of the spinal grey, namely in the
substantia gelatinosa and in ventro-intermediate and lateral nuclei
(refs. in 1,10,32). Functionally, these regions receive various
sensory inputs carried by fast-conducting axons in intermediate and
ventral layers and by slow Aδ and C fibres synapsing abundantly in

the external layers of the dorsal grey (5); hence it can be predicted that GABA-ergic synapses would ultimately be associated with
any type of primary aferents: either myelinated or unmyelinated.
That presynaptic GABA-ergic synapses are so widely distributed can
further be deduced from recent cytophysiological studies using
either autoradiographic labelling of GABA-receptor with ^{3}H-muscimol
(35) or ultrastructural immunocytochemistry based on the major
GABA-synthesizing enzyme, GAD (1).

Cytophysiological data may be a starting point for analyzing the
distribution of $GABA_A$ and $GABA_B$ receptors (38), even before one is
carried into the details of ionic mechanisms. One would first have
to know if there is indeed more than one population of sensory cells
affected by neurally-released GABA. By no means can it be predicted
that the mechanisms of presynaptic inhibition are essentially similar between one and another population of cells. In particular,
voltage-dependent Ca^{++}-currents are readily carried by Ca^{++}-depen-
dent action potentials in the vast majority of group C cells (also
in many Aδ cells: our results and others in 39), whereas they can
reasonably be assumed to be mainly distinguishable as delayed currents in fast-conducting axons (i.e., the population of large diameter group l_A afferents ; 1).

Intracellular Recordings of Group C and Aδ Sensory Cells

Experimental Procedures: They do not differ in any major respect
from previous means for recording intracellularly the largest
(> 30 µm) DRG neurones under microscopic vision (x 320) from ganglia
being mounted in a microperfusion chamber (200 µl; 2-5 ml.min^{-1}).

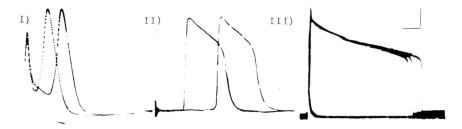

FIG. 1. Identification of Aδ and C neurones in DRG by means of
intracellularly-recorded spikes in a standard experiment: 7.5 mM
TEA continuously added to Ringer, cell impalement with $Cs_2 SO_4$ electrode, spike-latency upon a double fibre stimulation (scale: 20 mV).
I) Superimposed traces of Aδ spikes evoked from 2 stimulatory points
along the nerve: 6.5 and 15 mm from center of ganglion (conduction
velocity: 18 m.s.$^{-1}$; resting membrane potential: RP = -80 mV).
II) Same test as above with C neurone; stimulation on dorsal root
at 5 and 11 mm distance (conduction at 0.7 m.s.$^{-1}$; RP = -80 mV).
Immediately after cell penetration, C neurones most commonly show
slow spikes and a hump during repolarizing phase. III) Same cell,
but spikes prolonged as a result of additional block of K^+-current
(intracellularly-injected Cs^+). Time scales: 0.5 ms(I); 5 ms (II);
100 ms (III).

Methods for eliciting reproducible GABA responses, either by ionophoresis (Fig. 3) or by transient superfusion have also been described elsewhere (11,12). In rats, the lumbar DRG (L5) possess rather
smaller populations of sensory C cells than other ganglia (visceral
and cranial), but long segments of both central and distal nerve
fibres can be studied most favourably on a functional basis (Fig. 1).
Cytophysiological criteria for identifying small DRG cells (15-30 μm)
were rarely used, since we can rely on the electrophysiology. Thus,
any velocity of spikes below 2 m.s.$^{-1}$ (37°C) tended to be characteristic of C fibres (Aδ: 2.5-20 m.s.$^{-1}$). Other criteria were shapes
of either anti- or orthodromic action potentials (39) and the long
duration of any spike augmenting as a result of experimental block
of K$^+$-currents (Fig. 1,III and 2).
Ca^{++}-spikes of Aδ and C neurones: A detailed study of the various
configurations which action potentials can take has been made in the
DRG of the adult mouse by Yoshida (39); the basic characteristics of
TTX-resistent Ca^{++}-currents have been further elucidated by Kostyuk
et al (26), as they succeeded in using the most satisfactory techniques (voltage clamp and cell interior perfusion). We used the most
simple approach to unmask Ca^{++} components of the spikes, and always

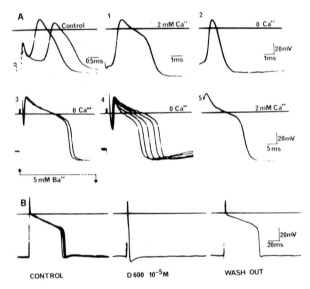

FIG. 2. A) Antidromic action potentials (evoked at 6 and 11 mm in
left trace) are prolonged by TEA and Cs$^+$ (trace number 1). 2) Plateau
phase is suppressed when Ca^{++} is replaced by Mg^{++}. 3) Plateau of
directly-evoked spikes being restored when Ba^{++} is then added to the
0 Ca^{++} medium. 4) Graded shortening as Ba^{++} is washed out. 5) Ca^{++}
added again, and final recovery (Vcond: 12 m.s.$^{-1}$; RP = -65 mV).
B) Superfusion of methoxy-verapamil (D 600) reversibly reduces Ca^{++}-
spike in a dose-dependent manner; maximal effect is shown on central
trace (Vcond:18 m.s.$^{-1}$; RP = -65 mV). TEA and Cs$^+$ were always present
except for control A (top left).

in a situation allowing antidromic spike propagation (no TTX added
to counteract Na^+). A consistent and stable increase in spike
duration was generally obtained by superfusing ganglia with 7.5 mM
TEA and by releasing Cs^+ intracellularly (Fig. 2). The magnitude of
this increase was kept stable, firstly by evoking spike depolarizations at a defined basal level of membrane potential (RP in Fig. 2),
and secondly by taking care to repeat stimulations slowly (1-min
time intervals).

In DRG neurones, as in other systems, the Ca^{++}-currents are
triggered by fast-inactivating Na^+-currents and switched off, not
so much by themselves as by outward K^+-currents causing repolariz-
ation (voltage-dependent and Ca^{++}-dependent K^+-channels). For a
variety of reasons we are still unable at this stage to know whether
the Ca^{++}-spikes we have seen in all C neurones and in about one-third
of Aδ correspond to those most frequently encountered in primary
cultures (16,21). This also complicates the comparison of pharmacological tests on $GABA_B$ receptors. However, for example, by maintaining ganglia under relatively stable conditions, as described
above, the prolongation of the antidromic action potential did not
differ in any major respect from that observed on locally-evoked
spikes: i.e., by means of brief (0.5-5 ms) depolarizing pulses
applied through recording electrode. As regards the use of these
spikes for identifying $GABA_B$ receptors (compare Figs. 2 and 5), the
above findings highlight the problems of interpreting the mechanisms
of drug action when technical difficulties are encountered for measuring "presynaptic membrane" currents under voltage clamp conditions.

$GABA_A$ receptor activation: In Aδ and C neurones, as in all large
diameter DRG cells, GABA caused transient conductance increases
leading to a complex sequence of membrane depolarization (Fig. 3).
As Aδ neurones are compared to C (continuing statistical analysis),
the latter display smaller voltage deflexion in response to GABA,

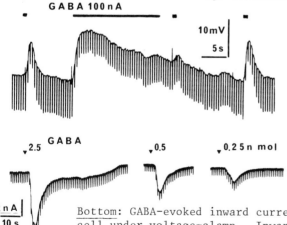

FIG. 3. Top: Aδ neurones
responding to brief (■)
and prolonged (line)
ionophoretic applica-
tions of GABA (100 nA);
note second pulse of
GABA being ineffective
and the final recovery
after desensitization
(right). Hyperpolariz-
ing current steps (0.5 nA,
60 ms) monitor membrane
resistance: 20 MΩ
(RP = -60 mV).

Bottom: GABA-evoked inward currents recorded from a Aδ
cell under voltage-clamp. Inward pulses (10 mV/100 ms)
monitor membrane conductance. Note increased conductance
at response peak, reflecting the opening of mainly Cl^-
channels. Clamp potential held at RP (-75 mV).

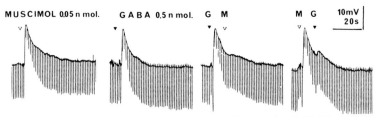

FIG. 4. Individual responses to GABA and muscimol followed by cross-desensitization test (Vcond 8 m.s.$^{-1}$; RP = 70 mV).

all pharmacological criteria being identical. These responses are dose-dependent and always diminish because of desensitization (Fig. 4). Results of greater depth of analysis have now also been obtained on the current flowing through the membrane of DRG cells with slow-conducting axons (Fig. 3, bottom). The major part of the conductance change corresponds to the opening of specific ionic channels, although the whole sequence of events may not be exclusively governed by the equilibrium potential of Cl$^-$. If any K$^+$-channels are going to close because of an additional population of extrasynaptic GABA receptors (like on crayfish muscle), this should firstly draw the reversal potential away from the high levels usually observed(-10 to -30 mV, as shown in 12; but see results on cultures: 7). Secondly, if any atypical effect on K$^+$ is involved in the late depolarizing phase of GABA responses (i.e., slight increase of membrane resistance following the initial decrease), this should also be noticeable as an increased duration of Ca^{++}-spikes. However, at doses of GABA below threshold for GABA$_A$ receptor activation (5-20 μM; also threshold for desensitization if continuously perfused; 11), the most frequent observation was a decreased duration of spikes (GABA$_B$ effect). At any rate, if one particular type of K$^+$-channel may close for some reason, the GABA-induced voltage deflexion can always reach amplitudes large enough to cause voltage-dependent K$^+$-channels to open. Indeed, in the DRG, we have already demonstrated a transient rise in extracellular K$^+$ being correlated with intracellularly-recorded depolarizations caused by GABA$_A$ receptor activation (13). This has now also been investigated in the neurohypophysis (Figs. 6-8).

GABA$_B$ receptor activation: No substantial desensitization effect having been observed, the ganglia could be superfused slowly in these experiments. Figure 5 exemplifies the means for detecting the presence of GABA$_B$ receptors on Aδ and C neurones, baclofen being the test substance. In a similar study on chick sensory ganglia in culture, GABA and (±)baclofen were also shown to markedly reduce the duration of Ca^{++}-spikes (16). The major differences to be emphasized are in the context of the specificity of agonists and antagonists. Firstly, as stated above, bicuculline is a favourable tool for competitively inhibiting GABA$_A$ receptors, and it can easily be used in biochemical assays to distinguish GABA$_A$ from GABA$_B$ binding sites (23). However, since this drug has a direct action on Ca^{++} spikes by some unknown mechanism (Fig. 5 and ref. 21), it is best used in a narrow range of doses. Secondly, clear evidence was

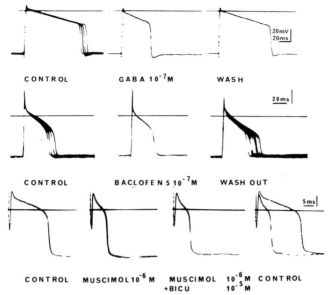

FIG. 5. <u>Top</u>: Reversible shortening of spike duration by GABA;
superimposed traces (left) show stability of control. <u>Middle</u>: Same
effect with (±)baclofen; serial traces display recovery (right).
<u>Bottom</u>: Muscimol also shortens the spike, and this effect is not
antagonized by bicuculline. Superimposed spikes on last trace show
control after washing out bicuculline (shortest spike) and after
washing out muscimol (longest spike). (Lines indicate potential
level 0 mV.) Note that a high dose of bicuculline may itself increase
spike duration.

obtained in our experiments that $GABA_B$ effects are bicuculline-re-
sistant; moreover, the most important observations are that isoguvacine does not shorten Ca^{++}-spikes, whereas muscimol, like GABA
and SL 75102, proved to be a mixed agonist.
    Finally, we are faced with physiological tests to be performed on
membranes where both types of GABA-receptors coexist, possibly with
uneven distribution patterns. We are also left with the argument
that desensitization more readily affects the receptors governing
transient conductance changes. In the following pages, we illu-
strate that this is unlikely to apply to GABA responses in neuroendocrine systems. In practice, the approach to the problem has
been statistical, as we have recorded the ionic movements involving
either a pool of neurosecretory axons or clusters of glandular cells.

GABA-RECEPTORS IN THE NEURO-INTERMEDIATE LOBE (NIL)

    Essentially, two <u>in vitro</u> models for GABA-ergic modulation of
Ca^{++}-dependent hormone release can be used. <u>Firstly, the pituitary
unmyelinated axons and nerve terminals in the neural lobe</u>; favourably, they provide a most homogeneous and large surface of "presynaptic" membranes in regard to receptor-mediated ionic exchange

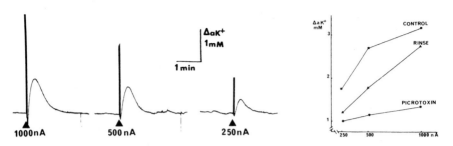

FIG. 6. Transients of elevated K^+ concentration (ΔaK) in neural lobe as elicited by ionophoretic pulses (1 Hz; 3s) of three doses of GABA (nA). Graph: Depression of responses by picrotoxin added to perfusate (5.10^{-5} M); final recovery: 2 h.

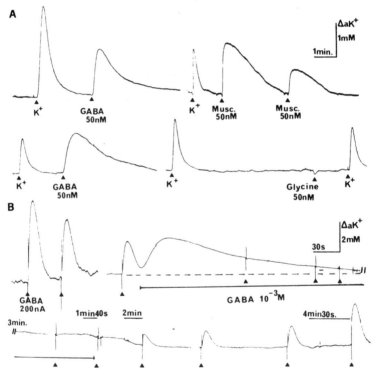

FIG. 7. Neural lobe recordings: A) Compounds applied by 5 µl drops directly into perfusion chamber (5 mM Hepes Ringer). Microperfusion was first calibrated by adding 500 nmol K^+ (5 µl drop). Depolarizing effect of GABA and muscimol as manifested by K^+ efflux. Compared to GABA, glycine (lower trace) elicits no K^+ efflux. B) Receptor desensitization shown when GABA is applied, first ionophoretically (arrow: GABA, 200 nA, 1s) at short time intervals, and second, by perfusion (10^{-3} M) whilst pulsing ionophoretic GABA (Δ). Initially, perfusion elicited an increase in extracellular K^+ which then faded with time, and ionophoretically-applied GABA ceased to elicit a K^+ efflux. Note that the phenomenon is reversible.

measures. As deduced from preceding results on sensory neurones, we have first investigated the K^+ efflux caused by $GABA_A$-mediated membrane depolarization (Figs. 6 and 7); these responses are antagonized by picrotoxin and by bicuculline. Most importantly, receptor-desensitization is also evident. Secondly, we used intermediate lobes of rats (Fig. 8), where GABA-ergic synapses have recently been demonstrated (GAD immunocytochemistry; 30,36) directly on the membranes of the set of cells secreting α-MSH and endorphins (refs. in 14,33). In this preparation, it is expected that Ca^{++}-currents in spikes of gland cells would be sensitive to $GABA_B$ agonists, the release of MSH being thereby depressed (for comparison, see results with dopamine: 14,34). In contrast, GABA-induced voltage deflexions, like K^+-induced membrane depolarization, may

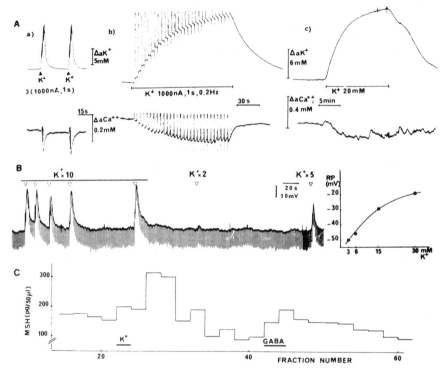

FIG. 8. A) In neural (a) and intermediate lobe (b,c), extracellular K^+ and Ca^{++} are monitored. K^+-induced depolarization is causing a Ca^{++} uptake which occurs rapidly (a), and persists when K^+ application is sustained either by ionophoresis (b) or perfusion (c). B) Intracellular recording of pars intermedia cells, illustrating the depolarizing effect of K^+ applied by the fast microperfusion technique (Fig. 7); numbers indicate fold increases in basal K^+ (3 mM). Membrane potential changes as indicated on the graph. C) Release of α-MSH (radioimmunoassay: ref. 33) caused by a 10-fold increase of K^+ in perfused NIL glands. A similar, but smaller release was obtained with GABA (10^{-4} M). Collection time was 3 min; concentrations are means of 2 fractions.

cause hormone release (Fig. 8, B,C).

Experiments have all been conducted in vitro under direct micro-scopic vision (x250), namely for placing K^+ and Ca^{++}-sensitive microelectrodes (calibrated as described in 12-35). The results are summarized by a set of figures. Interestingly, in view of correlating cell firing with hormone release, we show herein that the membrane of neurosecretory fibres (possibly also of gland cells) can become transiently shunted by the ionic channel governed by $GABA_A$ receptor.

CONCLUSIONS

The results show that on the membrane of sensory cells, as on that of neurosecretory axons, two targets exist for GABA: receptor-operated Cl^--channels which transiently open, and voltage-dependent Ca^{++}-channels which fail to operate. Evidence for the hypothesis that GABA functions as a presynaptic inhibitory transmitter on nociceptive primary afferents is presented. The activation of $GABA_A$ receptors may reflect phasic inhibition whose magnitude could de-pend on the degree to which the cells are refilled with Cl^-, and, most importantly, on a possible modulation of receptor-desensitiz-ation. A sustained component of presynaptic inhibition may be determined more reliably by $GABA_B$ receptor activation, which is almost insensitive to bicuculline antagonism and poorly subject to desensitization. This hypothesis implies that on unmyelinated primary afferents, and possibly also in neuroendocrine systems, GABA reduces the availability of extracellular Ca^{++}, either se-quentially and/or in relation with the various physiological means by which the concentration of extracellularly-free GABA is regulated.

We thank Mrs. S. Steible for assistance. Grants: CNRS (2581) and INSERM (PRC).

REFERENCES

1. Barber, R.P., Vaughn, J.E. and Roberts, E. (1982): Brain Res., 238: 305-328.
2. Barrett, E.F. and Barrett, J.N. (1982): J. Physiol. 323: 117-144.
3. Bowery, N.G., Doble, A., Hill, D.R., Hudson, A.L., Shaw, S.S., Turnbull, M.J. and Warrington, R. (1981): Eur. J. Pharmac. 71: 53-70.
4. Brown, D.A. and Marsh, S. (1978): Brain Res., 156: 187-191.
5. Brown, A.G. (1981): Organization in the Spinal Cord, Springer Verlag, Berlin.
6. Capek, R. and Esplin, B. (1982): Can. J. Physiol. Pharmac., 60: 160-166.
7. Choi, D.W. and Fischbach, G.D. (1981): J. Neurophysiol., 45: 605-620.
8. Collins, G.G.S., Anson, J. and Kelly, E.P. (1982): Brain Res., 238: 371-384.

9. Curtis, D.R. (1978): In: Amino Acids as Chemical Transmitters, edited by F. Fonnum, pp. 55-86, Plenum Press, New York.
10. Curtis, D.R. and Lodge, D. (1982): Exp. Brain Res., 46: 215-233.
11. Désarménien, M., Feltz, P. and Headley,P.M. (1980): J. Physiol. 307: 163-182.
12. Désarménien, M., Feltz, P., Headley, P.M. and Santangelo, F. (1981): Brit. J. Pharmac., 72: 355-364.
13. Deschenes, M. and Feltz, P. (1976): Brain Res., 118: 496-499.
14. Douglas, W.W. and Taraskevich, P.S. (1982): J. Physiol., 326: 201-212.
15. Dunlap, K. (1981): Brit. J. Pharmac., 74: 579-586.
16. Dunlap, K. and Fischbach, G.D. (1981): J. Physiol., 317: 519-535.
17. Fitzgerald, M. and Woolf, C.J. (1981): J. Physiol., 318: 25-40.
18. Fox, S., Krnjević, K., Morris, M.E., Puil, E. and Werman, R. (1978): Neuroscience, 3: 495-515.
19. Harmar, A. and Keen, P. (1982): Brain Res., 231: 379-386.
20. Headley, P.M., Désarménien, M., Linck, G., Santangelo, F. and Feltz, P. (1980): Brain Res. Bull., 5, suppl. 2: 77-81.
21. Heyer, E.J. and Macdonald, R.L. (1982): J. Neurophysiol., 47: 641-655.
22. Higashi, H. and Nishi, S. (1982): J. Physiol., 323: 543-567.
23. Hill, D.R. and Bowery, N.G. (1981): Nature, 290: 149-152.
24. Horn, J.P. and McAffee, D.A. (1980): J. Physiol., 301: 191-204.
25. Kato, K. and Kuba, K. (1980): J. Physiol., 298: 271-287.
26. Kostyuk, P.G., Veselovsky, N.S., Fedulova, S.A. and Tsyndrenko, A.Y. (1980): Neuroscience, 6: 2439-2444.
27. Levy, R.A. (1977): Prog. Neurobiol., 9: 211-267.
28. Llinas, R., Steinberg, J.Z. and Walton, K. (1981): Biophys. J., 33: 323-351.
29. Llinas, R., Sugimori, M. and Simon, S.M. (1982): Proc. Natl. Acad. Sci. U.S.A., 79: 2415-2419.
30. Nistri, A. and Constanti, A. (1979) Prog. Neurobiol., 13: 117-235.
31. Oertel, W.H., Mugnaini, E., Tappaz, M.L., Weise, V.K., Dahl, A.L., Schmechel, D.E. and Kopin, I.J. (1982): Proc. Natl. Acad. Sci. U.S.A., 79: 675-679.
32. Rudomin, P., Engberg, I. and Jimenez, I. (1981): J. Neurophysiol., 46: 532-548.
33. Schmitt, G., Briaud, C., Mialhe, C. and Stutinsky, F. (1979): Neuroendocrinology, 28: 297-301.
34. Sharman, D.F., Holzer, P. and Holzbauer, M. (1982): Neuroendocrinology, 34: 175-199.
35. Singer, E. and Placheta, P. (1980): Brain Res., 202: 484-487.
36. Tsien, R.Y. and Rink, T.J. (1980): Biochim. Biophys. Acta, 599: 623-638.
37. Vincent, S.R., Hökfelt, T. and Wu, J.Y. (1982): Neuroendocrinology, 34: 117-125.
38. Wilkin, G.P., Hudson, A.L., Hill, D.R. and Bowery, N.G. (1981): Nature, 294: 584-586.
39. Yoshida, S. and Matsuda, Y. (1979): J. Neurophysiol., 42: 1134-1145.
40. Zingg, H.H., Baertschi, A.J. and Dreifuss, J.J. (1979): Brain Res., 171: 453-459.

CNS Receptors—From Molecular
Pharmacology to Behavior, edited by
P. Mandel and F. V. Defeudis.
Raven Press, New York © 1983.

Anorexic and Analgesic Actions of THIP

F. V. Defeudis

Département de Biologie, U.P.S.A., 92506 Rueil-Malmaison Cedex, France

The inhibitory neurotransmitter γ-aminobutyric acid (GABA) is involved in the central regulation of food intake (12,26,32,36). In this regard, intracerebroventricularly-injected muscimol (33,34) and injections of GABA or muscimol into the ventromedial hypothalamus (VMH) of rats induced feeding behavior (18,24). Injections of muscimol into the dorsal raphé nucleus of satiated rats also stimulated feeding behavior by an action that was sensitive to bicuculline and picrotoxin (37). In contrast to results obtained with intracerebroventricular or intracerebral administration of GABA or muscimol, intraperitoneally-administered muscimol caused a dose-related decrease in milk consumption in rats (9).

Recent studies have indicated that GABA-ergic systems might also be involved in analgesia in various mammals (13). Parenteral or oral administration of potent, direct-acting GABA-agonists (e.g., muscimol or 4,5,6,7-tetrahydroisoxazolo[5,4-c]pyridin-3-ol (THIP)), inhibitors of GABA-α-oxoglutarate transaminase (e.g., γ-vinyl-GABA), or inhibitors of GABA uptake (e.g., nipecotic acid ethyl ester) induced antinociceptive actions in various mammals (21,25). As this analgesia was not reversed by naloxone or by bicuculline, it did not appear to be mediated by known endogenous opioid systems or by classic GABA-receptors.

The present report provides further evidence that parenteral or oral administration of THIP, an agent that penetrates the "blood-brain barrier" and which has negligible affinity for GABA-metabolizing enzymes or GABA transport systems (28,29), can produce anorexic and analgesic effects in rats or mice.

MATERIALS AND METHODS

Animals

For studies on food intake, male Sprague-Dawley rats (Charles River, France), 180 - 210 g, were used. The animals were housed singly in plastic cages (14 x 20 x 30 cm) containing litter. One week with food and water ad libitum was allowed for acclimatization of the animals to their new surroundings. A cycle of 12 hours of darkness (19.00 - 7.00 h) and 12 hours of light (7.00 - 19.00 h) was maintained throughout the experiments. For studies on analgesia, pathogen-free outbred mice (17 - 26 g) were used. Male CD_1 mice were obtained from Charles River; male OF_1 and male NMRI mice were obtained either from Iffa Credo (France) or from Evic-Ceba (France).

Drugs

The agents used were: (+)bicuculline (Sigma Chem. Co., St. Louis, Missouri); picrotoxin (J. Serigo, Paris); strychnine-SO_4 (Merck, Paris); γ-aminobutyric acid (GABA; Sigma Chem. Co.); pentylenetetrazol (K & K Labs, Inc., Plainview, New York); 4,5,6,7-tetrahydro-isoxazolo[5,4-c]pyridin-3-ol (THIP; kindly provided by Dr. P. Krogsgaard-Larsen and Dr. J. Arnt, Copenhagen); (+)bicuculline-methobromide (kindly provided by Dr. J.F. Collins, London, England); morphine-HCl (Coopération Pharmaceutique Française (C.P.F.), Melun, France); naloxone-HCl (Endo Labs, New York); phenyl-p-benzo-quinone (Sigma Chem. Co.); phentolamine-methanesulfonate (Ciba-Geigy, Rueil-Malmaison, France); atropine-SO_4 (Serlabo, Paris); methysergide-maleate (Sandoz, Rueil-Malmaison, France); d-amphetamine-SO_4 (C.P.F.); fenfluramine-HCl (Lab.Servier, Gidy, France); cocaine-HCl (C.P.F.).

For experiments on food intake, 0.9% NaCl was used as the vehicle for intravenous injections; water was the vehicle for oral administration. For experiments on analgesia, the different substances were administered as aqueous solutions, except for bicuculline which was dissolved in dilute HCl. Control animals received equivalent volumes of the respective drug vehicles.

Test for Food Intake

Rats were allowed to consume food between 11.00 - 15.00 h each day, while having free access to water. They received their cups of food (a mixture of 600 g of powdered standard rat chow (Union d'Alimentation Rationnelle) and 250 ml of soybean oil) in plastic cages (8.5 x 13 x 27 cm). Determinations made on Monday were not included in the final analysis, since the animals had received two pellets of standard rat chow per day on Saturday and Sunday. Determinations made on Tuesday and Wednesday were considered as "control" values ("Days 1 + 2"), drugs were tested on Thursday ("Day 3"), and determinations made on Friday ("Day 4") permitted evaluation of sustained effects of the drugs.

Animals were tested in groups of six. Using intragastric tubes, single oral doses of THIP, GABA, or other agents (1.0 ml/100 g body weight) were administered each week (on "Day 3") 30 minutes before presentation of food to the animals, the vehicle (water) being administered on the other days. Intravenous injections (0.25 ml/100 g body weight) were made immediately before presentation of food to the animals. For tests with possible antagonists, bicuculline (1 mg/kg), bicuculline-methobromide (1.5 mg/kg), strychnine-SO_4 (0.75 mg/kg), picrotoxin (1 mg/kg), or pentylenetetrazol (25 mg/kg) were administered subcutaneously 10 minutes before THIP. These agents did not produce convulsions or other noticeable behavioral changes at the doses used.

Hot-Plate Test

Batches of 10 - 30 mice of CD_1, OF_1, or NMRI strains were used for the hot-plate test (14). The animals were placed on a metal hot-plate that was maintained at 56°C or at 60°C. Reaction time (in seconds), characterized by licking of the forepaws or by jumping from the apparatus, was noted. Morphine or THIP was injected intraperitoneally (0.5 ml/20 g) 30 minutes or 20 minutes, respectively, before placing the animals on the hot-plate. Possible antagonists were administered subcutaneously (0.2 ml/20 g); naloxone was given simultaneously with morphine or THIP; bicuculline was given 10 minutes before, simultaneously with, or 10 minutes after THIP; phentolamine, atropine and methysergide were given 30 or 15 minutes before, or simultaneously with THIP. Mean reaction times were calculated for each batch of animals, the maximum reaction time being taken as 30 seconds.

ED_{50} values, representing the doses at which the antinociceptive effect was 50% of the maximal antinociceptive response, were determined by analyses of variance
of linear regression.

Antagonism of the Phenylbenzoquinone
Writhing Response

Painful responses were induced in batches of 12 CD_1
mice by intraperitoneal injection of 0.22 ml of a
hydro-alcoholic solution of 0.02% phenylbenzoquinone
(40). THIP or morphine (0.5 ml/20 g, i.p.) was injected 20 or 30 minutes, respectively, before phenylbenzoquinone. The mean number of writhing and stretching movements occurring from the fifth to the tenth
minute after phenylbenzoquinone injection, and the
percentage of inhibition of these responses for drug-
treated and control animals were calculated. ED_{50}
values, representing a 50% decrease in the number of
writhing and stretching movements, were determined by
analyses of variance of linear regression.

Evasion and Traction Tests

Batches of eight OF_1 mice received morphine (0.2 ml/
20 g, i.p.) 30 minutes before, or THIP (0.2 ml/20 g,
i.p.) 20 minutes before conducting the evasion test.
For the evasion test (7), the mice were divided randomly into groups of four, placed in cages (7.5 x
7.5 x 20.5 cm), and distinctively marked. After drug
treatment, each mouse was placed at the bottom of the
test apparatus. The apparatus consisted of an open
rectangular box which contained a sloping wooden board
covered with fine wire mesh. The slope was marked
with a horizontal line 2 cm below the point at which
it rested on the upper edge of the box. Any mouse
that crossed the line in an upward direction or jumped
directly from the bottom to the top of the box was
considered to have made an "exit". The mean numbers
of exits in five minutes were calculated, and ED_{50}
values were determined by analyses of variance of
linear regression.
For the traction test (10), which was performed
immediately after the evasion test, the mouse's forepaws were placed on a wire 2 mm in diameter, 25 cm
long, at a height of 30 cm. The mouse was released as
soon as its hindpaws gripped the wire. Normal mice
return to an upright position in less than five seconds.
The response was considered to be positive if the mouse
gripped the wire with one of its hindpaws within five
seconds. The mean numbers of mice displaying positive

TABLE 1. Inhibition of food intake in the rat by intravenous or oral administration of THIP

THIP (mg/kg)	Food intake (g)			
	During first hour		During four hours	
	Control	+ THIP	Control	+ THIP
Intravenous administration				
0.1	7.6±0.6	6.6±0.8	14.9±1.2	14.9±0.9
1.0	8.1±1.0	4.7±1.0 *	15.5±1.0	13.9±1.3
3.0	7.7±1.0	4.8±0.8 *	16.5±0.8	12.4±0.8 **
5.0	7.0±0.8	3.6±0.8 **	15.4±0.8	13.1±1.0
8.0	6.3±0.9	1.8±0.7 ***	15.6±0.9	10.4±1.1 **
10.0	6.2±0.8	0.8±0.3 ***	14.7±0.9	9.7±0.8 ***
Oral administration				
0.1	10.8±1.2	10.4±1.4	14.9±1.3	13.1±1.3
0.5	10.7±1.5	9.8±1.7	14.1±2.0	13.0±1.3
1.0	12.6±1.8	8.8±2.1	16.6±1.5	13.1±2.3
5.0	9.7±1.2	4.7±1.4 *	13.0±0.9	9.9±1.8
10.0	10.6±1.5	2.4±1.4 **	14.8±1.3	6.8±1.5 **

Control values were obtained during the two days prior to administration of THIP; no effects on food intake were evident on the day after THIP administration. Means ± S.E.M. of 6 - 24 values for control tests and of 3 - 12 values from the same animals for tests with THIP; *, ** and *** indicate, respectively, $p < 0.05$, $p < 0.01$ and $p < 0.001$ for comparisons between these values and corresponding control values; Student's t-test (two-tailed). THIP was administered intravenously immediately before presentation of food, or orally 30 minutes before presentation of food to the animals. Reproduced with permission from refs. 4 and 5.

TABLE 2. ED_{50} values for THIP and for other anorexic substances in the rat

Substance	ED_{50} (mg/kg)	
	i.v.	p.o.
THIP	1.5	3.0
d-Amphetamine-SO$_4$	0.1	0.3
Fenfluramine-HCl	0.6	0.7
Cocaine-HCl	1.0	9.0

These values were determined by log-probit analyses from the data obtained during the first hour after presentation of food to the animals. Reproduced with permission from refs. 4 - 6.

responses were noted for each batch, and ED_{50} values were determined by using the number of positive responses obtained per batch of mice (30).

RESULTS

Experiments on Food Intake

Intravenous or oral administration of THIP produced a dose-dependent decrease in food intake in the rat; this effect was more evident during the first hour of testing than during the total four-hour test period (refs 4 and 5; Table 1). A comparison of the ED_{50} values for this anorexic action of THIP and those for the anorexic actions of other substances is provided in Table 2. No marked influence on food intake was evident on the day following drug administration.
Results shown in Table 3 indicate that the anorexic effect of orally-administered THIP can be blocked by bicuculline, but not by bicuculline-methobromide (a quaternary bicuculline-analogue which is not expected to penetrate readily the "blood-brain barrier"), strychnine, picrotoxin, or pentylenetetrazol. Also, orally-administered bicuculline (1 - 10 mg/kg), or GABA (50 - 300 mg/kg) did not decrease food intake during the first hour of testing (ref. 3; data not shown).

TABLE 3. Effects of bicuculline, bicuculline-methobromide, strychnine, pentylenetetrazol or picrotoxin on the anorexic effect of orally-administered THIP

THIP (mg/kg, p.o.)	Food intake during first hour (g)		
	Days 1 + 2 [a]	Day 3 [a]	Day 4 [a]
Control (no convulsant)			
1	12.6±1.8	8.8±2.1	7.8±0.7
5	9.7±1.2	4.7±1.4 ✗	7.4±1.7
10	10.5±1.5	2.4±1.4 ✗✗	11.5±1.4 ✗✗
Bicuculline (1 mg/kg) before THIP			
1	8.4±1.2	9.7±1.1	9.2±1.0
5	10.1±0.9	7.7±0.5	9.0±1.3
10	9.9±0.8	7.8±1.3	11.6±0.9
Bicuculline-methobromide (1.5 mg/kg) before THIP			
1	11.8±1.3	12.4±2.1	10.9±1.5
5	11.4±1.1	5.3±1.6 ✗✗	12.4±1.5 ✗✗
10	12.7±1.3	1.0±0.5 ✗✗✗	13.6±1.7 ✗✗✗
Strychnine-SO₄ (0.75 mg/kg) before THIP			
1	9.9±0.9	9.1±1.7	9.4±1.4
5	9.1±0.7	6.9±1.8	9.9±1.2
10	9.8±0.8	4.0±1.6 ✗✗	11.2±1.8 ✗
Pentylenetetrazol (25 mg/kg) before THIP			
1	11.7±1.8	4.7±1.4 ✗	12.6±2.1 ✗
5	11.8±1.8	4.2±0.7 ✗✗	11.5±2.0 ✗✗
10	10.0±1.3	4.2±1.1 ✗✗✗	12.1±1.0 ✗✗✗
Picrotoxin (1 mg/kg) before THIP			
1	11.7±0.5	9.9±1.3	12.8±0.8
5	12.5±0.7	7.4±1.1 ✗✗✗	14.4±0.7 ✗✗✗
10	11.4±0.6	4.0±1.1 ✗✗✗	12.2±1.0 ✗✗✗

[a] Days 1 + 2 refers to the two days prior to drug administration; Day 3 refers to the day of drug administration; Day 4 refers to the day after drug administration.
THIP was administered 30 min before presentation of food; other agents were given subcutaneously 10 min before THIP. Means ± S.E.M. of 12 values from 6 animals for Days 1 + 2 and of 6 values from the same 6 animals for Day 3 and Day 4; ✗, ✗✗ and ✗✗✗ indicate, respectively, $p < 0.05$, $p < 0.01$ and $p < 0.001$ for paired t-tests; Days 1 + 2 were paired to Day 3 and Day 3 was paired to Day 4. Reproduced with permission from ref. 3.

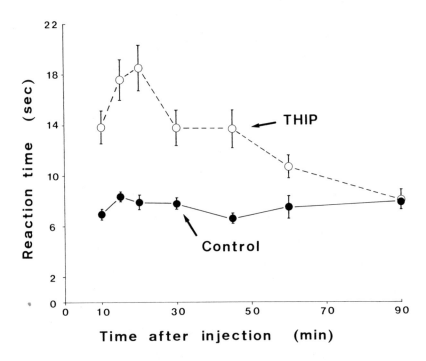

Time after injection (min)

FIG. 1. Time course of the analgesic action of intraperitoneally-injected THIP (3 mg/kg), determined using
the mouse hot-plate test at 56°C. Values for control
mice are also shown. Means ± S.E.M.; 10 - 30 Iffa
Credo OF_1 mice per dose; all values for THIP-treated
animals, except for the 90-minute value, differed significantly from corresponding control values
($p < 0.001$ or $p < 0.05$; Student's t-test; two-tailed);
unpublished data of A. Grognet, F. Hertz and F.V.
DeFeudis (1982).

___

Experiments on Analgesia

Using the hot-plate test at 56°C, THIP (3 mg/kg,
i.p.) produced a marked increase in reaction time in
OF_1 mice, this effect being maximal at about 15 - 20
minutes after injection (Fig. 1). In this test, ED_{50}
values differed for the antinociceptive effect of morphine in three mouse strains, whereas the ED_{50} values
for THIP did not differ significantly among mouse
strains (Table 4). Comparison of the results shown in
Figs. 2 and 3 indicates further that a high dose of
morphine overcame the difference in reaction time

TABLE 4. ED_{50} values (mg/kg) for the antinociceptive effects of intraperitoneally-administered THIP and morphine in three strains of mice, determined using the hot-plate test at $56°C$

Substance injected	Strain			
	Iffa Credo OF_1	Charles River CD_1	Iffa Credo NMRI	Evic-Ceba
THIP	4.0	3.8	3.7	5.1
	(3.3-4.8)	(3.5-4.2)	(3.2-4.2)	(4.5-5.8)
Morphine	6.8	16.9	27.6	30.2
	(5.9-7.9)	(14.1-20.2)	(22.6-33.8)	(25.2-36.2)

ED_{50} values were determined by analysis of variance of linear regression; 20 animals per dose; 3 - 5 doses of THIP or morphine and a control (vehicle-injected) group were used for each mouse strain. Mean values; 95% confidence limits in parentheses. From ref. 19 and unpublished results of A. Grognet, F. Hertz and F.V. DeFeudis (1982).

----

between hot-plate tests conducted at $56°C$ vs $60°C$, whereas a high dose of THIP increased the difference between the responses obtained at these two temperatures. On a mg/kg basis, THIP was more potent than morphine in all mouse strains tested (Table 4; Figs. 2 and 3). Increasing the dose of THIP led to sedation, whereas increasing the dose of morphine led to hyper-excitability.

Naloxone (0.1 - 5 mg/kg, s.c.), co-administered with either THIP (4 mg/kg, i.p.) or morphine (6 mg/kg, i.p.), abolished the antinociceptive effect of morphine, but did not affect the antinociception produced by THIP (19). Sub-convulsive doses of bicuculline (0.25 and 0.5 mg/kg, s.c.), given 10 minutes before, simultaneously with, or 10 minutes after THIP also did not affect the antinociceptive effect of THIP (19). The antinociceptive effect of THIP in the mouse hot-plate assay was also not affected by phentolamine (10 mg/kg, s.c.) or by methysergide (2 mg/kg, s.c.) when both agents

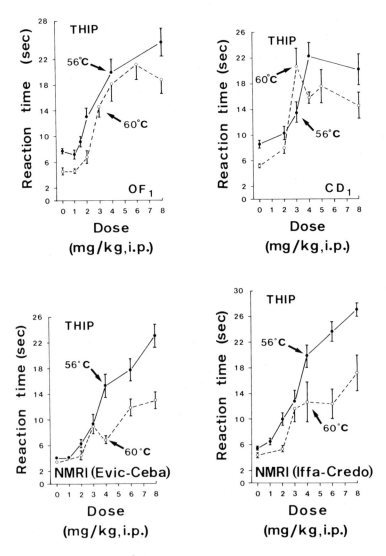

FIG. 2. Comparison of the antinociceptive actions of
intraperitoneally-injected THIP in three mouse strains
using the hot-plate assay at 56°C or 60°C. Means ±
S.E.M.; 20 mice for each dose at 56°C and 10 mice for
each dose at 60°C. Note that marked sedation was
evident with THIP at doses of 4 - 8 mg/kg in all
strains. ED_{50} values for the action of THIP at 56°C
are given in Table 4. Reproduced with permission from
ref. 20.

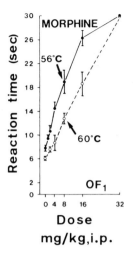

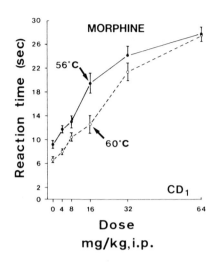

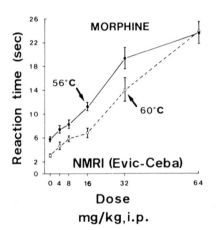

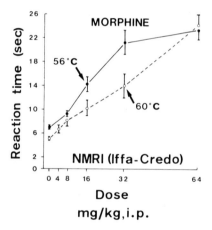

FIG. 3. Comparison of the antinociceptive actions of intraperitoneally-injected morphine in three mouse strains using the hot-plate assay at 56°C or 60°C. Means ± S.E.M.; 20 mice for each dose in all cases. Note that for all strains the reaction times for morphine were decreased at the higher temperature, but that reaction times were nearly identical at both temperatures for the 64 mg/kg dose of morphine. Reproduced with permission from ref. 20.

were given 15 or 30 minutes before THIP or simultaneously with THIP, but treatment with a high dose of atropine
(20 mg/kg, s.c.) partially reversed the antinociceptive
action of THIP (ref. 19 and unpublished data of A.
Grognet, F. Hertz and F.V. DeFeudis, 1982). In the
phenylbenzoquinone writhing test, evasion test and
traction test, THIP was also about equipotent or more
potent than morphine (unpublished results of A. Grognet,
F. Hertz and F.V. DeFeudis, 1982).

DISCUSSION

Experiments on Food Intake

The results presented herein have shown that intra-
venously- or orally-administered THIP decreases food
intake in the rat. On a mg/kg basis, intravenously-
administered THIP was about 15 times less potent than
$\underline{d}$-amphetamine-SO_4, about three times less potent than
fenfluramine-HCl, and nearly as potent as cocaine-HCl
as an inhibitor of food intake; orally-administered
THIP was about ten times less potent than $\underline{d}$-amphetamine-
SO_4, about four times less potent than fenfluramine-HCl,
and about three times more potent than cocaine-HCl in
reducing food intake (Table 2). The negligible anorexic
effect of GABA in the test system employed is likely
due to its difficulty in penetrating the "blood-brain
barrier" and to its rapid transport and catabolism by
extra-cerebral and cerebral tissues (15,29).
    Blockade of the anorexic effect of orally-adminis-
tered THIP was achieved with bicuculline (which readily penetrates the "blood-brain barrier"), but not with
bicuculline-methobromide (which is expected to affect
mainly extra-cerebral GABA-receptors), picrotoxin
(which probably interacts with GABA-regulated Cl^--
ionophores; ref. 41), strychnine (which has greater
affinity for glycine- or β-alanine-receptors than for
GABA-receptors; ref. 11) or pentylenetetrazol.
    It is of interest that intracerebroventricular and
intracerebral injections of GABA or GABA-agonists have
been shown to induce or stimulate feeding behavior
(1,18,24,33,34,37), whereas parenterally- and orally-
administered muscimol and THIP produce decreases in
food intake. The reason for this difference is not
clear, but it might be considered that intracerebroventricular or intracerebral administration of THIP or
muscimol inhibits satiety (e.g., VMH) mechanisms and
that peripheral administration of these GABA-agonists
causes mainly an inhibition of the lateral hypothalamic
"feeding center" (see also refs. 24,31). In any case,
the results presented here support the hypothesis that

the potent GABA-agonist THIP inhibits food intake by interacting with central GABA-receptors.

Experiments on Analgesia

The results presented herein have confirmed and extended those obtained in previous studies. Like morphine, THIP induced analgesia in the mouse, but in contrast to morphine, the analgesic effect of THIP was not reversed by naloxone (see also ref. 21). The antinociceptive effect of THIP was also not reversed by bicuculline, indicating a lack of involvement of bicuculline-sensitive GABA-receptors (see also ref. 21). As the analgesic effect of THIP was also not modified by treatment with phentolamine or methysergide, it does not appear to involve α-adrenergic or serotoninergic receptors. However, as a high dose of atropine did partially reverse the analgesic action of THIP, central cholinergic systems might be involved (see also ref. 25). Since the ED_{50} values for THIP, at least in OF_1 mice, were similar for hot-plate, evasion and traction tests, THIP's analgesic action might not be readily dissociated from its sedative (or myorelaxant) action.

The striking difference in the antinociceptive effects of THIP and morphine among three different strains of mice (Table 4) provides further evidence that the neural substrate for opiate action is under rigorous genetic control (see also 8,16,23,35,38), but that the neural substrate for THIP does not appear to possess this characteristic. Also, as THIP-induced analgesia was more sensitive than morphine-induced analgesia to changes in hot-plate temperature (cf. Figs. 2 and 3), this test might be useful for distinguishing between these two types of analgesia.

CONCLUDING COMMENTS

In addition to those anorexic agents that appear to act by influencing mechanisms associated with catecholamines or with serotonin (2,17,22,31,39), it now appears evident that THIP, a substance that influences GABA-ergic systems, also produces anorexic behavior. This action of THIP could be useful for treating human obesity. The analgesic effects produced by THIP differ markedly from those which involve opioid systems; thus, further research into the mechanisms underlying THIP-induced analgesia might lead to the development of an analgesic that does not produce tolerance/physical dependence in man (27). Taken together, the studies discussed above indicate that THIP might activate two different populations of GABA-receptors. If it is assumed that THIP is a selective GABA-agonist, then, its anorexic effect involves activation of bicuculline-sensitive GABA-receptors, whereas its analgesic effect involves activation of bicuculline-insensitive GABA-receptors.

REFERENCES

1. Arnt, J. and Scheel-Krüger, J. (1979): Life Sci., 25: 1351-1360.
2. Bedford, J.A., Borne, R.F. and Wilson, M.C. (1980): Pharmac. Biochem. Behav., 13: 69-75.
3. Blavet, N. and DeFeudis, F.V. (1982): Physiol. Behav., In press.
4. Blavet, N., DeFeudis, F.V. and Clostre, F. (1982): Behav. Neural Biol., 34: 109-112.
5. Blavet, N., DeFeudis, F.V. and Clostre, F. (1982): Psychopharmacology, 76: 75-78.
6. Blavet, N., DeFeudis, F.V. and Clostre, F. (1982): Gen. Pharmac., 13: 293-297.
7. Boissier, J.R., Simon, P., Lwoff, J.M. and Giudicelli, J.M. (1965): Thérapie, 20: 895-905.
8. Brase, D.A., Loh, H.H. and Way, E.L. (1977): J. Pharmac. Exp. Therapeut., 201: 368-374.
9. Cooper, B.R., Howard, J.L., White, H.L., Soroko, F., Ingold, K. and Maxwell, R.A. (1980): Life Sci., 26: 1997-2002.
10. Courvoisier, S. (1956): J. Clin. Exp. Psychopathol., 17, 25-37.
11. DeFeudis, F.V. (1977): Acta Physiol. Latinoamer., 27: 131-145.
12. DeFeudis, F.V. (1981): Neurochem. Int. 3: 273-279.
13. DeFeudis, F.V. (1982): Pharmac. Res. Commun., 14: 383-390.
14. Eddy, N.B., Touchberry, C.F. and Lieberman, J.E. (1950): J. Pharmac. Exp. Therapeut., 98: 121-137.
15. Elliott, K.A.C. and van Gelder, N.M. (1960): J. Physiol., 153: 423-432.
16. Eriksson, K. and Kiianama, K. (1971): Ann. Med. Exp. Fenn., 49: 73-78.
17. Garattini, S. (1980): Trends Pharmac. Sci., 1: 354-356.
18. Grandison, L. and Guidotti, A. (1977): Neuropharmacology, 16: 533-536.
19. Grognet, A., Hertz, F. and DeFeudis, F.V. (1982): Drug Alc. Dependence, 9: 269-272.
20. Grognet, A., Hertz, F. and DeFeudis, F.V. (1982): Pharmacol. Res. Commun., In press.

21. Hill, R.C., Maurer, R., Buescher, H-H. and Roemer, D. (1981): Eur. J. Pharmac., 69: 221-224.
22. Hoebel, B.G. (1977): In: Handbook of Psychopharmacology, edited by L.L. Iversen, S.D. Iversen and S.H. Snyder, pp. 55-129, Plenum Press, New York.
23. Jacob, J. and Barthelemy, C. (1967): Thérapie, 22: 1435-1448.
24. Kelly, J., Alheid, G.F., Newberg, A. and Grossman, S.P. (1977): Pharmac. Biochem. Behav., 7: 537-541.
25. Kendall, D.A., Browner, M. and Enna, S.J. (1982): J. Pharmac. Exp. Therapeut., 220: 482-487.
26. Kimura, H. and Kuriyama, K. (1975): J. Neurochem., 24: 903-907.
27. Krogsgaard-Larsen, P. (1981): J. Medic. Chem., 24: 1377-1383.
28. Krogsgaard-Larsen, P., Johnston, G.A.R., Lodge, D. and Curtis, D.R. (1977): Nature, 268: 53-55.
29. Krogsgaard-Larsen, P., Schultz, B., Mikkelsen, H., Aaes-Jørgensen, T. and Bøgesø, K.P. (1981): In: Amino Acid Neurotransmitters, edited by F.V. DeFeudis and P. Mandel, pp. 69-76, Raven Press, New York.
30. Litchfield, J.T. and Wilcoxon, F.J. (1949): J. Pharmac. Exp. Therapeut., 96: 99-113.
31. Lytle, L.D. (1977): In: Nutrition and the Brain, edited by R.J. Wurtman and J.J. Wurtman, pp. 1-145, Raven Press, New York.
32. Morley, J.E. (1980): Life Sci., 27: 355-368.
33. Morley, J.E., Levine, A.S. and Kneip, J. (1981): Life Sci., 29: 1213-1218.
34. Olgiati, V.R., Netti, C., Guidobono, F. and Pecile, A. (1980): Psychopharmacology, 68: 163-167.
35. Oliverio, A. and Castellano, C. (1974): Psychopharmacologia, 39: 13-22.
36. Panksepp, J., Bishop, P. and Rossi, J., III (1979): Psychoneuroendocrinology, 4: 89-106.
37. Przewlocka, B., Stala, L. and Scheel-Krüger, J. (1979): Life Sci. 25: 937-946.
38. Racagni, G., Bruno, F., Iuliano, E. and Paoletti, R. (1979): J. Pharmac. Exp. Therapeut., 209: 111-116.
39. Schmitt, H. (1979): Thérapie, 34: 155-179.
40. Siegmund, E., Cadmus, R. and Go, L.U. (1957): Proc. Soc. Exp. Biol. Med., 95: 729-731.
41. Ticku, M.K. (1977): Fed. Proc., 36: 751.

CNS Receptors—From Molecular
Pharmacology to Behavior, edited by
P. Mandel and F. V. DeFeudis.
Raven Press, New York © 1983.

Anterior Pituitary GABA Receptors in Relation to Prolactin Secretion

*,†G. Racagni, *,†J. A. Apud, *,†E. Iuliano, *D. Cocchi,
*V. Locatelli, and *E. E. Müller

*Institutes of *Pharmacology and †Pharmacognosy, University of Milan, Milan, Italy*

Anterior pituitary (AP) hormone secretion has been largely
known to be under the control of stimulating and inhibiting
neurohormones or neurotransmitters synthesized and released
from neural structures present in the hypothalamus (23). Among
the different hypothalamic structures, the medio-basal hypothalamus (MBH) and specifically the median eminence (ME) represents a privilaged site for the various neuroendocrine interactions between the different neurohormones and neurotransmitters. As for the release of many other AP hormones, prolactin
(PRL) secretion is a process involving the interactions of
several neuronal and hormonal components. Previous studies have
demonstrated that PRL is mainly under a tonic inhibitory dopaminergic control (20) exerted by neurons projecting from the
MBH to the ME and forming the tuberoinfundibular dopaminergic
(TIDA) system (13).

Dopamine (DA) released from TIDA system reaches the AP
through the hypothalamus-pituitary portal vessels (4) and inhibits PRL secretion by interacting with specific DA receptors
present on the lactotropes (8,10).

Recently, anatomical (32,33,35,36) and biochemical (5,27)
evidence has been accumulated supporting the existence also of
a tuberoinfundibular GABAergic (TI-GABA) system at the level of
the MBH. The evidence confirming the presence of the TI-GABA
are the following:

1) Autoradiographic studies have demonstrated the existence of
   neuronal elements which take up labelled GABA at the level of
   the external layer of the ME (33).

2) Immunohistochemical studies indicate the presence of GABA-

ergic nerve terminals in the external layer of the ME and
around the capillary loops (26,35).

3) Neurochemical studies have shown that GABA present in the AP
is not synthesized "in situ" but likely derives from central
nervous system structures, mainly from the MBH (5,27).
    In fact, activation of the hypothalamic GABAergic system
with ethanolamine-O-sulphate (EOS), a specific inhibitor of
GABA-T, the enzyme responsible for GABA catabolism, increases either AP (2,27) or portal plasma (authors unpublished results)
GABA concentrations. Moreover, the placement of the AP in a
site far remote from the sella turcica, e.g. under the kidney
capsule, results in a clear-cut decrease of AP-GABA content
(27).

    Recent pharmacological evidence has indicated that GABA
neurons exert a dual control on PRL secretion, one stimulatory
mediated by the TIDA system (5,18), the other inhibitory occurring at the level of the AP (5,27).
    The existence of a central stimulatory mechanism of GABA on
PRL release is supported by the fact that either GABA (25, 34)
or Muscimol (M)(18), a specific GABA agonist (9), administered
by intracerebroventricular (IVT) route increases plasma PRL
titers. This effect is completely suppressed by previous injection of the GABA antagonist bicuculline (18).
    An interaction between the dopaminergic and the GABAergic
system may be envisioned in this stimulatory component of GABA.
In fact, catecholaminergic system impairment,either by blockade
of DA synthesis with α-methyl-paratyrosine (α-Mpt) or by DA
depletion by reserpine, blocked the increase of plasma PRL
concentrations elicited by M (5). Moreover, IVT-injected M
decreases AP-DA concentrations (5), a reliable index of TIDA
function (1).
    Proof for the existence of an inhibitory component of GABA
on PRL release relies on the finding that either GABA (30) or M
(18) injected by systemic route decreases plasma PRL concentrations. Moreover, IVT administration of EOS, which increases
AP-GABA content (2,27) or i.v. injection of guvacine, a potent
inhibitor of GABA uptake (15), decreases plasma PRL titers
(17). This inhibitory effect of GABA and GABA-mimetic compounds doesn't seem to be mediated through the dopaminergic
system. In fact, both i.p.-injected M or IVT-administered EOS
are able to counteract the rise of plasma PRL elicited either
by blockade of the pre-synaptic DA function with α-Mpt (18) or

the post-synaptic receptors with domperidone (27), a specific DA- receptor blocking agent which does not cross the blood brain barrier (BBB), respectively. Instead, this inhibitory action of GABA would take place directly at AP level. In this context, i.v. administration of bicuculline-methiodide, a specific GABA antagonist which does not cross the BBB, completely blocks the inhibitory effect of peripherally-injected M on PRL release (5).

The purpose of this presentation is to give further evidence showing that the PRL-lowering effect of GABA is a receptor mediated event occurring directly at the level of the AP. Moreover, data will be presented demonstrating the plasticity of AP-GABA receptors which can be modulated in different physiological and pharmacological situations.

Evidence for the existence and the functional role of AP-GABA receptors in the rat

The evidence presented above strongly suggests the possibility that GABA agonists may directly inhibit PRL release from the AP. Table 1 shows that M (2.5×10^{-5} M) is effective in inhibiting PRL release from rat isolated pituitary halves, and this effect is selectively antagonized by co-incubation with picrotoxin, a GABA antagonist at ionophore level (31). On the contrary GABA (2.5×10^{-5} M) failed to modify PRL release from hemipituitaries "in vitro". Moreover, lower doses of GABA (10^{-6} M), close to physiological molar concentrations, are capable of inhibiting PRL release "in vitro", when in the incubation medium a GABA-T blocker (EOS) is added (Table 1). Based on this finding, previous reports on the failure of GABA itself to inhibit PRL release could be ascribed to a rapid degradation of the amino acid due to the high GABA-T activity present in the AP (27).

Logic corollary to the above results was the identification of GABA (14) and M binding sites in the AP. In crude P_2 membrane fractions prepared from rat AP, high and low affinity Na^+-independent M-binding sites have been detected (Table 2). Binding of ^{3}H-M to pituitary membranes was saturable and the Scatchard analysis indicated apparent dissociation constants of 2.93 and 37.71 nM and capacities of 27 and 132 fmol/ mg protein for the high and low affinity populations, respectively. The characteristics of ^{3}H-M binding to the AP tissue are similar to those of CNS tissue (11) since both possess high and low affinity recognition sites and the two populations are bicuculline-sensitive.

TABLE 1

EFFECT OF GABA, MUSCIMOL, PICROTOXIN OR ETHANOLAMINE-O-SULPHA-
TE (EOS) ON THE IN VITRO PROLACTIN RELEASE FROM INCUBATED PITUI-
TARIES OF MALE RATS

TREATMENT	PRL RELEASED (μg/ml/mg prot)
SALINE	0.46 ± 0.03
MUSCIMOL (2.5×10^{-5}M)	0.29 ± 0.02 *
PICROTOXIN (2.5×10^{-5}M)	0.35 ± 0.03
MUSCIMOL + PICROTOXIN	0.39 ± 0.07
SALINE	0.45 ± 0.03
GABA (10^{-6}M)	0.53 ± 0.08
EOS (10^{-6}M)	0.46 ± 0.04
GABA + EOS	0.37 ± 0.01 *

- Values represent the mean $\pm$ S.E.M. of at least 6 samples (2 experiments)

- Four hemisected pituitaries from male rats were incubated for 30 minutes in 2 ml of TC 199 and for 4 h in 2 ml of fresh TC 199 with or without the indicated concentration of drugs. Incubat-ions were done at 37°C under 95% CO_2 in a Dubnoff metabolic shaker.

* $p < 0.05$ vs. saline

TABLE 2

^{3}H-MUSCIMOL AND ^{3}H-GABA BINDING TO RAT ANTERIOR PITUITARY

	^{3}H-MUSCIMOL	^{3}H-GABA (a)
KD_1 (nM)	2.93	33.00
KD_2 (nM)	37.71	-
$Bmax_1$ (fmol/mg prot)	27.00	1,200
$Bmax_2$ (fmol/mg prot)	132.00	-
Bicuculline inhibition (IC 50)	3×10^{-4} M	5×10^{-5} M

- Binding assay was performed according to (14) with slight modifications

- (a) Taken from L. Grandison and A. Guidotti (14).

AP-GABA receptor modulation during physiological and pharmacological situations

a) AP-GABA receptors during long-term suckling

Lactation in the rat is one of the best-suited models to study biochemical and metabolic changes in neurons involved in the physiological neuroendocrine control of PRL. In this context, several lines of evidence support the proposition that DA and serotonin are the main transmitters involved in the PRL control during suckling (3,7,12,22,29). However, recently, evidence has been obtained suggesting that GABA could be involved in the regulation of PRL secretion during suckling. In fact, separation of the pups from their mothers for four hours and then reinstitution of suckling resulted in an increase of the MBH-AP GABAergic activity and of plasma PRL concentrations. Table 3 shows that AP-GABA concentrations, which represent a reliable index of the neurotransmitter released from the ME (28), is increased two hours after the onset of suckling, when PRL has already peaked in plasma and is decreasing. On the other hand, GAD activity in the MBH followed a different pattern. Significant activation of the enzyme, which represents an index of the rate of synthesis of GABA in the MBH, is observed already 30 minutes after the onset of suckling. The highest GABAergic activity in the MBH-AP area is detected during continuous suckling, when PRL concentrations in plasma have reached a steady-state with levels always above those present after 4 h separation.

TABLE 3

EFFECT OF SUCKLING ON GABAERGIC ACTIVITY IN THE MBH-AP AREA AND ON PLASMA PROLACTIN TITERS IN RATS PREVIOUSLY SEPARATED (4 hours) FROM THEIR PUPS

TIME	AP-GABA (nmol/mg prot)	MBH-GAD activity (nmol CO_2/mg prot/h)	PLASMA PRL (ng/ml)
0 min	0.50 ± 0.037	132.42 ± 9.80	15.83 ± 5.60
30 min	0.49 ± 0.060	275.90 ± 46.50*	123.50 ± 14.57**
120 min	0.75 ± 0.097*	–	98.75 ± 19.90**
(?)	1.10 ± 0.070**	320.10 ± 42.70**	40.80 ± 11.60

- Values represent the mean ± S.E.M. of at least 5 determinations

- GABA was determined by mass fragmentographic technique (27)

- GAD was determined by radioenzymatic assay (27)

- Plasma PRL was determined by radioimmunoassay

- Time (?) represent dams never separated from their pups

- * $p < 0.05$; ** $p < 0.01$ vs. time 0 (Dunnett's t test).

Analysis of the AP-GABA receptor population in lactating rats shows the presence only of the high affinity binding site component with complete disappearance of the low affinity recognition sites (Table 4).

TABLE 4

^{3}H-MUSCIMOL BINDING SITES IN ANTERIOR PITUITARY OF NORMAL
DIESTROUS AND LACTATING RATS

	DIESTROUS RATS	LACTATING RATS
KD_1 (nM)	3.26	3.20
KD_2 (nM)	49.74	not detectable
$Bmax_1$ (fmol/mg prot)	47.00	49.00
$Bmax_2$ (fmol/mg prot)	184.00	not detectable

- Values represent the mean of three individual determinations

- Binding assay was performed according to (14) with slight modifications.

As Table 4 shows, the characteristics of the high affinity component in lactating rats is similar to those observed for the same population in the normal diestrous rats.

To determine whether the high affinity binding sites for M are related to the receptors involved in the regulation of PRL secretion, M was injected by peripheral route. Intraperitoneal administration of M in lactating rats previously separated for two hours from their pups induced a significant decrease of plasma PRL concentrations. Similar results were obtained when M was injected into normal female rats in diestrous (Table 5).

b) AP-GABA receptors during acute and chronic estrogen treatment

Estrogens have been shown to potently affect PRL secretion in rodents; they increase the number of PRL-producing cells in vitro (19), cause an increase in PRL secretion (24), and administered chronically may even induce tumoral changes in the PRL secreting cells (21).

TABLE 5

EFFECT OF MUSCIMOL ADMINISTERED BY INTRAPERITONEAL ROUTE ON
PLASMA PRL CONCENTRATIONS IN NORMAL DIESTROUS AND LACTATING
RATS

GROUP	PLASMA PRL (ng/ml)	
	time 0'	time 90'
Normal diestrous rats (M, 2mg/kg)	26.30+7.50	0.80+0.30*
Lactating rats (M, 2mg/kg)	8.80+3.20	0.50+0.10*

- Values represent the mean ± S.E.M. of at least 5 determinations

- Plasma PRL was determined by radioimmunoassay

- *$p < 0.01$ vs. time 0 (Student's t test).

Recent data (6) have demonstrated that in rat chronic treatment with estrogens induces functional and morphological alterations in the TIDA system. However, no modifications seem to occur at post-synaptic level, implied from the findings that direct dopaminergic agonists (CB_{154}) were still able to decrease plasma PRL concentrations in chronically estrogen-treated rats (6).

In our study, either acute or chronic administration of estradiol valerate (EV) induced consistent changes at AP-GABA receptor level. Current studies are now under way to evaluate the effect of estrogens on the TI-GABA pathway.

As Table 6 indicates, Scatchard analysis of the ^{3}H-M binding sites in AP of rats treated with one dose of 2 mg EV shows the presence of a single high affinity recognition site with complete disappearence of the low affinity component. On the other hand, in chronically treated rats, i.e. rats treated five times at the dose of 2 mg EV at 3-week intervals, analysis of the Scatchard plot of AP-(^{3}H-M) binding sites   shows the   presence only of the low affinity component. In this model, the high affinity binding sites have disappeared.

TABLE 6

^{3}H-MUSCIMOL BINDING SITES TO RAT AP IN ANIMALS ACUTELY OR CHRO-
NICALLY TREATED WITH ESTRADIOL VALERATE (EV)

	DIESTROUS RATS	ACUTE EV	CHRONIC EV
KD_1 (nM)	3.0	2.85	n.d.
KD_2 (nM)	29.7	n.d.	27.6
$Bmax_1$ (fmol/mg prot)	36.0	30.0	n.d.
$Bmax_2$ (fmol/mg prot)	119.0	n.d.	125.0

- Binding assay was performed according to (24) with slight modifications

- In the acute experiment, EV was administered at the dose of 2 mg by s.c. route and binding was performed after 60 days

- In the chronic experiment, EV was injected by s.c. route five times at the dose of 2 mg at 3-week intervals and binding was performed 60 days after the last administration

- Values represent the mean of three separate determinations

- n.d. = not detectable.

    To determine the possible functional role of the high and low affinity binding sites of ^{3}H-M in the PRL lowering effect of GABA-mimetic drugs, M was injected either in acute or chronically estrogen-treated rats. As Table 7 shows, M is able to significantly decrease plasma PRL titers either in normal diestrous or in acutely-treated animals. On the contrary, in chronically-treated rats, M is ineffective in lowering plasma PRL concentrations.

TABLE 7

EFFECT OF MUSCIMOL ON PROLACTIN (PRL) SECRETION IN ESTROGEN
TREATED RATS AFTER ACUTE OR CHRONIC ADMINISTRATION OF ESTRADIOL
VALERATE (EV)

TREATMENT	PROLACTIN (ng/ml)		
	30'	60'	90'
SALINE	16.1 ± 5.5	19.7 ± 8.6	12.6 ± 5.8
MUSCIMOL (2 mg/kg, i.p.)	37.8 ± 7.2	7.4 ± 1.1^a	3.7 ± 0.6^a
ACUTE EV + SALINE	56.4 ± 7.2^a	77.1 ± 33.9^a	47.9 ± 2.2^a
ACUTE EV + MUSCIMOL	41.4 ± 9.9^a	18.1 ± 4.5^{ab}	19.4 ± 4.9^{ab}
CHRONIC EV + SALINE	888.0 ± 347.0^a	999.0 ± 354.0^a	800.0 ± 332.0^a
CHRONIC EV + MUSCIMOL	977.0 ± 275^a	839.0 ± 245.0^a	716.0 ± 194.0^a

- For details on the experimental schedule see Table 6

- Plasma PRL was determined by radioimmunoassay

- [a] $p < 0.01$ vs. saline-treated rats

- [b] $p < 0.01$ vs. acute EV-treated animals.

CONCLUDING REMARKS

The data presented herein   deserve the following considera-
tions:

1. In vivo and in vitro evidence support the view that the peripheral inhibitory effect of GABA is exerted at AP level.
This effect is mediated through specific GABAergic receptors
present in the gland.

2. The TI-GABA system, which is responsible for the synthe-

sis and release of the GABA present in the AP, would play a functional role on PRL secretion. This system would be involved in compensatory mechanisms preventing an exaggerated PRL output during continuous suckling stimulation.

3. The experiments in which binding assays were performed demonstrated that AP-GABA receptors present a certain degree of plasticity since they can be modulated by different physiological and/or pharmacological situations. However, the mechanisms underlying the changes in the various experimental models remain to be clarified.

4. The high affinity binding sites for M seem to be responsible for the PRL-lowering effect of the GABA agonists and GABA itself (this study and Ref. 16). In fact, when the high affinity component is present (suckling or acute estrogen treatment) M is effective in lowering plasma PRL concentrations. On the contrary, when the high affinity component has disappeared (chronic estrogen treatment), M fails to modify plasma PRL titers.

In all, these results demonstrate that GABA would be involved in the physiological regulation of PRL. Moreover, they confirm that the PRL-inhibiting effect of GABA is a receptor-mediated event.

REFERENCES

1. Apud, J.A., Cocchi, D., Iuliano, E., Casanueva, F. and Müller, E.E. (1980) Brain Res. 186:226-231.

2. Apud, J.A., Racagni, G., Iuliano, E., Cocchi, D., Casanueva, E. and Müller, E.E. (1981): Endocrinology 108:1505-1510.

3. Ben-Jonathan, N., Neill, M.A., Arbogast, L., Peters, L.L. and Hoefer, M.T. (1980): Endocrinology 106:690-696.

4. Ben-Jonathan, N., Oliver, C., Weiner, J., Mical R.S. and Porter, J.C. (1977): Endocrinology 100:452-458.

5. Casanueva, F., Apud, J.A., Locatelli, V., Martinez-Campos, A., Civati, C., Racagni, G., Cocchi, D. and Müller, E.E. (1981): Endocrinology 109:567-575.

6. Casanueva, F., Cocchi, D., Locatelli, V., Flauto, C., Zambotti, F., Bestetti, G., Rossi, G.L. and Müller, E.E. (1982): Endocrinology 110:590-599.

7. Chiocchio, S.R., Cannata, M.A., Cordero Funes, J.R. and Tramezzani, J.H. (1979): Endocrinology 105:544-547.

8. Cronin, J.M., Roberts, J.M. and Weiner, R. (1978): Endocrinology 103:302-309.

9. Curtis, D.R., Duggan, A.W., Felix, D. and Johnston, G.A.R. (1971): Brain Res 32:69-96.

10. De Camili, P., Macconi, D. and Spada, A. (1978): Nature (London) 278:252-254.

11. De Feudis, F.V. (1980): Neuroscience 5:675-688.

12. De Greef, W.J., Plotsky, P.M. and Neill, J.D. (1981): Neuroendocrinology 32:229-231.

13. Fuxe, K., Hökfelt, T., Jonsson, G. and Lofstrom, A. (1974): In: Neurosecretion. The Final Neuroendocrine Pathway, edited by F. Knowles and L. Vollrater, pp. 269-275 Springer-Verlag, Berlin.

14. Grandison, L. and Guidotti, A. (1979): Endocrinology 105: 754-759.

15. Johnston, G.A.R., Krogsgaard-Larsen, A. and Stephanson, A. (1975): Nature (London) 258:627-628.

16. Libertum, C., Arakelian, M.C., Larrea, G.A. and Foglia, V.G. (1979): Proc. Soc. Exptl. Biol. Med. 161:28-31.

17. Locatelli, V., Cocchi, D., Racagni, G., Cattabeni, F., Maggi, A., Krogsgaard-Larsen, P., Müller, E.E. (1978): Brain Res. 145:173-179.

18. Locatelli, V., Cocchi, D., Frigerio, C., Betti, R., Krogsgaard-Larsen, P., Racagni, G. and Müller, E.E. (1979): Endocrinology 105:778-785.

19. Lloyd, H.M., Meares, J.D., Jacobi, J. (1973): J. Endocrinol. 58:227-232.

20. MacLeod, R.M. and Lehemeyer, J.E. (1974): Endocrinology 103:200-203.

21. McEnen, C.S., Selye, H. and Collip, J.B. (1936): Lancet 230:775-776.

22. Mena, F., Enjalbert, A., Carbonell, L., Priam, M. and Kordon, C. (1976): Endocrinology 99:445-451.

23. Muller, E.E., Nisticò, G. and Scapagnini, U., editors

(1978): Neurotransmitters and Anterior Pituitary Function, Academic Press.

24. Neill, D. (1980): In: Frontiers in Neuroendocrinology, edited by L. Martini and W.F. Ganong, vol. 6:129-147.

25. Pass, K.A. and Ondo, J.C. (1977): Endocrinology 100:1437-1442.

26. Perez de la Mora, M., Possani, L.D., Tapia, R., Teran, L., Palacios, R., Fuxe, K., Hokfelt, T. and Lijungdahl (1981): Neuroscience 6:875-895.

27. Racagni, G., Apud, J.A., Locatelli, V., Cocchi, D., Nisticò, G., Di Giorgio, R.M., Muller, E.E. (1979): Nature 281: 575-578.

28. Racagni, G., Apud, J.A., Iuliano, E., Civati, C., Cocchi, D., Casanueva, F. and Muller, E.E. (1980): In: Central and Peripheral Regulation of Prolactin Function, edited by R.M. MacLeod and U. Scapagnini, pp. 321-325, Raven Press, New York.

29. Selmanoff, M. and Wise, P. (1981): Brain Res. 212:101-115.

30. Schally, A.V., Redding, T.W., Arimura, A., Dupont, A. and Linthicum (1977): Endocrinology 100:681-691.

31. Takeuchi, A. (1976): In: GABA in Nervous System Function, edited by E. Roberts, T.N. Chase and D.B. Tower, pp. 225-240, Raven Press, New York.

32. Tappaz, M.L. and Brownstein, M.J. (1977): Brain Res. 132: 95-106.

33. Tappaz, M.L., Aguera, M., Belin, N.F. and Pujol, J.F. (1980): Brain Res. 186:379-391.

34. Vijayan, E. and McCann, S.M. (1978): Brain Res. 155:35-43.

35. Vincent, R.S., Hokfelt, T. and Wu, J.Y. (1982): Neuroendocrinology 34:117-125.

36. Walaas, I. and Fonnum, F. (1978): Brain Res. 153:549-562.

CNS Receptors—From Molecular
Pharmacology to Behavior, edited by
P. Mandel and F. V. Defeudis.
Raven Press, New York © 1983.

Neurochemical and Neuropharmacological Indications for the Involvement of GABA and Glycine Receptors in Neuropsychiatric Disorders

*K. G. Lloyd, **G. DeMontis, †C. L. Broekkamp, *F. Thuret, and *P. Worms

*CNS Pharmacology Unit, L.E.R.S.-Synthélabo F-92220 Bagneux, France; **Second Department of Pharmacology, University of Cagliari, Cagliari, Italy; and †CNS Pharmacology Unit, Organon, Oss, The Netherlands

The role of inhibitory receptors in normal physiological function, in pathological dysfunction and in the mechanism of action of different pharmacological agents has received extensive attention in the past two decades. Thus, GABA receptors mediate inhibitory neurotransmission in such diverse regions as the spinal cord [31], dorsal Deiters'nucleus [31], substantia nigra [8], hippocampus [30], cerebral cortex [31] and cerebellar cortex [27]. In terms of neuropsychiatry, GABA receptors have been shown to undergo alterations in Parkinson's disease [22, 32], Huntington's disease [19, 28] and epilepsy [20]. The neuropharmacology of GABA receptors is related not only to the actions of agonists such as progabide [15, 36], muscimol [13, 35] or THIP [12, 34] but includes the actions of other drug classes such as the benzodiazepines and barbiturates which act within the GABA macromolecular receptor complex [5, 29].

Although GABA has been shown to be a very prevalent inhibitory neurotransmitter (one study estimated that 20-25 % of all cortical synapses are GABAergic [1], it is not the only inhibitory neurotransmitter in the central nervous system. Glycine, another inhibitory amino acid, has neurophysiologically well-demonstrated receptors in the spinal cord and brainstem [31]. There are some findings indicating that glycine receptors are involved in neurological disorders (see below), but the neuropharmacology of glycine receptors has received much less attention than GABA receptors.

The aim of the present study was to compare the distribution of GABA and glycine receptors in the human central nervous system, by means of radioligand binding techniques. The alterations in these inhibitory receptors in different neurological disorders is also considered and from these observations as well as from findings in animal models, the possible clinical applications of inhibitory neurotransmitter receptor agonists are discussed.

RELATIVE DISTRIBUTION OF GABA AND GLYCINE RECEPTORS IN THE HUMAN CNS

For this study an in-depth dissection (65-70 regions) of the human central nervous system (forebrain, brainstem and cervical spinal cord) was performed using rostral slices from two frozen human brains ("control" patients without known neurological or psychiatric disorders) as previously described (18). The distribution of GABA receptors (specific ^{3}H-GABA binding at 100 nM ^{3}H-GABA, no triton) and glycine receptors (specific ^{3}H-strychnine binding at 10 nM ^{3}H-strychnine) was determined by previously published techniques (6, 22) using the same whole tissue homogenate as the starting point for both assays. The results presented are the means of the two values which were usually in very good agreement (areas where there was poor agreement between the two brains are not included).

Figure 1 shows the binding of these two ligands (in fmol/mg protein) in 41 regions of the human central nervous system, the order being based on the number of ^{3}H-GABA binding sites found in the tissue. As can be seen in this figure, and in agreement with previous publications (10, 14), ^{3}H-GABA binding is greatest in the cerebellar, hippocampal and cortical regions. In these areas ^{3}H-strychnine binding was generally very low, although significantly above blank levels. However as one descends the neuraxis the number of ^{3}H-strychnine binding sites increases and the number of ^{3}H-GABA binding sites decreases. This is shown schematically in Figure 2, for a more limited number of areas. In Figure 2 the density of binding sites is expressed as the percentage of those in the pontine nuclei where ^{3}H-GABA and ^{3}H-strychnine binding sites occur in about equal numbers (50 and 45 fmol/mg protein, respectively).

The greatest density of ^{3}H-strychnine binding sites occurs in the spinal cord (dorsal horn), cranial nerve nuclei (especially N.X and N.XII) and throughout the brainstem. Of the forebrain regions studied, the anterior amygdala demonstrated the most ^{3}H-strychnine binding ; however this value (85 fmol/mg protein) was much lower than that of most of the lower brainstem regions and spinal cord (100-300 fmol/mg protein). This distribution is very similar to that observed for the neurophysiological potency of glycine application in different brain regions (cf. ref. 31).

From Figures 1 and 2 it can be seen that although there is not a mutually exclusive distribution of GABA (as represented by ^{3}H-GABA binding) and glycine (^{3}H-strychnine binding) receptors,

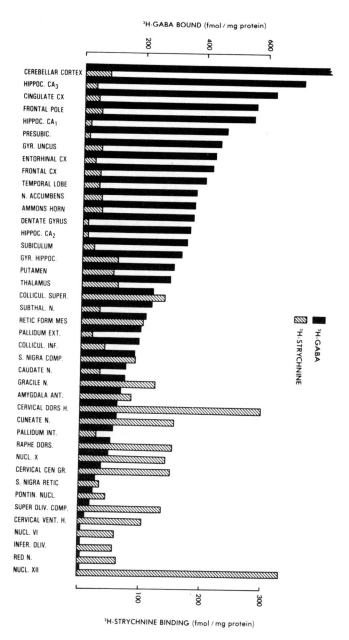

Figure 1. Distribution of ^{3}H-GABA and ^{3}H-Strychnine Binding in the Human CNS. Results are the means from two control brains using specific binding techniques. The aliquots from the same membrane preparation were not triton-treated and ^{3}H-GABA was present at 100nM and ^{3}H-strychnine at 10 nM using 1 mM GABA or gylcine respectively to control for non-specific binding.

Figure 2. Graphic Representation of ³H-GABA and ³H-Strychnine Binding in the Human CNS

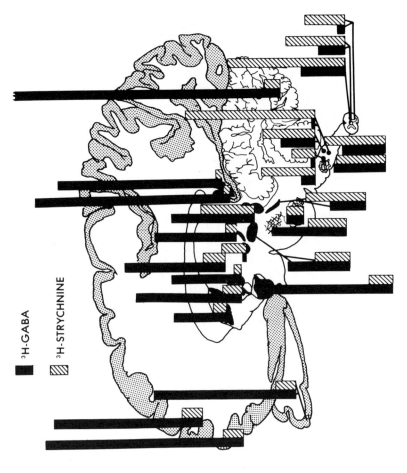

■ ³H-GABA

▨ ³H-STRYCHNINE

The data used are from Fig. 1.

there is a strong tendency for either one or the other to be present in much greater proportions. In fact there is a weak inverse correlation for the two parameters (r = - 0.31, p < 0.05, N = 41).

If the ratio of ^{3}H-GABA to ^{3}H-strychnine binding is calculated, the brain can be divided into 7 gross, but very distinct regions (Table 1). The ratios for all of these regions are statistically significantly different from one another (p < 0.01) except for the lower brainstem and spinal cord for which there is not a significant difference. Thus, in the regions of the cerebellar cortex, hippocampus (presubiculum, subiculum, CA_1, CA_2 and CA_3) and cerebral cortex (frontal pole, frontal cortex, temporal pole, cingulate cortex, entorhinal cortex) GABA receptors outnumber glycine receptors by a factor of at least 10 : 1. For the basal ganglia (caudate, putamen , thalamus, internal and external pallidum, subthalamic nucleus and accumbens) the ratio is about 5 : 1. When one descends into the brainstem (upper brainstem = mesenphalic reticular formation, superior and inferior colliculli, pars compacta and pars reticulata of the substantia nigra, pontine nuclei ; lower brainstem = superior and inferior olivary nuclei ; nuclei of VI, X and XII cranial nerves, gracile and cuneate nuclei) the ratio of GABA to glycine receptors is close to unity (2 : 1 - 1 : 2) and in the cervical spinal cord (ventral and dorsal horns, central grey) there is a predominance of glycine receptors (as reflected by ^{3}H-strychnine binding).

Table 1. Ratios of ^{3}H-GABA to ^{3}H-Strychnine Binding in Different Brain Areas

Area	Cerebellar Cortex	Hippocampus	Cerebral Cortex	Basal Ganglia
Ratio	50.4	28.8	10.2	6.0
$\dfrac{^3\text{H-GABA}}{^3\text{H-Strychnine}}$		± 4.3 (5)	± 1.1 (5)	± 0.8 (7)

Area	Brainstem Upper	Lower	Spinal Cord
Ratio	2.2	0.58	0.38
$\dfrac{^3\text{H-GABA}}{^3\text{H-Strychnine}}$	± 0.5 (6)	± 0.16 (7)	± 0.08 (3)

Data are expressed as mean ± S.E.M. The number of different distinct regions in each area is in parentheses.

It is not known if this distribution of receptors can be used as an accurate reflection of the sites of action for different classes of drugs. However, it is tempting to speculate that the action of compounds such as the specific receptor agonists would be related to this receptor distribution.

^{3}H-GABA AND ^{3}H-STRYCHNINE BINDING IN PARKINSON'S DISEASE AND HUNTINGTON'S CHOREA

One of those areas exhibiting a similar binding of both ^{3}H-GABA and ^{3}H-strychnine is the substantia nigra. As data are available on the binding of these ligands in the substantia nigra in different neurological conditions, it is of interest to compare the findings in these conditions and in their animal models.

As can be seen in Table 2, ^{3}H-GABA binding and ^{3}H-strychnine binding are both decreased in the substantia nigra in Parkinson's disease, and increased in Huntington's chorea (although statistically significant only for ^{3}H-GABA). In both cases the changes in ^{3}H-GABA binding were twice as large as were those for ^{3}H-strychnine binding. The data from the Parkinsonian material may indicate that there are relatively twice as many GABA receptors as glycine receptors on dopamine neurons and/or dendrites.

These findings are reproduced in the 6-hydroxy-dopamine model of Parkinson's disease (lesion of the ascending dopaminergic tract at the level of the median forebrain bundle, in the rat). Such a lesion (which lowered striatal tyrosine hydroxylase activity by at least 90 % in the same rats) decreased high affinity ^{3}H-GABA binding by 50 % (7) and ^{3}H-strychnine binding by 30 % (6).

From this it would appear that at least part of the GABA and glycine receptors in the substantia nigra are on dopamine neurons and/or dendrites. Furthermore, from neuropharmacological and neurophysiological evidence, it is very likely that these and possibly other GABA and glycine receptors are involved in the expression of "dopaminergic" activity (cf. refs 6 and 11).

A functional reflection of these receptors in the substantia nigra (and other regions of the basal ganglia) may be the anti-dyskinetic effect of GABA agonists, as shown in different animal models (16, 17). In rats which have been treated subacutely (10-14 days) with a neuroleptic such as haloperidol the animals develop a tolerance to the cataleptic effect of the neuroleptic, and after cessation of neuroleptic administration, the animals show a marked supersensitivity to the stereotypic effects of apomorphine. Both of these effects are thought to be due to the development of dopamine receptor supersensitivity and are used as a model for the tardive dyskinetic movements induced by neuroleptics. Co-administration of a GABAmimetic (eg. progabide or muscimol) with the neuroleptic greatly diminishes both the tolerance to the catalepsy and the apomorphine supersensitivity. In the cat apomorphine induces clear dyskinetic movements distinguished from stereotypic behavior. The GABA agonist progabide is very effective in blocking these dyskinetic movements.

Table 2. Alterations in ^{3}H-GABA and ^{3}H-Strychnine Binding in the Substantia Nigra in Parkinson's Disease and Huntington's Chorea

	^{3}H-GABA Binding (25 nm) (fmol/mg prot) Whole nigra	^{3}H-Strychnine Binding (10nM) (fmol/mg Prot)	
		Pars compacta	Pars reticulata
Parkinson's[1,2] Disease			
Controls	30.8 ± 5.0 (11)	127 ± 10 (13)	60 ± 12 (13)
Park. Dis.	9.7 ± 2.9** (6)	85 ± 9** (7)	30 ± 6* (7)
% Control	31	67	50
Huntington's[2,3] Disease			
Controls	18 ± 2 (8)	127 ± 10 (13)	60 ± 12 (13)
Hunt. Dis.	33 ± 7* (7)	189 ± 41 (4)	95 ± 22 (4)
% Control	183	149	158

Results expressed as mean with S.E.M. Number of patients in parentheses. $*p < 0.05$; $**p < 0.01$ vs controls.
1. Data from ref. 22 ; 2. Data from ref. 6 ; 3. Data from Ref. 9.

Furthermore in a monkey model of Parkinson's disease (bilateral destruction of the nigrostriatal dopamine path) dopaminomimetics (eg. L-DOPA, piribedil), not only reduce the parkinsonism but also induce dyskinetic behaviour similar to that observed in man. Progabide is effective in blocking the dyskinesia without altering the antitremor effect of dopaminomimetic.

From these data it appears that the activity of the GABA agonists on dopamine-related behaviours correlates well with the distribution of GABA receptors in the basal ganglia and their alterations in Parkinson's disease and Huntington's chorea.

GABA RECEPTOR FUNCTION IN EPILEPSY AND
CONVULSIONS

There is evidence available that GABA receptor alterations
are not limited to diseases of the basal ganglia, and that GABA
agonists have a wider application in neurology than to only move-
ment disorders. A case in point is at least certain forms of
epilepsy.
In a study of the neurochemistry of well defined epileptic
foci (by stereo EEG for non-tumour cases, by morphology for tumour
cases) removed during neurosurgical operations for untreatable
temporal lobe foci (20) it was observed that ^{3}H-GABA binding
was significantly decreased in some, but not all, of the material.
This finding together with the alterations (decrease) observed in
glutamic acid decarboxylase activity indicates that 60-70 percent of the patients studied exhibited a decreased GABA synaptic
function (Table 3) in the epileptic tissue. From this it seems
that there is a subpopulation of epileptic patients (in this
study mainly of temporal lobe origin) which fit into the hypothesis of a deficiency of GABAergic transmission in epilepsy.

Table 3. Alterations in ^{3}H-GABA Binding and L-Glutamic Acid
Decarboxylase (GAD) Activity in Epileptic Tissue Removed During
Neurosurgery.

	^{3}H-GABA BINDING		GAD ACTIVITY		^{3}H-GABA AND/OR GAD	
	Cases ↓ / Total Cases	%	Cases ↓ / Total Cases	%	Cases ↓ / Total Cases	%
Non-Tumour (Focus Stereo EEG definition)	10/18	56	9/19	47	14/23	61
Tumour (Morphological Definition)	3/7	43	4/5	80	5/7	71

Data taken from Ref. 20.

This data is supported by two different studies in animal models. The first is that convulsions are uniformly produced by
blockade of GABA synaptic function either by direct receptor block
(bicuculline), by blockade of the GABA-receptor mediated ion channel (picrotoxinin) or by inhibition of GABA synthesis (eg. by
allylglycine) (cf. Ref. 34). Secondly, enhancement of GABA receptor activity by agonists such as progabide, muscimol or THIP has
an anti-convulsant activity in most animal models (34). This includes those models in which seizures are due to GABA synaptic
dysfunction and also those in which GABA systems are apparently
not directly involved (eg. strychnine, electroshock). This anti-

convulsant activity is not limited to rodents (above models) but can also be shown in other species, including the cat (34) and the baboon, papio papio (3). It should be noted that in the latter model not all GABA agonists are equally effective (24).

However, a broad spectrum of anticonvulsant activities is not sufficient for a compound to qualify as a potential antiepileptic drug. Amongst other criteria, the induction of neurotoxic and other unwanted effects must be considered in relation to the anticonvulsant activity. In this regard, GABA agonists vary greatly (21). Muscimol exerts most of its anticonvulsant activities at doses which are equal to, or exceed, those which induce myorelaxation, ataxia and hypomotility. For THIP, the spectrum is more favorable with only the anti-electroshock and anti-picrotoxinin activities occurring at doses which induce undesirable secondary effects. For progabide, and its metabolite SL 75.102, the anticonvulsant doses are well below those found to induce myorelaxation, ataxia and hypomotility.

This difference between GABA agonists may be related to their different affinities for the GABA receptor. Muscimol and THIP are high affinity GABA agonists (12, 13) and at the doses given will likely displace ^{3}H-GABA from all of its binding sites (at least from the bicuculline-sensitive GABA receptors). On the other hand progabide and SL 75.102 have lower affinities than ^{3}H-GABA for the receptor (15). If the secondary effects of GABA agonists are due to the over-activation of GABA receptors, then it appears that the medium-low affinity compounds are the more advantageous as potential antiepileptics.

The most severe test is the activity of the compounds at the clinical level. To date the only clinical antiepileptic activity for a GABA agonist compound to be reported in the literature is for progabide. The antiepileptic activity of this drug has now been well-demonstrated in several reports (23, 25, 33).

THE USE OF INHIBITORY NEUROTRANSMITTER AGONISTS IN OTHER NEUROPSYCHIATRIC DISORDERS

Given the wide distribution of inhibitory neurotransmitter receptors (as indicated by ^{3}H-GABA and ^{3}H-strychnine binding) in the mammalian CNS (Figures 1 and 2), it is to be expected that inhibitory neurotransmitter agonists will have a varied use not only in neurology, but also in psychiatry. Although there are indications that GABA agonists have a potential anxiolytic effect (2, 4), the most exciting advances for the use of GABA agonists in psychiatry may be in depressive states.

The first indication came from the clinic where it was noted that progabide exerted an apparent antidepressant action during trials in other neuropsychiatric disorders. Following this observation, specific double-blind trials (vs imipramine) were performed in depressed patients. The results were clear and unequivocal: in these trials, progabide was equal to or superior to imipramine as an antidepressant agent (26).

Investigations in animal models support this view (K.G. Lloyd
and C.L.E. Broekkamp, unpublished results). Thus, in the olfactory
bulbectomy model for testing antidepressant drugs, both progabide
and muscimol reverse the passive avoidance deficit with a shorter
onset of action than imipramine. The action of at least progabide
is likely dependent on GABA receptor function as its activity is
completely reversed by bicuculline. Progabide functions as an
antidepressant in other animal models as well. In the learned
helplessness model progabide decreases the escape latency as does
imipramine, amitriptyline and other antidepressant drugs. In the
paradoxical sleep model, progabide specifically reduces paradoxical sleep in the manner of other antidepressant drugs
(H. Depoortere, personal communication).

SUMMARY AND CONCLUSIONS

From binding studies using ^{3}H-GABA and ^{3}H-strychnine in dissected human brain material, inhibitory amino acid neurotransmitter receptors have a widespead distribution in the human CNS.
Generally GABA receptors are predominant in the forebrain and
upper brainstem whereas glycine receptors are more localized in
the lower brainstem and spinal cord. Some areas (eg. the substantia
nigra) have appreciable quantities of both receptors.
    Although glycine receptors are altered in some pathological
conditions (eg. in Parkinson's disease, in the substantia nigra)
the neuropharmacology of the glycine system is still poorly understood. On the other hand the GABA system has been intensively
studied. Dysfunction of GABA receptors occurs in various neurological states, as epilepsy, Parkinson's disease and Huntington's
chorea. Furthermore GABA agonists are active in animal models
for dyskinesia, epilepsy and depression, amongst others. Clinical
studies with progabide confirm these findings in animal models,
and suggest that low-medium affinity GABA agonists are more
appropriate clinical agents than are high or very high affinity
GABA agonists.
    From these and many other findings there appears to be a very
large potential for creating new pharmacological agents for
different neuropsychiatric disorders based on agonist activity
at inhibitory amino-acid receptors. From the example of progabide
these compounds can be made not only specific for the receptor
involved, but also to have a lower incidence of neurotoxic effects
than presently available drugs.

REFERENCES

1. Bloom, E.E. and Iversen, L.L. (1971) : Nature, 229 : 628-630.
2. Bovier, Ph., Broekkamp, C.L.E. and Lloyd, K.G. (1981) : In :
   Biological Psychiatry 1981, edited by C. Perris, G. Struwe
   and B. Jansson, pp. 425-428. Elsevier, Amsterdam.
3. Cepeda, C., Worms, P., Lloyd, K.G. and Naquet, R. (1982) :
   Epilepsia, in press.

4. Costa, E. (1980) : Arzneim. Forsch., 30 : 858-860.
5. Costa, E. and Guidotti, A. (1979) : Ann. Rev. Pharmac. Toxic. 19 : 531-545.
6. DeMontis, G., Beaumont, K., Javoy-Agid, F., Agid, Y. Constantinidis, J., Lowenthal, A. and Lloyd, K.G. (1982) : J. Neurochem., 38 : 718-724.
7. DeMontis, G., Olianis, M.C., Mulas, G., Lloyd, K.G. and Tagliamonte, A. (1981) : Neurosci. Lett., 23 : 257-261.
8. Dray, A. and Straugham, D.W. (1976) : J. Pharm. Pharmac., 28 : 400-405.
9. Enna, S.J., Bennet, J.P., Bylund, D.B., Snyder, S.H., Bird, E.D. and Iversen, L.L. (1976) : Brain Res., 116 : 531-537.
10. Enna, S.J., Bennet J.P., Bylund, D.B., Creese, I., Burt, D.R. Charness, M.E., Yamamura, H.I. and Snyder, S.H. (1977) : J. Neurochem., 28 : 233-236.
11. James, T.A. and Starr, M.S. (1979) : Eur. J. Pharmac., 57 : 115-125.
12. Krogsgaard-Larsen, P., Hejds, H., Curtis, D.R., Lodge, D. and Johnston, G.A.R. (1979) : J. Neurochem., 32 :1717-1721.
13. Krogsgaard-Larsen, P., Johnston, G.A.R., Curtis, D.R., Game, C. and McCullough, J. (1975) : J. Neurochem., 25 : 803-809.
14. Lloyd, K.G. and Dreksler, S. (1979) : Brain Res., 163-77-87.
15. Lloyd, K.G., Arbilla, S., Beaumont, K., Briley, M. DeMontis, G. Scatton, B., Langer, S.Z. and Bartholini, G. (1982) : J. Pharmac. Exp. Therap. 220 : 672-677.
16. Lloyd, K.G., Broekkamp, C.L.E. and Worms, P. (1982) : In : Behavioural Pharmacology and Toxicology, edited by V. Cuomo, G. Racagni and G. Zbinden, in press. Raven Press, New York.
17. Lloyd, K.G., Broekkamp, C.L.E., Cathala, F., Worms, P. Goldstein, M. and Asano, T. (1981) : In : Apomorphine and other Dopaminomimetics, vol. 2., edited by G.U. Corsini and G.L. Gessa, pp. 123-133. Raven Press, New York.
18. Lloyd, K.G., Davidson, L. and Hornykiewicz, O.(1975) : J. Pharmac. Exp. Therap., 195 : 453-464.
19. Lloyd, K.G., Dreksler, S. and Bird, E.D. (1977) : Life Sci., 21 : 747-754.
20. Lloyd, K.G., Munari, C., Bossi, L., Stoeffels, C., Talairach, J., and Morselli, P.L. (1981) : In : Neurotransmitters, Seizures and Epilepsy, edited by P.L. Morselli, K.G. Lloyd, W. Löscher, B. Meldrum and E.H. Reynolds, pp 325-339. Raven Press, New York.
21. Lloyd, K.G., Munari, C., Worms, P., Bossi, L. and Morselli, P.L. (1982) : In : Recent Advances in Epilepsy, Edited by R. DiPerri, H. Meinardi and G. Nistico, Alan Liss, New York.
22. Lloyd, K.G., Shemen, L. and Hornykiewicz, O. (1977) : Brain Res. 127 : 269-278.
23. Loiseau, P., Cenraud, B., Bossi, L. and Morselli, P.L. (1981) : In : Proceedings of the 12th Epilepsy International Symposium, edited by M. Dam, L. Gram and J.K. Penry, pp. 135-140, Raven Press, New York.

24. Meldrum, B. (1981) : In : GABA and Benzodiazepine Receptors, Edited by E. Costa, G. DiChiara and G.L. Gessa, pp. 207-218 Raven Press, New York

25. Morselli, P.L., Bossi, L., Henry, J.F., Zarifian, E. and Bartholini, G. (1982) : Brain Res. Bullet., 5, suppl. 2 : 411-414.

26. Morselli, P.L., Henry, J.F., Macher, J.P., Bottin, P., Huber, J.P. and Van Landeghem, V.H. (1981) : In : Biological Psychiatry 1981, edited by C. Perris, G. Struwe and B. Jansson, pp. 440-443. Elsevier, Amsterdam.

27. Obata, K.C. (1972) : Int. Rev. Neurobiol., 15 : 167-187.

28. Olsen, R.W, Van Ness, P.C. and Tourtelotte, W.W. (1979) : In: Advances in Neurology, vol. 23. Edited by I.N. Chase, N.S. Wexler and A. Barbeau, pp. 697-704. Raven Press, New York.

29. Olsen, R.W. and Leeb-Lundberg, F. (1982) : In : Neurotransmitters, Seizures and Epilepsy, edited by P.L. Morselli, K.G. Lloyd, W. Löscher, B. Meldrum and E.H. Reynolds, pp. 151-163 Raven Press, New York.

30. Ozawa, S. and Okada, Y. (1976) : In : GABA and Nervous System Function, edited by E. Roberts, T.N. Chase and D.B. Tower, pp. 449-454. Raven Press, New York.

31. Phillis, J.W. (1970) : The Pharmacology of Synapses, Pergamon Press, New York.

32. Rinne, U.K., Koskinen, V., Laaksonen, H., Lönneberg, P. and Sonninen, V. (1978) : Life Sci., 22 : 2225-2228.

33. Van der Linden, G.J., Meinardi, H., Meijer, J.W.A., Bossi, L. and Gomeni, C. (1981) : In : Proceedings of the 12th Epilepsy International Symposium, edited by M. Dam, L. Gram and J.K. Penry, pp. 141-144. Raven Press, New York.

34. Worms, P. and Lloyd, K.G. (1982) : In : Neurotransmitters, Seizures and Epilepsy, edited by P.L. Morselli, K.G. Lloyd, W. Löscher, B. Meldrum and E.H. Reynolds, pp. 37-48. Raven Press, New York

35. Worms, P., Depoortere, H. and Lloyd, K.G. (1979) : Life Sci. 25 : 607-614

36. Worms, P., Depoortere, H., Durand, A., Morselli, P.L., Lloyd, K.G. and Bartholini, G. (1982) : J. Pharmac. Exp. Therap. 220 : 660-671.

CNS Receptors—From Molecular
Pharmacology to Behavior, edited by
P. Mandel and F. V. DeFeudis.
Raven Press, New York © 1983.

Comparison of the Effects of GABA-Mimetic Agents on Two Types of Aggressive Behavior

P. Mandel, E. Kempf, S. Simler, S. Puglisi, L. Ciesielski, and G. Mack

Centre de Neurochimie du CNRS, Université Louis Pasteur, 67084 Strasbourg Cedex, France

The goal of our presentation is to answer the following two questions: 1) Is a deficiency in inhibitory GABA neurotransmission involved in aggressive behaviour and does compensation of this deficiency block this behaviour? 2) What might be the preferred approach for compensating the deficiency in GABA neurotransmission in a complex behaviour such as aggressive behaviour: action on receptor sites using agonists, action on high affinity GABA uptake, or action on mechanisms of GABA degradation?

In order to answer these questions, we analyzed two types of aggressive behaviour: 1) interspecific mouse-killing by rats, described by Karli (1); 2) aggressive behaviour following social isolation, described by several authors (see ref. 2 for review).

CHEMICAL ALTERATIONS IN TWO TYPES
OF AGGRESSIVE BEHAVIOUR

Mouse-Killing Behaviour

It appears clear from lesion experiments performed by Karli and his colleagues (3) and by other workers that the olfactory pathway, the amygdala and the raphé are involved in modulation of mouse-killing by rats. Removal of the olfactory bulb induces killing behaviour in 60% of Wistar rats. Lesions of the raphé or para-chlorophenylalanine administration, which decrease the available serotonin in the CNS, increase the percentage of mouse-killers after removal of the the olfactory bulb to 95%, whereas specific lesions of the amygdala suppress this behaviour (4). Moreover, as we have shown recently, removal of the olfactory bulb by itself induces killing behaviour in about 95% of the inbred

August strain of rats which generally do not exhibit
mouse-killing behaviour.
    Investigations on the neurochemistry of the areas
involved in killing behaviour have shown (5,6):
1) lower values of GABA in the olfactory bulbs: non-
killer rats, 4.54 ± 0.40; killers, 2.92 ± 0.43 μ-moles/
g wet weight; p < 0.001; 2) lower values for the turnover of serotonin in the pons-medulla area: controls,
489 ± 59; killers, 322 ± 69 nanogrammes/g wet weight
(p < 0.001) and a significant decrease in serotonin
turnover in the raphé of animals which became killers
after ablation of the olfactory bulbs; 3) higher values
for choline acetyltransferase activity in spontaneous
killers or in animals which had become killers after
ablation of the olfactory bulbs; 4) higher values for
the turnover of dopamine in the olfactory tubercles of
killers, as compared to non-killers; however, this
alteration does not seem to be specific to aggressive
behaviour, since an increase in dopamine turnover in
this area was observed after olfactory bulb removal
whether or not the animals became killers. 5) When
GABA-mediated inhibition is experimentally decreased
by infusion into the olfactory bulbs of picrotoxin
(which blocks chloride channels), or bicuculline (which
blocks GABA receptors), or allylglycine (which decreases GABA synthesis), non-killers become killers.
    In addition, an involvement of genetic determinants
in killing behaviour has been demonstrated (6).

Aggressive Behaviour Induced by Psycho-Social Isolation

    The induction of aggressive behaviour by social
isolation has been extensively described (2,7,8).
Such behaviour appears to us to be strain-dependent.
For instance, C57/BL strains do not become aggressive
even after eight weeks of isolation, while the DBA/2
strain exhibits aggressive behaviour after four weeks
of isolation which increases markedly after eight
weeks of isolation (9). Recently, we observed lower
values for GABA levels in the olfactory bulbs of
grouped DBA/2 mice as compared to C57/BL mice. A decrease in GABA content of the olfactory bulbs of isolated C57 and DBA mice was also demonstrated. However,
this decrease was significant in DBA/2 mice which
became aggressive but not in C57/BL mice (9).
A decrease in GABA levels of the striatum and posterior colliculus in DBA/2 mice was also observed after
differential housing (9). Finally, it has also been
shown that glutamate decarboxylase activity was decreased in the olfactory bulbs and in the forebrains
of isolated mice (10). Thus, as in spontaneous

"killer" rats, a meaningful correlation appears between
the isolation-induced decrease in GABA-mediated inhibition in the olfactory bulbs and aggressive behaviour.
An involvement of alterations in serotonin neurotransmission in isolation-induced aggressive behaviour
in mice has been described (2,7,8). We have studied
brain serotonin turnover in grouped and isolated DBA/2
and C57/BL mice. Lower values of serotonin turnover
were observed in the raphé area, in the hypothalamus,
and in the amygdala of grouped DBA/2 mice, which become aggressive, as compared with grouped C57/BL, which
do not become aggressive (11). After isolation, serotonin turnover decreased in the raphé area, as well as
in the hypothalamus, in both strains. Only in the
lateral hypothalamus was the serotonin turnover of
isolated DBA/2 lower than that of isolated C57/BL mice.
No significant differences existed in the level of
serotonin of the amygdala, hypothalamus and pons-
medulla of the two strains. However, the level of
serotonin in the olfactory bulb was significantly lower
in the DBA mice, whether grouped or isolated. Thus,
several types of alterations of serotonin level or
turnover may be correlated with isolation-induced
aggressive behaviour.

EFFECTS OF GABA-MIMETIC COMPOUNDS ON
TWO TYPES OF AGGRESSIVE BEHAVIOUR

Interspecific Mouse-Killing Behaviour in Rats

Effects of local injections into the olfactory bulb

Compensation of the deficit in GABA-mediated inhibition by injecting GABA into the olfactory bulb
produces an immediate short-lasting inhibition of
killing behaviour (6). Since GABA-α-oxoglutarate
transaminase (GABA-T) activity is very pronounced in
the olfactory bulbs (12), it is highly probable that
the locally-injected GABA is rapidly degraded, thus
explaining the short duration of its effect.
Injection of valproic acid into the olfactory bulbs
produces, after a short latency, an inhibition of
mouse-killing behaviour; killing behaviour decreases
in parallel to an increase in GABA. After two hours,
when the GABA level begins to decrease again, probably
due to a diffusion or a disappearance of valproic acid
from the olfactory bulb, killing behaviour becomes
evident again (6). Moreover, local injection of GABA
together with valproic acid (which protects GABA
against degradation) produces an immediate inhibitory
effect on killing behaviour which lasts for several

TABLE 1. Effects of GABA-mimetic compounds injected into the olfactory bulb on muricidal behaviour

Compound (equimol. 25 μg/kg valproic acid)	Dose (μg/rat)	Efficiency of inhibition of killing behaviour during 4 hrs (conventional units)	Latency time (LT) for inhibition of killing behaviour (hrs) in 40% of rats	Duration of inhibition of killing behaviour in more than 40% of rats (hrs)
Muscimol-HBr	29	13	0.5 < LT < 1	⟩ 1
Valproic acid	25	49	0.5 < LT < 0.75	2.5
Nipecotic acid amide	36	21	1.0 < LT < 1.5	2.5

hours (6). Injection into the olfactory bulbs of either
nipecotic acid amide (a GABA uptake inhibitor) or muscimol (a GABA agonist) also blocked muricidal behaviour
(Table 1). Taken together, these data favour an involvement of GABA-ergic neurotransmission of the olfactory
bulb in killing behaviour, and thus offer an opportunity
for comparing the efficiencies of different types of
GABA-mimetic drugs in a situation characterized by a
deficiency in GABA-ergic neurotransmission.

Effects of intraperitoneal injection of GABA-mimetic
drugs

Intraperitoneal injections of valproic acid, muscimol
or nipecotic acid amide, which cross the blood-brain
barrier at the doses indicated (in a volume of 2 ml
saline solution/kg), produced dose-dependent suppression
of killing behaviour (Figs. 1-3). A similar effect was
produced by the GABA-agonists guvacine, isoguvacine and
THIP (Table 2), provided by Dr. P. Krogsgaard-Larsen.

TABLE 2.   Effects of GABA-mimetic compounds on
            muricidal behaviour   .

Compound (i.p., equimol. 500 μg/kg muscimol)	Latency time for 50% inhibition of killing behav. (hrs) by 50% of rats tested	Duration of inhibition of killing behav. in more than 50% of rats (hrs)
Muscimol-HBr	2.5	≥ 5.5
THIP-hydrate	2.0	4.5
Isoguvacine-HCl	2.15	≥ 5.5
Valproic acid	2.4	9.5
γ-Acetylenic-GABA	2.5	9.0
γ-Vinyl-GABA	2.75	8.0
Nipecotic acid amide	1.5	9.0

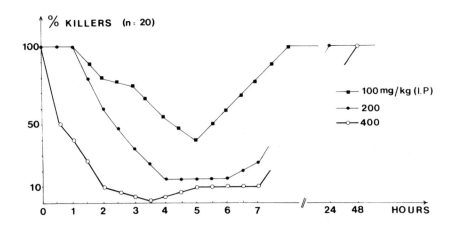

FIG. 1.   Effect of different doses of valproic acid
on killing behaviour.

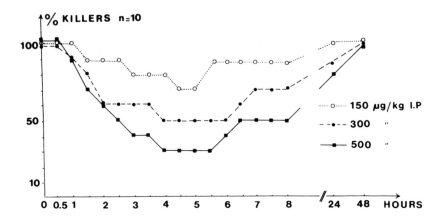

FIG. 2.   Effect of different doses of muscimol on
killing behaviour.

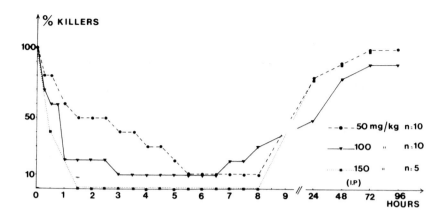

FIG. 3. Effect of different doses of nipecotic acid amide on killing behaviour.

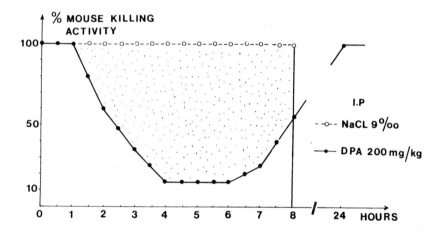

FIG. 4. Conventional evaluation of the suppression of killing behaviour during 8 hours, determined by measuring the surface area (∴∵∴∵∴) between a parallel to the abscissa that corresponds to the situation of controls that is 100% of killers and the curve which represents the decrease in the number of animals which still kill.

TABLE 3.　Effects of GABA-mimetic compounds on
muricidal behaviour

Compound	Efficiency (8 hours) Conven. units	Dose (mg/kg)	LD_{50} (mg/kg)
Muscimol	18	0.5	5.5
THIP	19	0.40	25
Isoguvacine	22	1.0	600
Nipecotic acid amide	25	50	700
Valproic acid	22	200	900
γ-Acetylenic-GABA	17	500	3000
γ-Vinyl-GABA	20	50	400

Concerning valproic acid, it is well established that
this substance produces a striking increase in GABA
content in different brain areas and mainly in the
olfactory bulbs (13,14). Thus, one might speculate
that intraperitoneally-administered GABA-mimetic drugs
act by increasing GABA-mediated neurotransmission in
the olfactory bulbs. To test this hypothesis, we examined the effects of GABA-mimetic drugs on the killing
behaviour of rats deprived of olfactory bulbs. After
bulbectomy the effects of all systemically-administered
GABA-mimetic drugs on killing behaviour was suppressed,
suggesting that the increase of GABA in the olfactory
bulb plays a critical role in blocking muricidal behaviour (6).

COMPARISON OF THE EFFICIENCIES OF GABA-MIMETIC
COMPOUNDS IN INHIBITING MURICIDAL BEHAVIOUR

The efficiencies of GABA agonists, GABA-T inhibitors,
and of an inhibitor of GABA uptake, administered either
intraperitoneally or locally into the olfactory bulbs,
were compared (Tables 1, 2, 3). The selected criteria
were: 1) the latency time to achieve inhibition of
killing behaviour and the duration of this inhibition
in more than 50% of rats after intraperitoneal injection, or in more than 40% of rats after local injection

into the olfactory bulb; 2) a conventional evaluation of the suppression of killing behaviour during eight hours after intraperitoneal or four hours after intra-olfactory bulb injection of the GABA-mimetic drugs. This evaluation was obtained by determining the surface area between a parallel to the abscissa that corresponds to the situation of controls, that is 100% of killers, and the curve which represents the decrease in the number of animals which still kill (Fig. 4).

After intraperitoneal injection, the latency for inhibition of killing by 50% of muricidal rats was quite similar for muscimol, valproic acid, γ-acetylenic-GABA and γ-vinyl-GABA at the doses used (2.4 - 2.75 hrs), and slightly lower for THIP and isoguvacine-HCl (2 - 2.15 hrs), although equimolar quantities were injected. A significantly lower value was obtained for nipecotic acid amide (1.5 hr). The duration of inhibition of killing behaviour in more than 50% of rats was greatest for valproic acid, nipecotic acid amide, γ-acetylenic-GABA, isoguvacine and γ-vinyl-GABA (8 - 9.5 hrs). Slightly lower values were obtained with muscimol and THIP (4.5 - 5.5 hrs). Thus, for both tests, nipecotic acid amide appeared to be the most efficient. Considering their shortest latency times and the long-lasting duration of their effects, valproic acid, γ-acetylenic-GABA and γ-vinyl-GABA (GABA-T inhibitors) appeared to be slightly less efficient, whereas for the other compounds the duration of the effect was strikingly shorter. Considering the "efficiency" in conventional units, nipecotic acid amide, valproic acid, and isoguvacine appeared to be slightly more efficient than γ-vinyl-GABA, THIP and muscimol, and the least effective agent was γ-acetylenic-GABA. Taking into account the ratio of dosage used/LD_{50}, the lowest value was obtained for iso-guvacine, followed by nipecotic acid amide, THIP, musci-mol, and then by γ-acetylenic-GABA, γ-vinyl-GABA and valproic acid.

Considering the effects of local injections into the olfactory bulbs of equimolar quantities of muscimol, valproic acid or nipecotic acid amide, the shortest latency time for inhibition of killing behaviour in 40% of rats was observed for valproic acid and muscimol; a slightly higher value was determined for nipecotic acid amide. A longer duration of inhibition of killing behaviour in more than 40% of rats was observed with val-proic acid and nipecotic acid amide than with muscimol. The most convenient agent, according to the efficiency (duration and latency time) was valproic acid, which had the lowest quotient : dosage administered/LD_{50}.

TABLE 4. Effects of GABA-mimetic compounds on the number of bites among isolated DBA/2 mice

Compound	Dose (mg/kg)	Decrease in number of bites (%)			LD_{50} (mg/kg)
		Day 1	Day 2	Day 3	
Muscimol-HBr	1.5	47	52	68	5.5
"	2.0	67	78	88	
Valproic acid	200	20	99	85	900
"	300	80	98	94	
Nipecotic acid amide	125	23	65	76	700
"	250	53	87	88	

COMPARISON OF THE EFFICIENCIES OF GABA-MIMETIC COMPOUNDS IN ISOLATION-INDUCED AGGRESSIVE BEHAVIOUR

Valproic acid, muscimol-hydrobromide and nipecotic acid amide were administered to male DBA/2 isolated-aggressive mice throughout three successive daily experimental sessions (15). Aggressive responses were assessed by analyzing biting behaviour between two mice and measured with an apparatus in which bites are recorded with a counter (16). In preliminary experiments the ranges of effective non-sedative doses of the three drugs were assessed. On the basis of these experiments, the following doses were selected: valproic acid, 200 and 300 mg/kg; muscimol-hydrobromide, 1.5 and 2 mg/kg; nipecotic acid amide, 125 and 250 mg/kg. Drugs were administered intraperitoneally (10 ml/kg in 0.9% saline) 30 minutes before testing, and the performance of each treated group was compared with that of the saline-injected group. Mean numbers of aggressive responses (bites) exhibited by experimental groups were calculated for all three 10-minute daily sessions. Table 4 shows the daily percentage of aggressive responses of drug-treated mice compared to that of saline-treated mice. One of the main points that has emerged from our results is that potentiation of GABA-ergic neurotransmission, either by inhibition of GABA-T, or by inhibition of GABA uptake, or by the action of a GABA

agonist, inhibits isolation-induced aggressive behaviour in mice. A trend analysis revealed the high significance of the effects (p < 0.01 or p < 0.001) at different sessions.
Taking into account the results obtained with the lower doses, which are easier to compare, muscimol appeared to be the most efficient on the first day of testing: 47% decrease in the number of bites, compared to 20% decrease with the other two drugs. On the second day, valproic acid appeared to be the most efficient, followed by nipecotic acid amide. The smallest effect was obtained with muscimol. On the third day, valproic acid again appeared to be the most efficient, followed by nipecotic acid amide and then very closely by muscimol. The dose/LD_{50} ratio was also lowest with valproic acid, followed closely by nipecotic acid amide. Thus, one might conclude that GABA-T inhibition by valproic acid is the most convenient approach for potentiation of GABA-mediated inhibition in this model of aggressive behaviour, followed by GABA uptake inhibition by nipecotic acid amide.

DISCUSSION

We have demonstrated, using two models of aggressive behaviour (mouse-killing by rats and isolation-induced aggressive behaviour), that a deficiency in GABA-mediated inhibition is involved in this behaviour. In muricidal behaviour a deficiency in GABA content of the olfactory bulbs seemed to play a fundamental role; compensation of these deficiencies by local or systemic treatment with GABA-mimetic drugs abolished muricidal behaviour, whereas decreases in the GABA content of the olfactory bulbs, using a receptor blocker or a glutamate decarboxylase inhibitor, induced aggressive behaviour (6). To overcome the deficiency in GABA-mediated inhibition and to inhibit aggressive behaviour, GABA-agonists, GABA-T inhibitors, or GABA uptake inhibitors were used. The most useful blocker of this type of aggressive behaviour would be a compound having a short latency time (onset of action), a long-lasting effect, a high efficiency, and a low toxicity. With regard to local injection, inhibition of GABA-T and GABA uptake appeared to be the most useful in view of the efficiency evaluation, the duration of the effect, and the dose/LD_{50} ratio. An action on the receptor site with muscimol seems less useful.
After intraperitoneal injections, grading of the different GABA-mimetic compounds, as a function of their efficiency and the dose/LD_{50} ratio, appears rather difficult. Nipecotic acid amide (i.e., the GABA

uptake inhibitor used) presents the most favourable
efficiency and latency time, and has a long-lasting
duration and quite a satisfactory dose/LD_{50} ratio
(1/12). Among the other compounds, the agonists isoguvacine and THIP offer a favourable latency time and
dose/LD_{50} ratio, whereas the GABA-T inhibitors, with
a less favourable dose/LD_{50} ratio, are efficient for a
longer period of time. It is noteworthy that all agonists have the shortest duration of the effect. Finally,
regarding isolation-induced aggressive behaviour,
valproic acid and nipecotic acid amide appear to be the
most efficient agents on the second and third days of
treatment, regardless of the criterion that is used.

In conclusion, a lack of GABA-mediated inhibition
appears to be one of the basic phenomena that underlie
aggressive behaviour. Compensation of this deficiency
can overcome the expression of aggressive behaviour.
Thus, the question is raised: What is the best approach
for promoting GABA-mediated inhibition: GABA agonists,
GABA uptake inhibitors, or GABA-T inhibitors? It seems
difficult to draw a conclusion at the present time.
As a first approximation, inhibition of GABA uptake
and GABA-T appear most favourable with local treatment
(intra-olfactory bulb injections) and with systemic
treatment of isolation-induced aggressive behaviour.
When the drugs that were used are administered intraperitoneally in muricidal rats, grading is more difficult. Inhibition of GABA uptake by nipecotic acid amide
seems the most efficient. The answer is not consistent
with respect to the different criteria. Moreover, it
appears that some new GABA agonists are rather promising in terms of their ability to inhibit aggressive
behaviour. A suppression of changes in serotonin turnover by the GABA-mimetic drug in the two forms of aggressive behaviour also has to be considered. Valproic
acid appeared to be efficient in this respect. The effects of the other GABA-mimetic drugs is under investigation. Finally, more studies have to be conducted on
the side-effects of the drugs used before concluding
whether an action at the receptor site or on GABA metabolism is the most convenient.

REFERENCES

1. Karli, P. (1956): Behaviour, 10: 81-103.
2. Valzelli, L. (1974): In: Determinants and Origins
   of Aggressive Behaviour, edited by J. De Witt and
   W.W. Hartup, pp. 299-308, Mouton, The Hague.
3. Karli, P., Vergnes, M. and Didiergeorges, F. (1969):
   In: Aggressive Behaviour, edited by S. Garattini
   and E.B. Sigg, pp. 47-53, Excerpta Medica, Amsterdam.

4. Karli, P. Vergnes, M., Eclancher, F., Schmitt, P. and Chaurand, J.P. (1972): In: Neurobiology of the Amygdala, edited by B.E. Eleftheriou, PP. 553-580, Plenum Press, New York.
5. Mandel, P., Mack, G., Kempf, E., Ebel, A. and Simler, S. (1978): In: Interactions Between Putative Neurotransmitters in the Brain, edited by S. Garattini, J.F. Pujol and R. Samanin, pp. 285-303, Raven Press, New York.
6. Mandel, P., Mack, G. and Kempf, E. (1979): In: Psychopharmacology of Aggression, edited by M. Sandler, pp. 95-110, Raven Press, New York.
7. Valzelli, L. and Garattini, S. (1972): Neuropharmacology, 11: 17-22.
8. Valzelli, L. and Bernasconi, S. (1979): Neuropsychobiology, 5: 129-135.
9. Simler, S., Puglisi-Allegra, S. and Mandel, P. (1982): Pharmacol. Biochem. Behav. 16: 57-61.
10. Blindermann, J.M., DeFeudis, F.V., Maitre, M., Misslin, R., Wolff, P. and Mandel, P. (1979): J. Neurochem. 32: 1357-1359.
11. Kempf, E., Puglisi-Allegra, S., Schleef, C. and Mandel, P. (1982): (Submitted for publication).
12. Austin, L., Recasens, M. and Mandel, P. (1979): J. Neurochem. 32: 1473-1474.
13. Simler, S., Gensburger, C., Ciesielski, L. and Mandel, P. (1978): Commun. Psychopharmacol. 2: 123-130.
14. Simler, S., Gensburger, C., Ciesielski, L. et Mandel, P. (1976): C.R. Soc. Biol. 170: 1285.
15. Puglisi-Allegra, S. and Mandel, P. (1980): Psychopharmacology, 70: 287-290.
16. Puglisi-Allegra, S. and Renzi, P. (1977): Behav. Res. Meth. and Instr. 9: 503-504.

CNS Receptors—From Molecular
Pharmacology to Behavior, edited by
P. Mandel and F. V. Defeudis.
Raven Press, New York © 1983.

Pharmacology of the Excitatory Actions of Sulphonic and Sulphinic Amino Acids

*K. N. Mewett, **D. J. Oakes, *H. J. Olverman, *D. A. S. Smith, and **J. C. Watkins

*Departments of *Pharmacology and **Physiology, The Medical School, Bristol, BS8 1TD, England*

Several acidic amino acids containing sulphonic and sulphinic acid groups have been compared with respect to their effectiveness as excitants of frog and immature rat spinal neurones, their susceptibility to the actions of selective excitatory amino acid antagonists and their ability to displace [^{3}H]L-glutamate from binding sites on rat brain membranes. The compounds tested comprised the D and L forms of each of cysteine sulphinic acid, cysteic acid, homocysteine sulphinic acid, homocysteic acid and S-sulphocysteine.

The depolarizing potency of the compounds spanned a range of two orders of magnitude. The L and D forms of cysteate and cysteine sulphinate, at the low end of the range, had a potency similar to that of L- and D-aspartate. At the high end of the range, D-homocysteine sulphinate had a potency equal to or higher than that of N-methyl-D-aspartate (NMDA) and comparable with that of quisqualate and kainate.

D-Homocysteine sulphinate appeared to have a highly selective action at N-methylaspartate (NMA) receptors in that the responses it produced were abolished by low concentrations of D(-)-2-amino-5-phosphonopentanoate (AP5). A high proportion of the actions of L-homocysteate, S-sulpho-L-cysteine, and D-cysteate was also sensitive in each case to antagonism by AP5. Other sulphur containing excitants showed intermediate susceptibility to AP5, the most resistant substance being S-sulpho-D-cysteine.

Several of the substances were very effective inhibitors of the binding of [^{3}H]L-glutamate to brain membranes measured in a Na$^+$-free medium, which is considered to reflect affinity for an excitatory amino acid depolarizing receptor site. The most potent inhibitors of this mode of [^{3}H]L-glutamate binding were the L forms of S-sulphocysteine, homocysteate and homocysteine sulphinate. L-Cysteate, L-cysteine sulphinate, D-cysteine sulphinate, and to a lesser extent, D-cysteate, were effective inhibitors of the binding of [3H]L-glutamate measured in the presence of a high (100 mM) Na+ concentration, considered to reflect interaction with high affinity L-glutamate uptake sites. The D forms of S-sulphocysteine, homocysteate and homocysteine sulphinate had potent and selective effects as inhibitors of the binding of [3H]L-glutamate measured in a Na-free medium while being without significant effect on [3H]L-glutamate binding measured in a high-Na medium.

The results presented indicate that sulphur-containing amino acids should be considered as candidates for excitatory transmitter function in the mammalian central nervous system.

INTRODUCTION

L-Glutamate and L-aspartate have long been considered as transmitter candidates in the mammalian central nervous system[9,14] and this possibility has recently received strong support from the synaptic blocking activity of newly developed amino acid antagonists of high specificity [38]. However, several sulphur containing amino acids with excitatory properties similar to those of glutamate and aspartate are known to exist in brain and/or have been reported to be formed in other tissues in normal or pathological states. Such substances include L-cysteine sulphinate[6], L-cysteate[29,30], L-homocysteate and L-homocysteine sulphinate[28,31] and S-sulpho-L-cysteine[25]. The structures of these amino acids are shown in Fig. 1.

The excitatory action of sulphur-containing amino acids has been known for many years. Thus, L-cysteate was included with L-glutamate and L-aspartate in the first descriptions of the excitatory actions of acidic amino acids on single neurones in the mammalian central nervous system[10]. The actions of L-cysteine sulphinate, DL-homocysteine sulphinate and DL-, D- and L-homocysteate were reported soon thereafter[11-13]. L-Cysteine sulphinate was shown to have a similar potency to that of L-glutamate, L-aspartate and L-cysteate, while DL-homocysteine sulphinate and DL-homocysteate (especially) were found to be somewhat more potent. Highest potency was shown by D-homocysteate, which also had a considerably longer time course of action compared with the other substances[13]. More recently, S-sulpho-L-cysteine, which is a close structural analogue of L-homocysteate, was shown to have comparable excitatory activity to the latter amino acid[8,37].

The candidature of endogenous excitants as transmitters is strengthened by evidence of a means for their rapid removal from the vicinity of receptor sites to terminate their action. For acidic amino acids such inactivation is probably by uptake[9]. The finding that high and low affinity uptake of [3H]L-glutamate[27] is inhibited by L-cysteate and L-cysteine sulphinate[2,3] probably indicates that uptake of these sulphur-containing acidic amino acids takes place at least partially via dicarboxylic amino acid carriers. Direct evidence for efficient uptake of [35S] L-homocysteate[7] and [35S] L-cysteine sulphinate[33] has also been presented, such uptake being inhibited by dicarboxylic amino acids in accordance with the concept of common acidic amino acid uptake

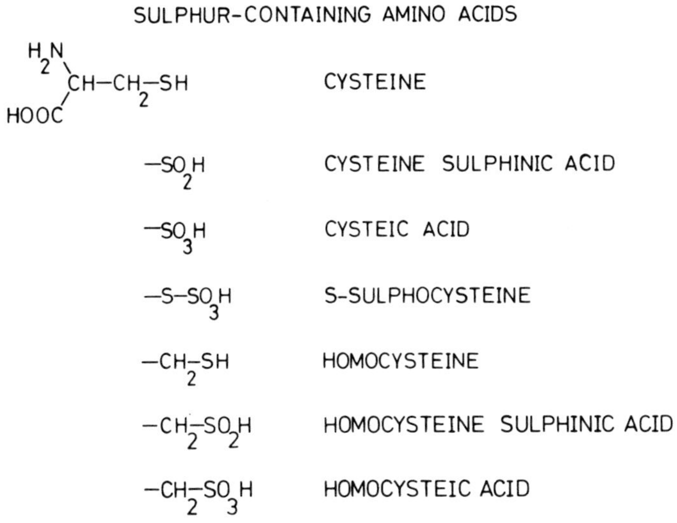

SULPHUR-CONTAINING AMINO ACIDS

$$\begin{array}{l} H_2N \\ \quad\diagdown \\ \qquad CH-CH_2-SH \\ \quad\diagup \\ HOOC \end{array}$$ CYSTEINE

$-SO_2H$ CYSTEINE SULPHINIC ACID

$-SO_3H$ CYSTEIC ACID

$-S-SO_3H$ S-SULPHOCYSTEINE

$-CH_2-SH$ HOMOCYSTEINE

$-CH_2-SO_2H$ HOMOCYSTEINE SULPHINIC ACID

$-CH_2-SO_3H$ HOMOCYSTEIC ACID

Fig.1.   Structures of sulphur-containing amino acids.

mechanisms. L-Cysteine sulphinate also inhibits the binding of [^{3}H]L-glutamate to brain membranes in the presence of a high Na$^+$ concentration in the medium, which is considered to reflect interaction with high affinity L-glutamate uptake sites[4,36]. However, L-homocysteate and L-homocysteine sulphinate may also be taken up by a system with a different ionic mechanism[7,21,39], and it is significant that β-(p-chlorophenyl)-glutamic acid inhibits the uptake of L-homocysteate (and enhances depolarizing responses produced by this amino acid) without affecting the uptake or actions of L-glutamate[38].

Sulphur-containing acidic amino acids also inhibit binding of [^{3}H]L-glutamate to brain membranes in the absence of Na$^+$ in the medium; in particular, DL-homocysteate is a potent inhibitor of this mode of L-glutamate binding[4,24,34,35]. The binding sites involved in this type of binding are believed to be receptor sites mediating at least part of the excitatory (depolarizing) effects of L-glutamate on neurones. Direct measurements have indicated that [^{35}S]L-cysteine sulphinate also binds to whole rat brain membranes in the absence of Na$^+$ and that this binding is inhibited by L-glutamate and by DL-cysteate, but very much less effectively by DL-homocysteate[33]. Thus, more than one site may have affinity for excitatory sulphur-containing amino acids.

Different types of excitatory amino acid receptors have recently been described[38]. L-Cysteate and L-cysteine sulphinate both appear to have a similar susceptibility to the actions of specific NMA receptor antagonists to that of L-aspartate and L-glutamate. Although the actions of both these latter two amino acids can be partially blocked by NMA receptor antagonists, a considerable proportion of the depolarizing responses they produce in each case appears to be resistant to such antagonists[15,38], reflecting a substantial involvement of non-NMA type receptors in these responses. On the other hand, most of the action of L-homocysteate and S-sulpho-L-cysteine in the mammalian and amphibian spinal cord is mediated by NMA receptors[17,19,22]. D-Homocysteate and L-homocysteine sulphinate show a sensitivity to NMA antagonists which is intermediate between that of L-homocysteate and L-cysteate[17,19,22]

On the basis of this evidence L-cysteate and L-cysteine sulphinate would appear to warrant consideration as possible transmitters at non-NMA receptors while L-homocysteate, L-homocysteine sulphinate and S-sulpho-L-cysteine might be considered as possible transmitters at either NMA or non-NMA receptors. Although these latter three amino acids have yet to be identified as normal brain constituents, their formation from L-homocysteine or L-cysteine (in the case of S-sulpho-L-cysteine) would not be surprising. Therefore we have made a detailed study of the excitatory potency, the depolarizing receptor type preference, and the affinity for [³H]L-glutamate binding sites in the presence and absence of Na^+ of each of the enantiomeric forms of cysteate, cysteine sulphinate, homocysteate, homocysteine sulphinate and S-sulphocysteine.

METHODS

N-Methyl-D-aspartic acid and all the sulphur-containing amino acids used in this study except L-cysteic acid were prepared in our laboratory. All the other amino acids were obtained from commercial sources (Sigma and Cambridge Research Biochemicals).

Relative potencies of excitants were determined on isolated hemisected spinal cords of frogs or 4-8 day old rats from the concentrations of the excitants required to produce equal-magnitude motoneuronal depolarizations, measured from ventral roots[19,20].

Where not known from previous experiments[1,15,19,22] the extent of the participation of NMA receptors in the responses produced by the excitants were assessed from the degree of antagonism produced by D(-)-2-amino-5-phosphonopentanoate (AP5). In these experiments the superfusion medium contained tetrodotoxin (10^{-7}M) to abolish indirect effects of the excitants on motoneurones. After control responses of approximately equal magnitude were obtained for a series of excitants, AP5 (25 μM) was added to the medium, and responses in the presence of the antagonist measured 15 min later. This level of AP5 abolished responses to NMDA (10-30 μM), but had little effect on responses to quisqualate (5-10 μM) these two amino acids being used as standard agonists with highly susceptible and resistant actions, respectively[20].

The binding of [³H]L-glutamate to whole brain membranes was measured by a modification of the method described by Foster & Roberts[24]. Rat brains (minus brain stems and cerebella) were homogenized in 60 volumes of ice cold 50 mM Tris-HCl buffer, pH 7.2 and centrifuged at 50,000 g for 10 min. The pellets were resuspended in

TABLE 1. Neuro-excitatory actions of acidic amino acids.

	Approximate Potency Relative to L-Glu = 1.0*	Relative Sensitivity to NMA Antagonists**
L-Aspartate	1	+
D-Aspartate	1	+
L-Glutamate	1	+
D-Glutamate	5	++
L-Cysteine sulphinate	1	+
D-Cysteine sulphinate	1	+
L-Cysteate	1	+
D-Cysteate	1	++
L-Homocysteine sulphinate	4	++
D-Homocysteine sulphinate	100	+++
L-Homocysteate	15	++
D-Homocysteate	30	+
S-Sulpho-L-cysteine	15	++
S-Sulpho-D-cysteine	3	+
NMDA	70	+++
Kainate	150	-
Quisqualate	200	-

* Determined on isolated spinal cord preparations of the immature rat.
** The number of symbols gives an approximate indication of the degree of depression produced by a concentration of an NMDA antagonist (e.g. AP5, 25 μm) sufficient to abolish depolarizations of frog motoneurones induced by NMDA (10-30 μm).

TABLE 2. Inhibitory effects of acidic amino acids on [^{3}H]L-glutamate binding to brain membranes

	IC$_{50}$ Values (μM)	
	100 mM Na$^+$	Na$^+$-free
L-Aspartate	5.1	56
D-Aspartate	3.8	250
L-Glutamate	3.8	1.2
D-Glutamate	100	180
L-Cysteine sulphinate	4.2	19
D-Cysteine sulphinate	6.3	28
L-Cysteate	2.1	24
D-Cysteate	20	71
L-Homocysteine sulphinate	41	1.6
D-Homocysteine sulphinate	1000	7.1
L-Homocysteate	300	0.7
D-Homocysteate	>1000	3.2
S-Sulpho-L-cysteine	200	0.5
S-Sulpho-D-cysteine	>1000	1.0
NMDA	>1000	>1000
Kainate	560	>1000
Quisqualate	>1000	0.5

the same volume of cold Tris buffer, incubated at 37°C for 30 min, and again centrifuged at 50,000 g for 10 min. Pellets were washed once by resuspension and centrifugation in Tris buffer and the final pellets were resuspended in 80 volumes of 50 mM Tris-HCl buffer. For [³H]L-glutamate binding, 0.5 ml samples of membrane suspension were preincubated for 3 min at 25°C with drug or Tris buffer before addition of [³H]L-glutamate (35 Ci/mmol), final concentration 0.1 μM, and the incubation continued for 20 min. Binding was terminated by high speed centrifugation (20,000 g; 1 min). The resultant membrane pellets were washed with 0.5 ml Tris buffer, then digested with 100 μl 20M formic acid and the bound radioactivity determined by liquid scintillation counting. Specific binding of [³H]L-glutamate was calculated by subtracting from the total binding in control samples, the non-specific component of binding which remained in samples containing 1mM unlabelled L-glutamate.

RESULTS

The results obtained are summarized in Tables 1 and 2 and are described in detail below:

Excitatory Potency

When tested on the isolated spinal cord of the frog or immature rat, D-cysteate and D-cysteine sulphinate had depolarizing actions very similar in potency and time course to their L counterparts and also to D and L forms of both glutamate and aspartate (Table 1). L-Homocysteine sulphinate and S-sulpho-D-cysteine comprised a pair of somewhat more potent excitants while S-sulpho-L-cysteine, L-homocysteate, D-homocysteate and D-homocysteine sulphinate (especially) constituted a further group of yet more potent excitants. On the spinal cord of the immature rat, D-homocysteine sulphinate had a potency which was equal to or higher than that of NMDA and comparable with that of the non-NMA receptor agonists, quisqualate and kainate. The time courses of action of D-homocysteate and S-sulpho-D-cysteine were longer than those of the other sulphur-containing amino acids. Representative examples of the excitatory actions of these substances are illustrated in Fig.2.

Antagonism of Excitant Actions

The effects of the highly specific NMA receptor antagonist AP5[16,18,20] showed several interesting features (Table 1). The degree of antagonism of the responses by AP5 at a concentration sufficient to abolish responses to NMDA spanned a considerable range from around 50% or less (S-sulpho-D-cysteine, L-cysteate, D- and L-cysteine

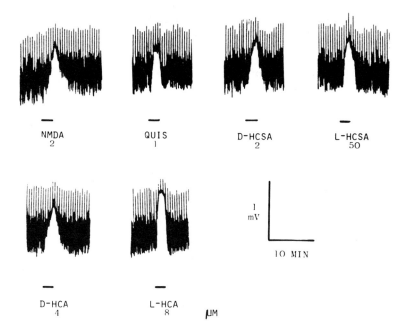

Fig. 2. Actions of a range of amino acid excitants
in the isolated spinal cord of the immature rat. The
figure shows dorsal root-evoked potentials of motoneurones,
recorded on a chart recorder (regular responses, 2 stimuli
per min) and spontaneous activity (irregular activity, dark
region of records), recorded from ventral roots. Depolarizing
potentials were also produced by 2ml volumes of superfusion
medium (flow rate, 1 ml/min) containing excitatory amino acids
at the concentrations (µM) shown. NMDA, N-methyl-D-aspartate;
QUIS, quisqualate; HCSA, homocysteine sulphinate; HCA,
homocysteate.

sulphinate), through an intermediate range (D-homocysteate, L-
homocysteine sulphinate), to marked antagonism (80-100%) in the case
of D-cysteate, L-homocysteate, S-sulpho-L-cysteine and D-
homocysteine sulphinate. Responses to D-homocysteine sulphinate
were abolished by AP5, suggesting that this amino acid has a selectivity
for NMA receptors similar to that of NMDA itself. Fig.3 is
representative of the range of effects observed.

Binding Studies

Inhibition of [^{3}H]L-glutamate binding in a high (100 mM) Na$^+$-
containing medium (Table 2) indicated that all sulphur-containing

excitatory amino acids of the L configuration had higher inhibitory potency than the corresponding D amino acids, except in the case of D- and L-cysteine sulphinate which were approximately equi-effective. These latter two amino acids, together with both L-cysteate (especially) and D-cysteate, were the most effective inhibitors among the sulphur-containing amino acids, while L-homocysteine sulphinate also showed significant activity.

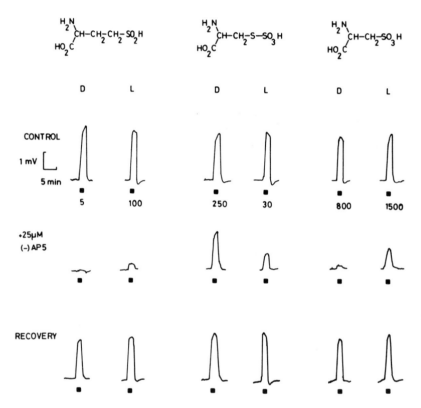

Fig. 3. Action of D(-)-2-amino-5-phosphonopentanoate (AP5) on depolarizing responses produced by a range of amino acids (enantiomeric pairs) in the tetrodotoxin $(10^{-7}M)$-blocked isolated spinal cord of the frog. Approximately equal magnitude depolarizing responses were produced, at the concentration (µM) shown, by the D and L forms of: left hand panel, homocysteine sulphinate; middle panel, S-sulpho-cysteine; right hand panel, cysteate. AP5 abolished the response to D-homocysteine sulphinate, and reduced the responses produced by the other amino acids to varying extents, the response to S-sulpho-D-cysteine being the least affected.

When binding of $[^3H]$L-glutamate was measured in a Na^+-free medium, several of the sulphur-containing amino acids showed potent inhibitory activity (Table 2). Again L forms of the amino acids were more effective than the D forms although the two enantiomeric cysteine sulphinates and S-sulphocysteines showed lower stereoselectivity. Four substances had inhibitory potencies which were similar to, or greater than that of L-glutamate itself, namely L-homocysteine sulphinate, L-homocysteate, and both D- and L- S-sulphocysteines. D-Homocysteine sulphinate and D-homocysteate also showed relatively high inhibitory potency. The D and L forms of both cysteine sulphinate and cysteate all showed considerably lower activity.

DISCUSSION

The relatively low excitatory potencies of D and L forms of both cysteine sulphinate and cysteate are, like those of L-glutamate and L-aspartate[3], probably due, at least partially, to their effective uptake on the glutamate/aspartate transport carrier(s). All four of these sulphur amino acids were potent inhibitors of Na^+-dependent binding of [^{3}H]L-glutamate, though D-cysteate was less effective in this respect than the other three substances. Such inhibitory effects on Na^+-dependent binding have been previously reported in the case of L-cysteine sulphinate[4,36]. Also the uptake of [^{35}S]L-cysteine sulphinate is stimulated by high Na^+ concentrations in the medium, and this uptake, which may be mediated by the high affinity L-glutamate carrier, is inhibited by D-cysteine sulphinate and by DL-cysteate[33] suggesting common uptake mechanisms for these sulphur-containing amino acids.

A major finding of the present work is that D-homocysteine sulphinate is one of the most potent excitatory amino acids yet tested in the mammalian or amphibian central nervous systems, ranking in effectiveness with quisqualate, kainate, NMDA[37], ODAP[32,37], AMPA[26] and bromowillardine[15]. The high potency of D-homocysteine sulphinate was not unexpected in view of its close structural similarity to D-homocysteate. It is considered that a major factor in the high potency of D-homocysteate is the lack of efficient uptake mechanisms for this amino acid[7]. The fact that D-homocysteine sulphinate, like D-homocysteate, was not an effective inhibitor of Na^+-dependent binding of [^{3}H]L-glutamate is consistent with lack of uptake of either amino acid on the high affinity L-glutamate carrier. However, the offset of action of D-homocysteine sulphinate is faster than that of D-homocysteate, suggesting a more rapid inactivation of the former compound, or a faster dissociation from receptors. It is possible that D-homocysteine sulphinate is inactivated by a similar mechanism to that responsible for the rapid termination of the excitatory action of D-glutamate[7], another amino acid that has little effect on Na^+ dependent binding of [^{3}H]L-glutamate (refs 4, 34, 36 and present work). D-Glutamate is transported by a high capacity low affinity system[5]. The lower excitatory potency of L-homocysteine sulphinate, compared with the D form, may be due to uptake of the L isomer by both high and low affinity systems. Thus, L-homocysteine sulphinate, which has a fast offset of action, inhibits the Na^+-dependent binding of [^{3}H]L-glutamate (present work), and also the low affinity uptake of L-homocysteate[7].

S-Sulpho-L-cysteine resembled its close structural analogue L-homocysteate (Fig.1) in potency and time course of action. The high potency of S-sulpho-L-cysteine is of considerable interest in view of its known formation in human tissues in sulphite oxidase deficiency[25] and hence the possibility that it may occur, at least in low concentration, also as a normal constituent in brain and perhaps function as a transmitter substance. S-Sulpho-L-cysteine is a thio-ester and as such could perhaps be subject to the action of esterases to terminate its action. Recovery from the depolarizing action of this substance is indeed quite rapid, though this might be because of an uptake mechanism, similar to that considered to participate in the termination of the action of L-homocysteate[7,21,39]. That such a mechanism is different from that mediating high affinity L-glutamate uptake is indicated by the relatively weak inhibitory effect of both S-sulpho-L-cysteine and L-homocysteate on Na+-dependent binding of [3H]L-glutamate.

Correlation of the binding data observed in a Na-free medium with the electrophysiological effects poses certain problems. Clearly the relative potencies of the substances inhibiting the Na+-free binding of [3H]L-glutamate bears little relation to the depolarizing effects of the excitants mediated by NMA receptors. Thus, NMDA had no effect on such binding, and D-homocysteine sulphinate, the most potent and selective NMA agonist of all the sulphur-containing amino acids tested, was not as effective in inhibiting binding as the less selective L-homocysteine sulphinate, L-homocysteate or S-sulpho-L-cysteine. It is suggested that the observed potencies for inhibition of Na-free binding of [3H]L-glutamate reflects the affinities of the substances for the quisqualate type of excitatory amino acid receptor. Thus, quisqualate was a very effective inhibitor of this mode of [3H]L-glutamate binding in conformity with the results of other investigations[4,24,35]. The quisqualate type of receptor is considered to show a preference for L-amino acids[15] and it is noteworthy that the most potent inhibitors of Na-free [3H]L-glutamate binding in the present work were all L amino acids. Furthermore, the most effective inhibitors had a similar chain length to that of L-glutamate, which is another structural feature of agonists showing a preference for the quisqualate type of receptor[15]. An apparent paradox is that the D forms of these amino acids also had relatively high potency as inhibitors of the Na-free [3H]L-glutamate binding. Yet, with the exception of S-sulpho-D-cysteine these substances produced most of their depolarizing effects via the NMA type of receptors. This paradox can be resolved by proposing that the depolarizing effects of the substances at quisqualate receptors were obscured by an even greater potency of the substances at NMA receptors and/or by the presence in the spinal cord of a greater proportion of NMA receptors over quisqualate receptors compared with brain membranes on which the binding studies were conducted.

The availability of potent and specific NMA receptor antagonists such as AP5 and AP7 provides a means of estimating potency ratios for actions of excitants at non-NMA receptors[15]. Such experiments, which are currently in progress, may provide a better correlation between binding and electrophysiological data. In any event, the present results indicate that sulphur-containing amino acids strongly warrant further consideration as transmitter candidates.

This work was supported by the Wellcome Trust and the Medical Research Council.

REFERENCES

1. Ault, B., Evans, R.H., Francis, A.A., Oakes, D.J. and Watkins, J.C. (1980) J. Physiol. (Lond), 307: 413-428.
2. Balcar, V.J. and Johnston, G.A.R. (1972a) J. Neurochem. 19: 2657-2666.
3. Balcar, V.J. and Johnston, G.A.R. (1972b) J. Neurobiol. 3 : 295-301.
4. Baudry, M. and Lynch, G. (1981) J. Neurochem., 36:295-301.
5. Benjaman, A.M. and Quastel, J.H. (1976) J. Neurochem., 26 : 431-441.
6. Bergeret, B. and Chatagne, F. (1954) Biochim. Biophys Acta (Amst.)., 14 : 297.
7. Cox, D.W.G., Headey, P.M. and Watkins, J.C. (1977) J. Neurochem. 29 : 579-588.
8. Curtis, D.R., Felix, D. and Watkins, J.C. (1971) unpublished observations.
9. Curtis, D.R. and Johnston, G.A.R. (1974) Ergebn. Physiol. 69 : 97-188.
10. Curtis, D.R., Phillis, J.. and Watkins, J.C. (1960) J. Physiol. (Lond) 150 : 656-682.
11. Curtis, D.R., Phillis, J.W. and Watkins, J.C. (1961) Br. J. Pharmacol. 16 : 262-283.
12. Curtis, D.R. and Watkins, J.C. (1960) J. Neurochem., 6 ; 117-141.
13. Curtis, D.R. and Watkins, J.C. (1963) J. Physiol. (Lond) 166 : 1-14.
14. Curtis, D.R. and Watkins, J.C. (1965) Pharmacol. Rev., 17 : 347-391.
15. Davies, J., Evans, R.H., Jones, A.W., Smith, D.A.S. and Watkins, J.C. (1982) Comp. Biochem. Physiol. C.72 : 211-224.
16. Davies, J., Francis, A.A., Jones, A.W. and Watkins, J.C. (1981) Neurosci. Lett. 21 : 77-81.
17. Davies, J. and Watkins, J.C. (1979) J. Physiol. (Lond) 197 : 621-635.
18. Davies, J. and Watkins, J.C. (1982) Brain Res. 235 : 378-386.
19. Evans, R.H., Francis, A.A., Hunt, K., Oakes, D.J. and Watkins, J.C. (1979). Br. J. Pharmac. 67 : 591-603.
20. Evans, R.H., Francis, A.A., Jones, A.W., Smith, D.A.S. and Watkins, J.C., (1982) Br. J. Pharmac., 75: 65-75.
21. Evans, R.H., Francis, A.A. and Watkins, J.C. (1977) Experientia (Basel), 33 : 246-248
22. Evans, R.H., Francis, A.A. and Watkins, J.C. (1977) Experientia (Basel) 33 : 489-491
23. Evans, R.H., Francis, A.A. and Watkins, J.C. (1978) Brain Res., 148 : 536-542.

24. Foster, A.C. & Roberts, P.J. (1978) J. Neurochem., 31 : 1467-1477.
25. Irreverre, F., Mudd, S.H., Heizer, W.D. and Laster, L. (1967) Biochem. Med., 1 : 187-217.
26. Krogsgaard-Larsen, P., Honore, T., Hansen, J.J., Curtis, D.R. and Lodge, D. (1980) Nature (Lond) 284 : 64-66
27. Logan, W.J. and Snyder, S.H. (1972) Brain Res., 42 : 413-431.
28. McCully, K.S. (1971) Nature (Lond), 231 : 391-392.
29. Mandel, P. and Mark, J. (1965) J. Neurochem. 12 : 987-992.
30. Mussini, E. and Marcucci, F. (1962) In: Amino Acid Pools, edited by J.T. Holden, pp 486-492, Elsevier/Amsterdam.
31. Ohmori, S. (1975) Hoppe-Seyler's Z. Physiol. Chem., 356 : 1369-1373.
32. Pearson, S. and Nunn, P.B. (1981) Brain Res., 206 : 178-182.
33. Recasens, M., Varga, V., Nanopoulos, D., Saadoun, F., Vincendon, G., and Benavides, J. (1982) Brain Res., 239 : 153-173.
34. Roberts, P.J. (1974) Nature (Lond) 252 : 399-401
35. Roberts, P.J. and Sharif, N.A. (1981) In: Glutamate as a Neurotransmitter, edited by G. Di Chiara and G.L.Gessa, pp 295-305, Raven Press, New York.
36. Vincent, S.R. and McGeer, E.G. (1980) Brain Res., 184 : 99-108.
37. Watkins, J.C. (1978) In: Kainic Acid as a Tool in Neurobiology, edited by E.G. McGeer et al., pp. 37-69.
38. Watkins, J.C. and Evans, R.H. (1981) Ann. Rev. Pharmacol. Toxicol., 21 : 165-204.
39. Watkins, J.C., Evans, R.H., Headley, P.M. Cox, D.W.G., Francis, A.A. & Oakes, D.J. (1978) In: Iontophoresis and Transmitter Mechanisms in the Mammalian Central Nervous System, edited by R.W.Ryall and J.S. Kelly, pp. 397-399, Elsevier-North Holland, Amsterdam.

CNS Receptors—From Molecular
Pharmacology to Behavior, edited by
P. Mandel and F. V. Defeudis.
Raven Press, New York © 1983.

Excitatory Amino Acid Receptor Stimulation: Involvement of Cyclic GMP?

G. A. Foster and P. J. Roberts

Department of Physiology and Pharmacology, School of Biochemical and Physiological Sciences, University of Southampton, Southampton SO9 3TU, England

Considerable research effort has been expended in recent years to demonstrate a neurotransmitter role in the mammalian central nervous system for a number of acidic amino acids, most notably L-glutamate (L-glu) and L-aspartate (L-asp) (2,10,21,31,41). The literature surrounding the post-synaptic effects of these compounds is dominated by electrophysiological investigations in whole tissue (9,22) and by binding studies in severely disrupted material (13,26). Both of these preparations have inherent disadvantages, and in an attempt to overcome some of these, we have used a slicing technique, whereafter the tissue environment can be altered at will, and yet a high degree of physiological and morphological preservation may be maintained (20).

Cyclic GMP has been implicated in the actions of excitatory amino acids in the rat cerebellum (12) and changes in response to in vivo stimulation or inhibition of the two excitatory pathways, namely the parallel and the climbing fibres, are well documented (3,4,32). Indeed, glutamate, and glutamate/aspartate have been suggested to be the respective neurotransmitters of these two fibre systems (25,33).

PHARMACOLOGY OF RECEPTORS MEDIATING CHANGES IN CYCLIC GMP

Garthwaite and Balazs (19) first described the massive increase in cyclic GMP in response to addition of L-glutamate to neonatal rat cerebellar slices. Although the reasons for the supersensitivity at this age are unclear, we elected to conduct our initial experiments in this preparation. Full details of our methods have been published (15).

Agonists

The effects of over forty putative agonist analogues closely related to glutamate have been studied for their ability to raise cyclic GMP concentrations. Glutamate itself caused a 200-fold stimulation over basal levels, with an EC50 of 1.2mM and a maximal effect at 3mM. Where comparative electrophysiological data have been available, the potencies of these compounds, both in absolute terms (39) and relative to L-glutamate (36) are very similar to those that we have observed in vitro (14). The only exception to this was kainic acid, which despite being between 8 -80 times more potent than glutamate in depolarising spinal neurones (5), is only equipotent with glutamate in stimulating cyclic GMP. However, the zenith of kainate's efficacy in increasing cyclic GMP occurs at 15-20 days post-natal, some 7-12 days later than that for glutamate, and it may well be that the variation in its ontogenetic manifestation is responsible for this discrepancy.

Antagonists

Since the advent of some of the newer acidic amino acid antagonists, such as 2-aminophosphonovalerate (2-APV), γ-D-glutamylglycine (γ-DGG) and cis-piperidine-2,3-dicarboxylate (cis-PD), it has proved possible to effect a more discrete and selective characterisation of the receptors mediating neuronal excitation. We have studied these and other antagonists for their ability to inhibit the cyclic GMP response to either glutamate, N-methyl-D-aspartate (NMDA) or kainate. Each of these agonists possessed a different pharmacological profile (Table 1), which in the first two cases coincided with observations in the frog spinal cord (37).

TABLE 1. Inhibition of the stimulation of cyclic GMP by excitant amino acids[a]

| Antagonist | Agonist | | | | |
	L-glu(1mM)	L-asp(1mM)	NMDA(0.3mM)	$(\pm)$-ibo(1mM)	Kain(1mM)
GDEE	0.25	1.0	>1.0	>3.0	0.1
APB	2.9	>3.0	>3.0	>3.0	>3.0
DαAA	>3.0	>3.0	>3.0	2.0	NT
2-APV	3.2	0.25	0.054	0.08	0.01
γ-DGG	>3.0	0.25	0.55	1.0	0.074
cis-PD	>3.0	3.0	1.2	0.3	0.3
HA966	>3.0	1.3	0.19	0.95	0.25

[a]Values are the concentrations of antagonist producing 50% inhibition. APB=2-amino-4-phosphonobutyrate, DαAA=D-α-aminoadipate, HA966=3-amino-1-hydroxypyrrolidone, $(\pm)$-ibo=ibotenate, NT = not tested. Other abbreviations are as in the text.

The most potent inhibitor of glutamate was glutamate diethylester (GDEE) with an apparent K_i of 1mM. In contrast, the effects of NMDA were antagonised most successfully by 2-APV, with an apparent K_i of approximately 15μM. However, as well as exhibiting anomalous agonist activity, kainate also showed an extraordinary sensitivity to inhibition by nearly all the antagonists tested, and closer analysis revealed its totally non-competitive nature (15). We have subsequently demonstrated, instead, the ability of Ca^{2+} to overcome the inhibition of the kainate response by, for example, 2-APV (15) or GDEE. It is not clear whether this reflects an effect of these drugs at or near a calcium-binding site, or whether they are able to induce a conformational change which inhibits calcium binding indirectly. What is obvious, though, is that kainate is not acting directly at an NMDA- or glutamate-type receptor. Of the other agonists studied, aspartate appeared similar to glutamate in its sensitivity to antagonists, and ibotenate closely resembled NMDA.

Ionic dependence of stimulation of cyclic GMP

A number of ion-channel antagonists and manipulations of the external medium were used to examine the ionic dependence of the cyclic GMP response to glutamate. Tetrodotoxin, which blocks Na^{+}-channels was without effect up to 0.3mM, whereas the Ca^{2+}-channel antagonist verapamil (0.01-1mM), or calcium-free medium completely abolished the response. Surprisingly, Mg^{2+} (2mM) was almost inactive and Mn^{2+} (10mM) caused only a 50% reduction in the stimulation by glutamate. This last cation has been shown to totally prevent the opening of the voltage-dependent Ca^{2+}-channel in Purkinje cells at concentrations considerably lower than we used (23), implying that the stimulation of cyclic GMP is contingent on binding of Ca^{2+} at an external voltage-independent site on the membrane. Evidence for precisely this sort of Ca^{2+}-channel, whose opening depends on glutamate but not on voltage, has been provided by Nicoll and Alger (29). Merely raising the intra-cellular Ca^{2+}, using the calcium ionophore A23187, or the mitochondrial Ca^{2+} uptake inhibitor ruthenium red, is insufficient stimulus alone to cause a major increase in cyclic GMP. For example, the maximal effect of A23187, which occurred at 10μM, was less than one tenth of that seen with glutamate. It appears, therefore, that the dependence on Ca^{2+} occurs at a membrane rather than an intra-cellular locale.

Depolarisation-induced stimulation of cyclic GMP

We have used the depolarising agent protoveratrine (PTV) as a tool to investigate the nature of the endogenous transmitter(s) capable of eliciting changes in cyclic GMP. PTV prevents the closing of voltage-dependent Na^{+}-channels, which exist in neuronal,but not glial membranes. This has been suggested to be the basis for its selective release of transmitter substances only from neuronal compartments (30). In 8-day old animals PTV was signally ineffective in enhancing cyclic GMP levels, whereas by 16 days of age it provoked a stimulation as high as that caused by glutamate (15). It is perhaps germane that the depolarisation-evoked, Ca^{2+}-dependent release of endogenous glutamate from cerebellar slices only becomes apparent at this age (18). In addition the dose-response to PTV in stimulating cyclic GMP corresponded extremely well with its ability to release amino acids from rat brain slices (27), and was potently inhibited by Mn^{2+} (IC50=1mM) with a potency similar to that known to antagonise pre-synaptic Ca^{2+} entry (6). For these reasons it is likely that PTV is stimulating cyclic GMP not directly, but via release of an endogenous transmitter substance.

The response to 100μM PTV is markedly attenuated by the glutamate-type receptor antagonist GDEE (IC50=1.0mM), but is not significantly affected by the NMDA-type receptor antagonists 2-APV or DL-∝-aminosuberate (38) up to a concentration of 3mM (15). 2-APV had previously been shown to inhibit the cyclic GMP response to kainate also (Table 1). It seems,therefore, that the substance released by PTV, and subsequently interacting with cyclic GMP accumulating sites, is glutamate-like in nature.

CELLULAR LOCALISATION OF THE CYCLIC GMP RESPONSE

We have now shown a close similarity between the types of receptors mediating the cyclic GMP response in cerebellar slices and those involved in glutamate/aspartate-induced depolarisations measured electrophysiologically. We now need to know whether the sites responsible for the stimulation of cyclic GMP also receive one or more afferents utilising an excitatory amino acid as its transmitter, and also whether this localisation is compatible with previously published findings.

Earlier attempts to localise within the cerebellum cyclic GMP (7,8), its synthetic enzyme guanylate cyclase (1,42) or the protein kinase for which it is a selective cofactor (24) have all used immunocytochemical techniques in fixed tissue. Conclusions drawn from these experiments have differed substantially, and the important disadvantage of them all is that chemically sensitive sites are not distinguished from those merely exhibiting basal activity. We have attempted to surmount this problem by the use of the large number of toxins or X-irradiation schedules which permit selective ablation of individual cell-types in the cerebellum.

Depletion of granule cells

Irradiation of the rat cerebellum between 8 and 15 days post-natal (8-15X) resulted in a large reduction in the granule cell population. The density of these cells within the granular layer of irradiated animals varied from one folium to another, whereas in the controls there was a more uniform distribution throughout. The volume of the granular layer was estimated using a camera lucida and a Digiplot area calculator in serial sections of the whole cerebellum (Table 2). The X-irradiation regime caused at least a 69% depletion in the granule cell population. Concomitantly, in agreement with Sandoval and Cotman (33), there was a small but non-significant decrease in the uptake of ^{3}H-D-aspartate into a P_2 fraction, when measured on a protein basis. In addition, there was a 60% attenuation of the K^+-induced, Ca^{2+}-dependent release of endogenous glutamate from perfused cerebellar slices (Table 2).

TABLE 2.   Effects of X-irradiation in rat cerebellum[a]

	Control	8-15X
Granule cell density ($cells/1000\mu m^3$)	3.3	2.1-3.3
Volume of granular layer (cm^3)	6.4×10^{-2}	2.4×10^{-2}
Granule cell population (cells/cerebellum)	2.6×10^8	$< 8.0 \times 10^7$
Uptake of ^{3}H-D-aspartate (nmol/mg prot/3 min)	0.95	0.72 NS (8)
Release of endogenous glutamate in response to 50mM K^+ (nmol/mg prot/5 min)	8.47	3.68 P<0.02 (8)

[a]Significance values are shown, with the number of observations in parentheses.

The effects of glutamate on cyclic GMP levels in 16-day old degranulated rats did not differ from controls over the whole dose-response. Moreover, kainate (3.0mM) caused the same increase in cyclic GMP concentrations in both groups. However, there was a consistent reduction in the ability of PTV to stimulate cyclic GMP (Fig. 1), with levels at maximally stimulating concentrations of PTV some 45% lower than normal. These data demonstrate that the stimulation of cyclic GMP by glutamate does not occur on the fraction of the granule cell population which is destroyed by 8-15X, although it does not conclusively exclude those granule cells formed before 8 days. However, the diminution of the response via the endogenous substance released by PTV indicates that this substance emanates from the parallel fibre terminals. The earlier demonstration that this endogenous transmitter is glutamate-like in its actions, and that glutamate release is attenuated after the same X-irradiation procedure supports the hypothesis that glutamate is indeed the transmitter of the parallel fibres. We cannot as yet, however, discriminate which target cells are responsible for the cyclic GMP accumulation.

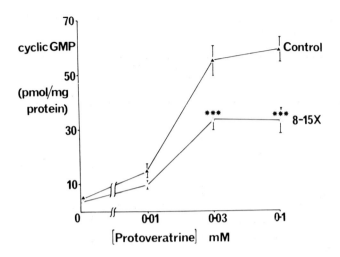

FIG. 1.   Effects of protoveratrine in stimulating levels of
cyclic GMP in cerebellar slices taken from 16 day
old X-irradiated rats (8-15X).

Ablation of the climbing fibres

3-acetylpyridine (3-AP) has been used extensively as a selective agent for the complete destruction of the rat inferior olive
(11,25), the sole source of climbing fibres, which course to the
cerebellum (28).

TABLE 3.   Effects of 3-acetylpyridine (3-AP) in rat cerebellum[a]

	Control	3-AP
Uptake of ^{3}H-D-aspartate (nmol/mg prot/3 min)	0.87	0.53 P<0.001 (8)
Release of endogenous aspartate in response to 50mM K$^+$ (16d) nmol/mg prot/5 min)	0.35	0.3 NS (8)
Release of endogenous glutamate in response to 50mM K$^+$ (16d) (nmol/mg prot/5 min)	1.89	1.83 NS (24)

[a]Significance values are shown, with the number of observations
in parentheses.

2-3 days after administration of 3-AP (65mg/kg,ip), the uptake of ^{3}H-D-aspartate into a P_2 fraction from cerebellum is diminished by 40% (Table 3), but there is no change in the K$^+$-stimulated, Ca^{2+}-dependent release of either endogenous glutamate or aspartate. However, the loss of the climbing fibre input did result in a 40% decrease in the maximal effect of PTV in stimulating cyclic GMP (Fig. 2) with no change in the EC50.

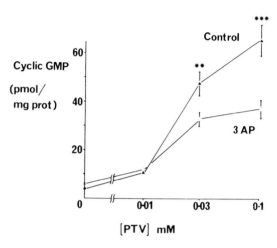

FIG. 2. Effects of protoveratrine in stimulating levels of cyclic GMP in cerebellar slices taken from 16-day old rats previously treated with 3-acetylpyridine (3-AP).

Again, no difference was observed in the dose-response to glutamate, indicating that the stimulation of cyclic GMP does not occur on the climbing fibres themselves. It does appear,however, that PTV is releasing an endogenous glutamate-like substance from the climbing fibre terminals, which interacts with the only target structure, namely the Purkinje cell dendrites. The previously described uptake and release parameters (Table 3) would imply that although this endogenous transmitter is glutamate-like in its actions, it is probably not glutamate itself, nor aspartate. However, some caution needs to be exerted in drawing any firmer conclusions than these, as we cannot discount the possibility that the release of glutamate or aspartate from other sources may greatly exceed, and thus mask, that from the climbing fibres (17).

Glial ablation

The nicotinamide antagonist 6-aminonicotinamide (6-AN) has been reported to selectively destroy Bergmann glia and other astrocytes after a single dose (34), by blocking the pentose phosphate pathway, upon which glia are more heavily dependent. Two days after administration of 8mg/kg ip, we observed a general behavioural syndrome typical of that seen with other cerebellar

dysfunction - ataxia, particularly in the hindlimbs, combined
with uncoordinated motor control and an impaired righting reflex.
The accumulation of ^{3}H-β-alanine into cerebellar slices was used
as a marker for the remaining glia, as this compound is a selective substrate for the astrocytic GABA transport system (35).
The V_{max} for ^{3}H-β-alanine uptake was approximately 37% lower in
lesioned animals (P<0.005), with no apparent change in K_m.   The
cyclic GMP response to glutamate in these 16-day old animals was
enhanced (Fig. 3a), while the kainate response was unmodified
except at the lowest concentrations examined (Fig. 3b).

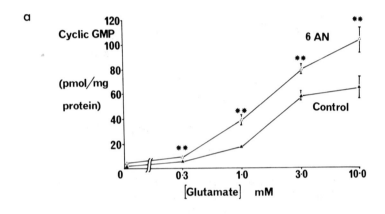

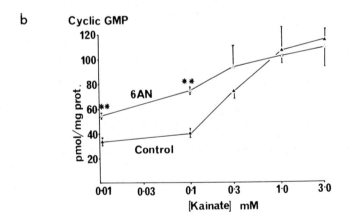

FIG. 3a.   Effects of glutamate and 3b.   of kainate on cyclic GMP
levels in cerebellar slices taken from 16-day old rats previously
treated with 6-aminonicotinamide (6-AN).

Assuming that the proportional loss of β-alanine accumulating glia reflects the loss of glia in general, and of those able to take up glutamate in particular, it is tempting to suggest that not only does the glutamate stimulation of cyclic GMP not occur in these cells, but that they represent a barrier to the diffusion of glutamate into or out of the synaptic cleft. This latter hypothesis coincides with autoradiographic evidence from cerebellar slices incubated with ^{3}H-D-aspartate, where grain density over glia was 4-5 times higher than over neuronal structures (40).

DISCUSSION

We have demonstrated that excitatory amino acids are capable of eliciting increases in cyclic GMP in neonatal rat cerebellar slices via receptors similar to those characterised electrophysiologically. The stimulation is highly dependent on external Ca^{2+}, but voltage-dependent calcium-channels do not seem to be involved. The enhancement of cyclic GMP concentrations by depolarising stimuli is similarly calcium-dependent, but is almost certainly mediated by one or more endogenous substances, which appear to be predominantly glutamate-like in their pharmacological profile.

The lesioning studies have revealed that the major proportion of the cyclic GMP response to PTV is accounted for by release of transmitter from the parallel and the climbing fibres. In the former, it is likely that the transmitter is indeed glutamate, but in the case of the climbing fibres, the lack of attenuation of either glutamate or aspartate release after lesioning argues against a transmitter role in this particular afferent system. However, in the absence of positive evidence against an involvement of glutamate/aspartate, this possibility still remains.

One, if not the sole post-synaptic site involved in cerebellar cyclic GMP production is the Purkinje cell dendritic tree, the only target structure of the climbing fibres. Microdissection techniques (32) and immunocytochemical studies (1,7,8,24,42) have localised cyclic GMP, guanylate cyclase or the cyclic GMP dependent protein kinase to Purkinje cells, amongst others, and thus support our findings.

The role of excitatory amino acid-stimulated cyclic GMP production in the cerebellum is unknown. It is improbable that it mediates the depolarisation evoked by afferent stimulation, because the time-course of events would not coincide. It is more possible, however, that it mediates changes in neuronal sensitivity by regulating various intra-membrane or intracellular events.

Whatever the function cyclic GMP fulfils, its measurement does provide a useful model for assessing the stimulation of excitatory amino acid receptors: as such it has already provided us with clues to the mode of action of kainic acid (16), a pharmacological paradigm of several progressive neurodegenerative disorders.

REFERENCES

1. Ariano, M.A., Lewicki, J.A., Brandwein, H.J. and Murad, F.
   (1982): Proc. Natl. Acad. Sci. USA, 79: 1316-1320.
2. Balcar, V.J. and Johnston, G.A.R. (1972): J. Neurochem.,
   36: 501-505.
3. Biggio, G., Costa, E. and Guidotti, A. (1977): J. Pharm. Exp.
   Therap., 200: 207-215.
4. Biggio, G. and Giudotti, A. (1976): Brain Res., 107: 365-375.
5. Biscoe, T.J., Evans, R.H., Headley, P.M., Martin, M.R. and
   Watkins, J.C. (1976): Brit. J. Pharmacol., 58: 373-382.
6. Blaustein, M.P. (1975): J. Physiol.(Lond.), 247: 617-655.
7. Chan-Palay, V. and Palay, S.L. (1979): Proc. Natl. Acad.
   Sci. USA, 76: 1485-1488.
8. Cumming, R., Arbuthnott, G. and Steiner, A.L. (1979):
   J. Cyclic Nucleotide Res., 5: 463-467.
9. Curtis, D.R., Duggan, A.W., Felix, D., Johnston, G.A.R.,
   Tebecis, A.K. and Watkins, J.C. (1972): Brain Res., 41:
   283-301.
10. Curtis, D.R. and Watkins, J.C. (1960): J. Neurochem., 6:
    117-141.
11. Desclin, J.C. and Escubi, J. (1974): Brain Res., 77: 349-364.
12. Ferrendelli, J.A., Chang, M.M. and Kinscherf, D.A. (1974):
    J. Neurochem., 22: 535-540.
13. Foster, A.C. and Roberts, P.J. (1978): J. Neurochem., 31:
    1467-1477.
14. Foster, G.A. and Roberts, P.J. (1980): Life Sci., 27: 215-221.
15. Foster, G.A. and Roberts, P.J. (1981): Brit. J. Pharmacol.,
    74: 723-729.
16. Foster, G.A. and Roberts, P.J. (1981): Neuroscience Lett.,
    23: 67-70.
17. Foster, G.A. and Roberts, P.J. (1982): Neuroscience, in press.
18. Foster, G.A., Roberts, P.J., Rowlands, G.J. and Sharif, N.A.
    (1981): Brit. J. Pharmacol., 173: 235P.
19. Garthwaite, J. and Balazs, R. (1978): Nature (Lond.), 275:
    328-329.
20. Garthwaite, J., Woodhams, P.L., Collins, M.J. and Balazs, R.
    (1979): Brain Res., 173: 373-377.
21. Katz, R.I., Chase, T.N. and Kopin, I.J. (1969): J. Neurochem.,
    16: 961-967.
22. Krnjević, K. and Phillis, J.W. (1967): J. Physiol.(Lond.),
    165: 274-304.
23. Llinas, R. and Sugimori, M. (1980): J. Physiol.(Lond.), 305:
    197-213.
24. Lohmann, S.M., Walter, U., Miller, P.E., Greengard, P. and
    de Camilli, P. (1981): Proc. Natl. Acad. Sci. USA, 78: 653-
    657.
25. McBride, W.J., Rea, M.A. and Nadi, N.S. (1978): Neurochem.
    Res., 3: 793-801.

26. Michaelis, E.K., Michaelis, M.L. and Boyarsky, L.L. (1974): Biochim. Biophys. Acta., 367: 338-348.
27. Minchin, M.C.W. (1980): Biochem. J., 190: 333-339.
28. Montarolo, P.G., Raschi, F. and Strata, P. (1980): Pflügers Arch., 383: 137-142.
29. Nicoll, R.A. and Alger, B.E. (1981): Science, 212: 957-959.
30. Orrego, F. (1979): Neuroscience, 4: 1037-1057.
31. Roberts, P.J. (1974): Nature (Lond.), 252: 399-401.
32. Rubin, E.H. and Ferrendelli, J.A. (1977): J. Neurochem., 29: 43-51.
33. Sandoval, M.E. and Cotman, C.W. (1978): Neuroscience, 3: 199-206.
34. Schaarschmidt, W. (1975): Acta anat., 91: 362-375.
35. Schon, F. and Kelly, J.S. (1974): Brain Res., 66: 289-300.
36. Watkins, J.C. (1978): In: Kainic Acid as a Tool in Neuro-biology, edited by E.G. McGeer, J.W. Olney and P.L. McGeer, pp 37 -69. Raven Press, New York.
37. Watkins, J.C. (1981): In: Glutamate: Transmitter in the Central Nervous System, edited by P.J. Roberts, J. Storm-Mathisen and G.A.R. Johnston, pp 1-24. J. Wiley and Sons, London.
38. Watkins, J.C., Davies, J., Evans, R.H., Francis, A.A. and Jones, A.W. (1981): In: Glutamate as a Neurotransmitter, edited by G. di Chiara and G.L. Gessa, pp 263-273. Raven Press, New York.
39. Wheal, H.W. Personal communication.
40. Wilkin, G.P., Garthwaite, J. and Balazs, R. (1982): Brain Res., 244: 69-83.
41. Wong, P.T.-H., McGeer, E.G. and McGeer, P.L. (1981): J. Neurochem., 36: 501-505.
42. Zwiller, J., Ghandour, M.S., Revel, M.O. and Basset, P. (1981): Neuroscience Lett., 23: 31-36.

CNS Receptors—From Molecular
Pharmacology to Behavior, edited by
P. Mandel and F. V. Defedis.
Raven Press, New York © 1983.

Development of Specific Binding Sites for [3H]kainic Acid and [3H]muscimol in the Chick Optic Tectum: Modulation by Early Changes in Visual Input

Galo Ramírez, Ana Barat, Javier Gómez-Barriocanal,
Esteban Manrique, and Alicia Batuecas

Centro de Biología Molecular, CSIC-UAM, Madrid-34, Spain

The sequence of events leading to the establishment of function in the chick retinotectal visual system is fairly well understood (see 17 for a review and additional references on this topic). From a neurochemical standpoint, this maturation process involves the appearance and progressive accumulation of a variety of neurotransmission-related macromolecules that will later support neuronal communication at specific synaptic (and other) sites. Since eye-opening entails the sudden exposure of the system to visual stimuli, we have been trying to ascertain the existence of some kind of developmental coordination between excitatory (permissive) and inhibitory (signal-blocking) synaptic mechanisms, which would be of help in handling the arrival to the visual centers of the first light-derived electrical signals.

In this context, we have attempted a comparative analysis, in chick optic tectum membranes, of the developmental profiles of specific binding sites for (3H)kainic acid and (3H)muscimol, used here, tentatively, as representative ligands for glutamate-related excitatory neurotransmission (6,12) and GABA-related inhibitory neurotransmission (1,4,14), respectively, and we have further characterized the regulatory effects of early changes in visual input on the postnatal development of the above receptor populations.

EXPERIMENTAL

Tecta from embryos or young chicks (kept on a 12-hour light/ 12-hour darkness schedule) were homogenized in 20 vol of 1mM potassium phosphate, pH 7, containing 0.32M sucrose and 1mM $MgCl_2$. In the case of kainic acid binding this homogenate was first centrifuged at 1000g, and the resulting pellet was washed and discarded (6,12). In the case of muscimol binding, however, the presence of a high concentration of receptor sites in the 1000g pellet forced us to process the whole homogenate without further fractionation. Both the 1000g supernatants (kainic acid) and the homogenate (muscimol) were next centrifuged at 72,000g for 30 min. The resulting pellets were lysed (by osmotic shock) in 40 vol of 1mM potassium phosphate, pH 7, for 30 min, and centrifuged again at 72,000g. For the kainic acid binding assay this pellet was washed twice in the lysis buffer. In the case of the muscimol binding assay the pellet was frozen for at least 24h and, after thawing, it was either washed twice as above or extracted with 0.05% (v/v) Triton X-100, at 37°C,for 30 min, prior to washing. The final membrane preparations were, in all cases, resuspended in 10mM potassium phosphate, pH 7, and used as such for the binding studies. Except where otherwise stated, all this preparative procedure was carried out at 4°C.

Binding assays were performed , at 4°C, in small polycarbonate tubes containing, in a total volume of 1ml, 0.5mg of membrane protein and the radioactive ligand ((G-^{3}H)kainic acid, 2.6Ci/mmol; or (methylamine-^{3}H)muscimol, 19Ci/mmol), with or without the displacer. The concentrations of radioligand used in each case are given in the text and figure legends. Other details concerning incubation, termination of the binding process, and measurement of the amount of radioligand bound specifically to tectal membranes have been fully described in previous publications (6,12).Specific binding is defined as that part of total binding displaced by a concentration of non-labelled ligand 10[4] times the radioligand concentration.

The general properties of the kainic acid specific, saturable binding to chick tectal membranes have been the subject of a previous paper (6). Many of these properties are shared by tectal muscimol receptors, as we will discuss elsewhere. Consistent and reproducible results were obtained, for muscimol binding, in membranes prepared with or without detergent; detergent extraction, however, enhances the affinity of muscimol for its putative receptors, as we will discuss later. At the above-mentioned displacer concentrations, both GABA and bicuculline were as efficient as non-labelled muscimol in displacing (^{3}H)muscimol specific binding.

To assess the effects of changes in visual input (both deprivation and stimulation) on postnatal receptor development in the chick optic tectum, the right eye of some chicks was either covered with a light-proof patch, just prior to hatching, or subjected from birth to daily 10-min sessions of stroboscopic stimulation (6,12). In these visually-deprived or stimulated chicks the densities of kainic acid and muscimol binding sites were measured independently in the left (experimental) and right (control) tectal lobes. Both the left and right cerebellar halves from these experimental chicks, and pooled tectal lobes (of both sides) from chicks of the same hatch, raised under standard conditions, were used as further controls.

The curves and developmental profiles shown in the figures are the means of at least 3 independent experiments, with 12 embryos or 6 chicks for each point. All standard deviation bars have been omitted to make figures simpler.

RESULTS

Developmental properties of the chick tectal membrane fractions used for the binding assays

Fig.1 shows the developmental changes in the amount of protein measured in the membrane preparations used for the binding assays, both in absolute terms (panel A), and expressed as % of the total homogenate protein (panel B). The lower protein content of the preparation used for kainic acid binding (●) reflects the absence of the 1000g pellet material. In the case of muscimol binding, extraction by Triton X-100 (Δ) results in a loss of 25-35% of the protein, relative to the simply frozen-thawed/washed material (o).

Saturation kinetics of (^{3}H)kainic acid and (^{3}H)muscimol binding to chick tectal membranes

Figs. 2 and 3 summarize the kinetic properties of the tectal membrane binding sites for kainic acid and muscimol. Only one statistically homogeneous population of high affinity binding sites, increasing in density with maturation, is revealed in each case, either in embryonic or postnatal tissues. When using (^{3}H)muscimol as the radioligand we have analyzed the effect of membrane extraction with 0.05% Triton X-100 on both the apparent affinity constant (K_d) and the density of binding sites at saturation (B_{max}). From the Eadie-Scatchard plots in Fig.3 we can conclude that the effect of Triton X-100, in the case of our tectal membrane preparation, appears to be limited to an increase of about 10 times in ligand-receptor affinity, without significant changes in the number of binding sites (the increases in B_{max} in the Triton X-100-treated membranes is more than offset by the associated loss of protein).

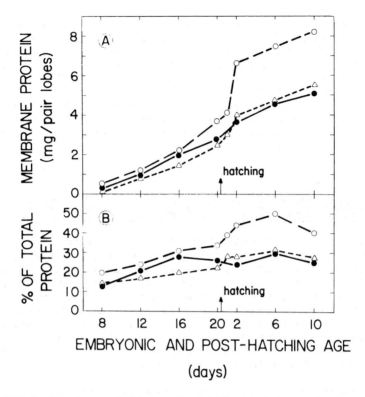

FIG.1. Developmental changes in the protein contents of
the chick tectal membrane preparations used to assay for
kainic acid and muscimol binding sites. A: Absolute results in mg of protein/pair of tectal lobes. B: Percent
of the total protein measured in the respective homogenates. (●) Membrane preparation used for kainic acid
binding. (o) Membrane preparation used for muscimol binding, without detergent extraction. (Δ) Membrane preparation used for muscimol binding, extracted with 0.05% Triton X-100, as described in Experimental.

Developmental profiles of the specific
(^{3}H)kainic acid and (^{3}H)muscimol
binding to chick tectal membranes

     Fig.4 shows the maturation-related changes in recep-
tor density (panel A: kainic acid or muscimol bound
per mg of membrane protein), and in the accumulated re
ceptor population (panel B: radioligand bound by the
membrane material obtained from a pair of tectal lobes
-Fig.1-). In the case of kainic acid (●) the assays
were performed with a 40nM concentration of radioli-

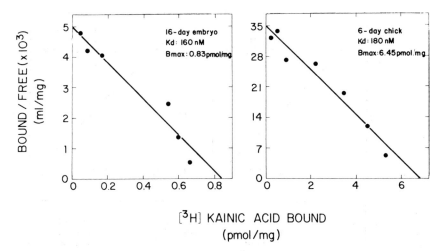

[³H] KAINIC ACID BOUND
(pmol/mg)

FIG.2. Eadie-Scatchard plots of (³H)kainic acid binding to
chick tectal membranes in 16-day embryos (left) and 6-day
chicks (right). The kinetic parameters K_d (apparent dissociation constant) and B_{max} (maximal binding capacity) are given
in the top right corner of each panel.

gand, while in the case of muscimol the assays were
carried out either at 40nM radioligand in frozen-thaw-
ed/washed membranes (o) or at 4nM in detergent-extracted membranes (Δ), taking into account the results in
Fig.3. The close similarity between the muscimol receptor density profiles (Fig.4A), under the two conditions, is consistent with the effect of Triton X-100
on muscimol binding sites being simply a change in ligand-receptor affinity.

The postnatal stabilization in muscimol receptor
density (Fig.4A) is confirmed by the results obtained
20 days after hatching, about 0.7pmol/mg (not shown in
the curve); conversely, by that age, kainic acid binding reaches a value of 2.1pmol/mg (that is, 5 times
the value at hatching). This marked divergence in receptor developmental profiles will be taken up again
in the Discussion.

Influence of early visual function
on postnatal receptor development

The fact that kainic acid receptor accumulation takes place mainly after birth, while the maturation of
muscimol binding sites is almost complete at the time
of eye-opening (Fig.4), suggested to us the possibility
that early changes in visual input levels might affect
and modulate the postnatal evolution of both receptor

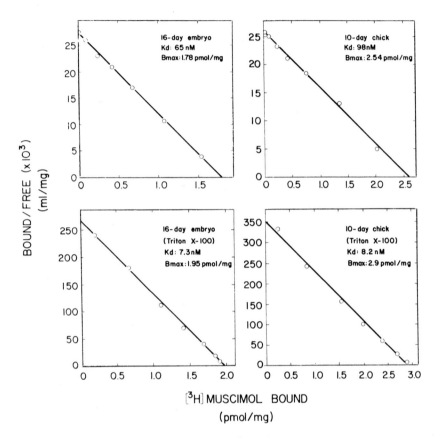

[3H] MUSCIMOL BOUND
(pmol/mg)

FIG.3. Eadie-Scatchard plots of (^{3}H)muscimol binding to chick
tectal membranes, either frozen-thawed and washed (above),or
additionally extracted with Triton X-100 (below), in 16-day
embryos (left) and 10-day chicks (right). K_d and B_{max} are given in the top right corner of each panel.

populations in a different way. Fig.5 summarizes the
results of a series of experiments exploring the effects of both monoocular deprivation and stimulation
on the postnatal development of kainic acid and muscimol binding sites in the contralateral optic lobe. The
curves in Fig.5 show that while kainic acid binding sites are rather strongly modulated by visual input (●,■),
during at least 20 days after hatching, the density
of muscimol receptors is only sensitive to light deprivation (o) the first few days after eye-opening. Interestingly, receptor densities appear to be regulated by
visual input only at times when a physiological increase in the number of binding sites is taking place (Fig.
4: note that muscimol receptor density reaches a peak

by day 1-2 after birth).
   No significant differences were observed, in kainic acid and muscimol binding sites, between left and right cerebellar halves, in the same chicks.

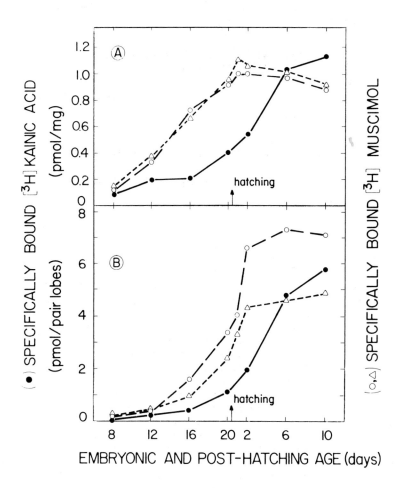

FIG.4. Developmental profiles of the densities (per mg of protein: A) and the total populations (per pair of tectal lobes: B) of receptor sites specifically labelled in chick tectal membranes by fixed concentrations of (^{3}H)kainic acid and (^{3}H) muscimol. (●) Receptor sites labelled by 40nM (^{3}H)kainic acid. (o) Receptor sites labelled by 40nM (^{3}H)muscimol (frozen-thawed/washed membranes). (Δ) Receptor sites labelled by 4nM (^{3}H) muscimol (Triton X-100-extracted membranes). The curves in B were obtained from the experimental data in A and the protein data given in Fig.1.

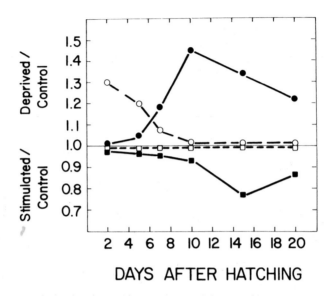

DAYS AFTER HATCHING

FIG.5. Effects of monoocular light deprivation and stimulation
on the postnatal development of specific binding sites for (^{3}H)
kainic acid and (^{3}H)muscimol in chick tectal membranes prepared
from the optic lobe opposite to the experimental eye. The right
eye in several series of chicks was either occluded with a
light-proof patch, just prior to hatching, or stimulated daily,
from birth, with a flashing light (10-min sessions). The ratios
between the densities of binding sites measured in the tectal
lobe opposite to the experimental eye and in the ipsilateral
lobe, at different times after birth, have been plotted in the
figure. (•) (^{3}H)kainic acid binding sites, deprivation experiments. (■) (^{3}H)kainic acid binding sites, stimulation experiments. (o) (^{3}H)muscimol binding sites, deprivation experiments.
(□) (^{3}H)muscimol binding sites, stimulation experiments. In the
case of (^{3}H)muscimol binding, extraction of the membranes with
Triton X-100 did not influence the ratios. The results obtained
in the ipsilateral control lobes of the experimental chicks
were not significantly different from the standard control values (tectal lobes of both sides) measured in normally-raised
chicks from the same lots. Ratios over 1.15 or below 0.9 are
statistically significant.

DISCUSSION

We have carried out a comparative analysis of the
developmental profiles of two populations of binding

sites, potentially specific for (glutamate-related) ex
citatory and (GABA-related) inhibitory amino acid
transmitters, labelled by (^{3}H)kainic acid and (^{3}H)mus-
cimol, respectively. The choice of kainic acid as the
excitatory ligand has been justified elsewhere (6,12).
In the case of inhibitory amino acid binding sites, it
is possible to use (^{3}H)GABA instead of (^{3}H)muscimol
with practically the same results (our unpublished data). However, (^{3}H)GABA binding seems to be more sensitive to minor variations in the experimental procedure,
as suggested by a considerable dispersion in the quantitative results of comparable experiments. Moreover,
the use of conformationally-restricted analogues as
radioligands has the potential advantage of a higher
target selectivity.

A number of published studies on both GABA and muscimol binding in membrane preparations from mammalian
central nervous system tissues, with or without detergent extraction, have revealed some heterogeneity of
the binding sites (1,4,7,8,10,15). This heterogeneity
is not dependent on the use of detergent-extracted mem
branes (1,8,10). In the chick tectal membrane preparations used in this study we have detected only single
binding modes for both kainic acid and muscimol (Figs.
2 and 3), with apparent dissociation constants (K_d)
that remain fairly stable from embryonic to postnatal
life, while the maximal binding capacities (at saturation: B_{max}) increase with development in keeping with
the maturation profiles in Fig.4. In the case of muscimol binding, extraction of the membranes with 0.05%
Triton X-100 increases the affinity of the radioligand
for its binding site by a factor of 10 (Fig.3). This
is clearly exemplified in the developmental profiles
in Fig.4A where 4nM (^{3}H)muscimol shows the same recep
tor-labelling efficiency in detergent-extracted membra
nes (Δ) as 40nM (^{3}H)muscimol in simply frozen-thawed/
washed membranes (o). The changes in GABA and muscimol
binding properties upon membrane treatment with Triton
X-100 have been alternatively ascribed to the more efficient removal of endogenous GABA (9), and of phospho
lipid or protein inhibitors (4,15,16). In our case,
however, further removal of GABA seems an unlikely cau
se since prolonged dialysis of frozen-thawed membranes
did not modify binding efficiency; on the other hand,
if endogenous modulators are responsible for the obser
ved changes, we must accept that these substances only
hamper, but do not completely block, the access of the
radioligand to the recognition site since we have registered an increase in affinity without any modification in the number of binding sites. Thus, at least in
the case of the chick tectum, it seems more appropria-

te to talk about a structural modification (by detergent) of the binding site environment leading to a fa-
cilitated access of the ligand and/or to a more efficient molecular interaction between ligand and receptor.

Perhaps the most interesting results presented in
this report refer to the different time-courses of maturation of the excitatory (kainic acid) and inhibitory (muscimol) amino acid binding sites, and the associated differences in the postnatal response of the
two receptor populations to changing levels of visual
input. As seen in Fig.4, while the chick tectal membra
nes reach the highest level of muscimol receptor densi
ty in the 24-48h that follow eye-opening (that is, the
GABAergic inhibitory or controlling system is mature -
from this point of view- almost before hatching), excitatory amino acid recognition sites (as represented by
kainic acid binding sites) start to visibly increase in
density just at hatching, and the growing density trend
is still noticeable after 20 days of postnatal life.

There is some evidence that in central motor and as-
sociative neuronal networks excitatory (permissive)
connections precede the onset of tonic inhibition (2,
13). From a functional point of view this translates
into an early appearance of spontaneous motility that
is only later 'refined' by adequate controlling (i.e.
inhibitory) mechanisms. Interestingly, the available
data on the time-course of development of glutamate,
GABA and muscimol binding sites in rat and mouse cerebellum are consistent with the above notion (3,5,11).
However, the situation in a sensory system (such as the
retinotectal visual system in the chick) makes it perhaps desirable to have an adequately developed and func
tionally ready controlling system before visual stimuli
(that do not appear gradually, as is the case with
motility, but suddenly at hatching) are free to penetra
te the excitatory pathways distributing sensory informa
tion throughout the central nervous system. The results
given in Fig.4 are compatible with this hypothetical
priority.

The differences between the regulatory effects of
both eye-opening and visual experience on the postnatal
ly measured densities of kainic acid and muscimol recep
tors (Fig.5) are similarly consistent with the general
views expressed in the previous paragraph. If we assume that the program responsible for the accumulation
of excitatory receptors in tectal membranes is triggered by some embryonic events (there are some receptor si
tes before hatching) it seems quite clear, from the results in Fig.5, that exposure to light (that is, sustained visual experience) plays a crucial role in the

postnatal modulation and progressive shutting-off of
that program: hence the higher and lower than normal
kainic acid receptor densities in signal-deprived (●)
and overstimulated (■) tectal lobes, respectively. On
the other hand, eye-opening (that is, acute visual experience) may act as a triggering factor to stop inhibitory receptor accumulation in tectal membranes, as
suggested by the developmental profiles in Fig.4 (o,Δ).
Light-deprivation is thus associated with higher muscimol receptor densities immediately after birth, although the deprived optic lobe seems to learn quite
soon that the receptor-accumulating program is to be
stopped, probably through commissural and other indirect influences (Fig.5, (o)). A similar mechanism may
help to explain the apparent 'habituation' observed in
the case of the light-regulation of kainic acid binding sites (Fig.5) where both deprived/control (●) and
stimulated/control (■) ratios become progressively clo
ser to 1.0 after two weeks of altered visual input.
    All the above results do furthermore confirm that
the chick retinotectal visual system is a convenient
and fruitful model to study the mutual regulatory influences between the maturation of neural communication (including synaptic) mechanisms and the onset and
development of function, as well as the associated phe
nomena of synaptic validation and experience-mediated
plasticity.

ACKNOWLEDGEMENTS

    This work was supported by grants from the 'Comi-
sión Asesora de Investigación Científica y Técnica',
the 'Plan Nacional de Prevención de la Subnormalidad',
and the 'Fundación Eugenio Rodríguez Pascual'

REFERENCES

1. Beaumont, K., Chilton, W.S., Yamamura, H.I., and Enna, S.J.
   (1978): Brain Res., 148:153-162.
2. Crain, S.M., and Bornstein, M.B. (1974): Brain Res., 68:351-
   357.
3. DeBarry, J., Vincendon, G., and Gombos, G. (1980): FEBS Lett.,
   109:175-179.
4. DeFeudis, F.V. (1980): Neuroscience, 5:675-688.
5. East, J.M., and Dutton, G.R. (1981): FEBS Lett., 123:307-311.
6. Gómez-Barriocanal, J., Barat, A., and Ramírez, G. (1982):
   Neurochem. Int., 4:157-166.
7. Herschel, M., and Baldessarini, R.J. (1979): Life Sci., 24:
   1849-1854.

8. Jordan, C.C., Matus, A.I., Piotrowski, W., and Wilkinson, D. (1982): J.Neurochem., 39:52-58.
9. Napias, C., Bergman, M.O., Van Ness, P.C., Greenlee, D.V., and Olsen, R.W. (1980): Life Sci., 27:1001-1011.
10. Olsen, R.W., Bergman, M.O., Van Ness, P.C., Lummis, S.C., Watkins, A.E., Napias, C., and Greenlee, D.V. (1981): Molec. Pharmacol., 19:217-227.
11. Palacios, J.M., Niehoff, D.L., and Kuhar, M.J. (1979): Brain Res., 179:390-395.
12. Ramírez, G., Gómez-Barriocanal, J., Escudero, E., Fernández-Quero, S., and Barat, A. (1981): In: Amino Acid Neurotransmitters, edited by F.V.DeFeudis and P.Mandel, pp. 467-474. Raven Press, New York.
13. Roberts, E. (1976): In: GABA in Nervous System Function, edited by E.Roberts, T.N.Chase and D.B.Tower, pp. 515-539, Raven Press, New York.
14. Snodgrass, S.R. (1978): Nature, 273:392-394.
15. Toffano, G., Guidotti, A., and Costa, E. (1978): Proc. Natl. Acad. Sci. USA, 75:4024-4028.
16. Toffano, G., Aldinio, C., Balzano, M., Leon, A., and Savoini, G. (1981): Brain Res., 222:95-102.
17. Villafruela, M.J., Barat, A., Manrique, E., Villa, S., and Ramírez, G. (1981): Dev. Neurosci., 4:25-36.

CNS Receptors—From Molecular
Pharmacology to Behavior, edited by
P. Mandel and F. V. DeFeudis.
Raven Press, New York © 1983.

L-Glutamate Receptor Populations in Synaptic Membranes: Effects of Ions and Pharmacological Characteristics

*Graham E. Fagg, E. Edward Mena, and Carl W. Cotman

Department of Psychobiology, University of California, Irvine, California 92717

Acidic amino acids are thought to function as synaptic transmitters at many sites in the mammalian central nervous system
(CNS)(3,16,32), and studies of their receptors are a prerequisite
for understanding both the function and dysfunction of the CNS,
and for the rational development of pharmacological agents with
which to combat neurological disorders. Electrophysiological
examination of a large number of excitants and their sensitivity
to antagonism by D-α-aminoadipate (DαAA) and glutamate diethyl
ester has led to a '3-receptor' classification scheme for excitatory amino acids based on the most selective agonists, N-methyl-
D-aspartate (NMDA), quisqualate and kainate; L-glutamate and L-
aspartate are less specific but show some preference for the
quisqualate and NMDA receptor types, respectively (3,32). A
number of authors have recently described an additional receptor
type which is present at some acidic amino acid-using synapses,
is highly sensitive to the glutamate analogue L-2-amino-4-
phosphonobutyrate (APB), and apparently does not conform to the
'3-receptor' scheme previously outlined (5,7,15,24,29).
 Parallel biochemical studies are more limited, partly due to
the lack of a wide range of radiolabeled ligands, although
distinct binding sites for L-glutamate, L-aspartate and kainate
have recently been identified in synaptic plasma membrane (SPM)
fractions isolated from brain tissue (10,11,17,21,28). However,
pharmacological analyses have demonstrated a number of anomalies
between the sites labeled in binding assays and those examined
electrophysiologically (see ref. 27), and it has proven difficult
to equate conclusively binding sites with physiological synaptic
receptors.
 The goal of our research has been to identify and study the

---

*Present address: Friedrich Miescher Institut, P.O. Box 273, CH-
4002 Basel, Switzerland.

properties of excitatory amino acid receptors in SPMS in vitro
and, to this end, we have focused our attention on methodological
discrepancies between electrophysiological and ligand binding
experiments. One notable difference is the composition of the
medium employed in these two types of study, binding assays are
commonly conducted using simple buffer systems (e.g., Tris-Cl,
Tris-acetate), whereas electrophysiological investigations util-
ize a complex medium of similar ionic composition to that occurring in the extracellular space of the CNS. This is of particular
significance in view of recent reports that a number of ions are
capable of modifying the interaction between receptor agonists/
antagonists and their binding sites (see refs. 14,25,30). Here we
report that Cl^- and Ca^{2+} regulate the expression of distinct L-
glutamate binding sites in SPMs and further, that the pharmacological properties of Cl^-/Ca^{2+}-dependent and -independent sites
closely resemble those of the L-APB and NMDA receptor populations
identified using electrophysiological techniques.

EXPERIMENTAL OBSERVATIONS

Effects of ions on L-glutamate binding

Cl^- and Ca^{2+} ions. Earlier studies from this laboratory demonstrated that the inclusion of 2.5 mM $CaCl_2$ in a HEPES-KOH assay
buffer markedly increased the number of binding sites for L-[^{3}H]-
glutamate in rat brain SPMs, with no change in the apparent
affinity of the interaction (11). Recent experiments show that
both Ca^{2+} and Cl^- are involved in this response (19,20). In the
absence of exogenous Ca^{2+}, Cl^- (added as Tris-Cl or NH_4Cl) caused
a pronounced increase in the binding of L-glutamate (50 nM concentration), achieving a maximum effect of 2.4 ± 0.3 times the
basal level at a concentration of about 10 mM; this stimulation
exhibited saturation kinetics, with a K_d of 3.8 ± 0.2 mM Cl^-. As
in the case of $CaCl_2$ (11), the effect of Cl^- appeared to involve
an increase in the number of L-glutamate binding sites and no
change in affinity (Fagg et al., unpublished observations).
Experiments with a range of anions indicated that Br^-, NO_3^-
and $HCOO^-$ also were able to stimulate L-glutamate binding, but
ions such as F^-, acetate, propionate, SO_4^{2-} and PO_4^{3-} could not
(Mena et al., submitted; see Fig. 1).
In contrast to Cl^-, Ca^{2+} alone (added as the acetate salt)
had little effect on L-glutamate binding (0.8 ± 0.2 times basal
binding at 10 mM Ca^{2+}). However, in the presence of an 'active'
anion (such as Cl^- or NO_3^-), Ca^{2+} augmented L-glutamate binding
to a greater level than that caused by the anion alone; thus, inclusion of 10 mM $CaCl_2$ in the assay buffer increased L-glutamate
binding to 3.3 ± 0.3 times the basal level (19).
Cl^-/Ca^{2+} interactions. The interaction between Ca^{2+} and Cl^-
in enhancing L-glutamate binding was studied by constructing
dose-response curves for each ion in the presence of varying concentrations of the other (using a fixed 50 nM L-[^{3}H]glutamate
concentration). Scatchard analyses of these curves demonstrated

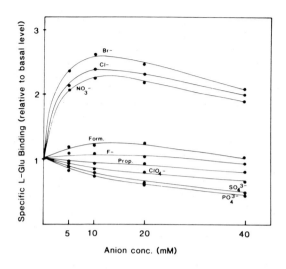

FIG. 1. Effect of various anions on the binding of L-[^{3}H]glutamate to rat forebrain SPMs. Binding was assayed using 0.2-0.3 mg SPM protein and 50 nM L-[^{3}H]glutamate; incubations (30°C, 20 min) were terminated by centrifugation for 3 min in a Microfuge (Beckman)(12). The level of glutamate binding in the presence of each anion is expressed relative to the basal level (=1; measured in Tris-acetate buffer pH 7.2). Values are means from 3-4 separate experiments (data from Mena et al., submitted).

that raising the Ca^{2+} concentration of the assay buffer increased the B_{max} for Cl^--enhancement of L-glutamate binding without affecting the K_d. Hence, in the presence of 5 mM EGTA the K_d for Cl^- was 3.8 ± 0.6 mM and the B_{max} 1.8 ± 0.4 pmol glutamate bound/mg protein, while in the presence of 1 mM Ca^{2+} the K_d was 3.6 ± 0.6 mM and the B_{max} 6.8 ± 1.2 pmol/mg protein. On the other hand, as the Cl^- concentration was increased from 5 mM to 42 mM, the K_d for Ca^{2+}-enhancement of L-glutamate binding progressively decreased (from 182 ± 42 µM to 29 ± 15 µM) and the B_{max} increased (from 4.7 ± 0.4 to 9.0 ± 1.9 pmol/mg protein). In all cases, Hill plots indicated an absence of cooperativity (20; Mena et al., submitted).

Are the Cl^- and Ca^{2+} effects reversible? A number of authors have suggested that Ca^{2+} stimulates L-glutamate binding to SPMs by activating a membrane-bound protease which irreversibly unmasks additional binding sites (1,31). We examined the reversibility of both the Cl^- and the Ca^{2+} effects using the following approaches. (1) SPMs were incubated (30°C, 30 min) in Tris-Cl buffer (42 mM Cl^-) containing 1 mM Ca^{2+}, and were subsequently washed free of these ions by 3-fold resuspension and centrifugation in Tris-acetate buffer. When assayed in Tris-acetate buffer, the level of L-glutamate binding in these membranes was effectively unchanged from that in untreated membranes, as was the magnitude of the $CaCl_2$ stimulation. (2) The binding of L-glutamate to SPMs was assayed in 50 mM Tris-Cl containing 0.5 mM Ca^{2+}. Addition of 5 mM EGTA 2 min prior to termination of the 20 min assay reduced the amount of L-glutamate bound essentially to the level measured when EGTA was added prior to initiation of the assay. These observations indicate that, when adequate procedures are employed to remove ions from treated SPMs, both Cl^- and Ca^{2+} enhancements of L-glutamate binding exhibit a reversibility not expected of a protease-mediated process (20, Mena et al., submitted).

Na^+ ions. Na^+ has been reported to exert a biphasic effect on the binding of L-glutamate to SPMs, being inhibitory at concentrations below 5 mM and stimulatory at concentrations greater than 40 mM (stimulation is thought to result from the binding of glutamate to Na^+-dependent transport sites, see ref. 2). Our data indicate that a biphasic curve is apparent only when SPMs are assayed in Cl^--containing buffers, whereas in the absence of this anion a single stimulatory component is observed (19, Mena et al., unpublished observations). Hence, low concentrations of Na^+ appear to inhibit specifically that portion of L-glutamate binding introduced by Cl^-.

Pharmacological specificity of L-glutamate binding

Effects of Cl^- and Ca^{2+} ions. The effects of Cl^- and Ca^{2+} on the pharmacological properties of L-$[^3H]$glutamate binding to SPMs were examined initially using a homologous series of acidic amino acid analogues - the α-amino-ω-phosphonic acid derivatives of propionic (APP), butyric (APB) and valeric (APV) acids. Inclusion

TABLE 1. Pharmacological   specificity of L-glutamate binding in the presence and absence of Cl^- and Ca^{2+}: phosphonic acid analogues

Compound[a]	Percent inhibition of L-glutamate binding	
	Zero $CaCl_2$	2.5 mM $CaCl_2$
DL-APP	5 ± 5	8 ± 3
L-APB	5 ± 8	60 ± 6
D-APB	9 ± 12	21 ± 5
DL-APV	42 ± 13	53 ± 6
DL-APHX	22 ± 8	64 ± 7
L-APH	28 ± 6	60 ± 7
D-APH	50 ± 3	53 ± 10

[a]Compounds were included in the assay buffer to give a final concentration of 100 µM, except the L and D isomers of APB and APH, which were used at 50 µM. Abbreviations are defined in the text. Values are means ± S.E.M. from 4-6 separate experiments (data are from ref. 8 and Fagg et al., submitted).

of $CaCl_2$ in the assay buffer markedly altered the relative inhibitory potencies of these three compounds; in the absence of $CaCl_2$ APV was more effective than APB and APP as a displacer of L-glutamate binding, whereas APB was most potent in the presence of these ions (8; see Table 2).

Kinetic analyses in the presence of $CaCl_2$ demonstrated that APB inhibited L-glutamate binding competitively (8), and that DL-APB, its stereoisomers, and DL-APV all competed with different affinities for the same L-glutamate binding site, which represented about 80% of the L-glutamate bound (Fig. 2a). The K_i values calculated from these plots showed that the order of potency for inhibition of L-glutamate binding was APB > APV > APP, with L-APB 15-fold more effective than its enantiomer (Table 2). Moreover, with the exception of APV, which appears to be a potent inhibitor of NMDA-induced neuronal excitation (32), these values are in close agreement with those determined for the antagonism of perforant path-evoked field potentials in the outer molecular layer of the rat dentate gyrus _in vitro_ (15; see Table 2).

Are APB-insensitive binding sites identical to Cl^-/Ca^{2+}-independent sites? In order to determine whether the approximately 20% APB-resistant L-glutamate binding sites observed in the presence of $CaCl_2$ could be equated with the Cl^-/Ca^{2+}-independent sites, a comparison was made of the residual L-glutamate binding after inhibition by APB in the two assay conditions ($\pm$ $CaCl_2$).

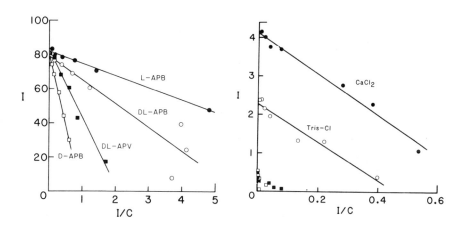

FIG. 2. (a) Scatchard plots describing the inhibition of L-[^{3}H]-glutamate binding by L-APB ($\bullet$), D-APB ($\square$), DL-APB ($\circ$) and DL-APV ($\blacksquare$) in the presence of 2.5 mM $CaCl_2$. I is the percent inhibition of specific L-glutamate binding, and C the inhibitor concentration (1-1000 μM). (b) Scatchard plots of the inhibition of L-[^{3}H]glutamate binding by DL-APB in buffer alone ($\square$), or in the presence of 2.5 mM Ca^{2+} (acetate, $\blacksquare$), of 5 mM Cl^- (Tris-Cl, $\circ$), or of 2.5 mM $CaCl_2$ ($\bullet$). I is the amount (pmol/mg protein) of APB-sensitive L-glutamate binding determined at concentrations of DL-APB from 1 to 500 μM. (Data are from ref. 8).

TABLE 2. Kinetic parameters[a] for the inhibition of L-glutamate binding and of synaptically-evoked responses: phosphonic acid analogues

Compound	Synaptic response[b]	L-glutamate binding	
	K_i (μM)	K_i (μM)	I_{max} (%)
DL-APP	5000	>1000	ND
L-APB	2.5	5 ± 1	81 ± 3
D-APB	100	75 ± 15	80 ± 4
DL-APV	250	39 (37,40)	84 (83,85)
DL-APHX	ND	5 ± 3	82 ± 1
L-APH	ND	12 ± 6	86 ± 3
D-APH	ND	48 ± 20	89 ± 1

[a]Apparent K_i and I_{max} (maximum percent inhibition) values were determined by Scatchard analyses (see Fig. 2a), and K_i values were corrected for the L-[^{3}H]glutamate concentration in the assay (50 nM). Values are means ± S.E.M. from 2-5 separate experiments (data from ref. 8 and from Fagg et al., submitted). [b]Apparent K_i values for antagonism of lateral perforant path-evoked field potentials in the rat dentate gyrus in vitro (calculated from ref. 15). ND, not determined.

In the presence of 0.1 mM L-APB (a concentration giving near maximal inhibition), the amount of L-glutamate bound to SPMs was similar whether $CaCl_2$ was included in the assay buffer or not (zero $CaCl_2$, 1.5 ± 0.5 pmol/mg protein; 2.5 mM $CaCl_2$, 1.7 ± 0.5 pmol/mg protein) despite the observation that the specific L-glutamate binding was augmented more than 3-fold by these ions (8). Hence, the increase in L-glutamate binding induced by Cl^- and Ca^{2+} appears to represent the introduction of a new population of L-glutamate binding sites which are selectively sensitive to inhibition by APB.

Do both Cl^- and Ca^{2+} expose APB-sensitive L-glutamate binding sites? The observations presented above indicate that Cl^- stimulates L-glutamate binding to SPMs and that Ca^{2+} acts only in the presence of Cl^- to enhance this response further. The pharmacological studies described in the preceding section were conducted in the presence of both Cl^- and Ca^{2+} (as $CaCl_2$), and these investigations demonstrated that the additional binding sites revealed by these ions in combination were of the APB-sensitive type. Further experiments to define the role of each ion revealed that the K_i values for the inhibition of L-glutamate binding by APB were similar (parallel lines in Scatchard plots) both when 5 mM Cl^- and 2.5 mM $CaCl_2$ were included in the assay buffer (Fig. 2b). However, almost 2-fold more APB-sensitive sites were apparent in the presence of $CaCl_2$ than in the presence of Cl^- alone. In the presence of only 2.5 mM Ca^{2+} or in the absence of added ions, a small number of APB-sensitive L-glutamate binding sites were detected (Fig. 2b), possibly due to the presence of residual Cl⁻ and/or Ca^{2+} in the SPM preparation.

Additional experiments indicated that pretreatment of SPMs with EDTA or inclusion of 10 mM EDTA in the assay buffer (a) abolished the small degree of APB sensitivity observed in the absence of added ions and (b) reduced (but did not abolish) the number of APB-sensitive sites introduced by 5 mM Cl⁻ (8). These data suggest that Cl⁻ is necessary to unmask the APB-sensitive population of L-glutamate binding sites in SPMs and that Ca^{2+}, possibly by binding to the receptor molecule, is required to reveal the full extent of this response.

Effects of Na⁺. The data presented earlier in this chapter indicated that low concentrations (1-5 mM) of Na⁺ specifically inhibit the Cl⁻-stimulated component of L-glutamate binding, and therefore one would predict that there should be no APB-sensitive binding in the presence of this cation. Assays conducted in the presence of 5 mM Na⁺ (in addition to Cl⁻ and Ca^{2+}) verified that this was indeed so. Essentially no displacement of L-glutamate binding was observed when using concentrations of DL-APB (up to 200 µM) sufficient to give near-maximal inhibition of Cl⁻/Ca^{2+}-dependent binding in the absence of Na⁺ (Fagg et al., unpublished observations).

General pharmacological properties of Cl⁻/Ca^{2+}-dependent and -independent L-glutamate binding. In addition to the phosphonic acid derivatives, the pharmacological specificities of Cl⁻/Ca^{2+}-dependent and -independent L-glutamate binding sites were assessed using analogues which, through electrophysiological analyses, have been proposed as agonists or antagonists of the various excitatory amino acid receptor classes (32). Inhibition studies demonstrated that, although L-glutamate was of similar potency at both sites, other compounds displayed remarkable differences in potency at Cl⁻/Ca^{2+}-dependent and -independent binding sites (Fagg et al., submitted, see Table 3). L-aspartate was some 10-fold more potent at Cl⁻/Ca^{2+}-independent than at -dependent sites, whereas the D isomers of both aspartate and glutamate exhibited the opposite trend. DαAA inhibited Cl⁻/Ca^{2+}-dependent L-glutamate binding with a K_i of 1µM but was much less effective in the absence of these ions (24 ± 1% inhibition at 1 mM). This compound maximally inhibited about 80% of Cl⁻/Ca^{2+}-dependent binding sites, and experiments using 0.1 mM DαAA and 0.5 mM DL-APB alone and in combination indicated that their effects were not additive (% inhibition: 78 ± 5, 79 ± 6 and 81 ± 6, respectively). Hence, both APB and DαAA appear to bind principally to the Cl⁻/Ca^{2+}-dependent population of sites.

The heterocyclic excitants, quisqualate and ibotenate, were unusual in exhibiting curvilinear Scatchard plots in the presence of $CaCl_2$. Computer analyses indicated that these two compounds maximally inhibited 70-75% of Cl⁻/Ca^{2+}-dependent binding with K_i values in the nanomolar range, and the remaining 25% with lower affinity (Table 3). In the absence of Cl⁻ and Ca^{2+}, only low affinity inhibition components were observed. Another cyclic analogue, DL-cis-2,3-piperidine dicarboxylate (cis-2,3-PDA) was

TABLE 4. Kinetic parameters[a] for the inhibition of L-glutamate
binding to Cl^-/Ca^{2+}-dependent and -independent sites

Compound	Zero $CaCl_2$		2.5 mM $CaCl_2$	
	K_i (μM)	I_{max} (%)	K_i (μM)	I_{max} (%)
L-aspartate	0.813 ± 0.041	98 ± 3	11 ± 2	84 ± 11
D-aspartate	270 ± 9	75 ± 2	27 ± 6	79 ± 3
L-glutamate	0.388 ± 0.001	99 ± 3	0.445 ± 0.029	99 ± 1
D-glutamate	244 ± 92	66 ± 3	9 ± 1	90 ± 6
DαAA	ND	ND	1.2 ± 0.3	78 ± 6
DL-quisqualate	89 ± 22	94 ± 3	0.103 ± 0.035	72 ± 7
			41 ± 20	23 ± 6
DL-ibotenate	117 ± 23	99 ± 6	0.494 ± 0.076	74 ± 7
			76 ± 26	24 ± 6
DL-cis-2,3-PDA	471 ± 56	92 ± 2	ND	ND

[a]Kinetic parameters were determined by non-linear least squares
curve fitting of untransformed data (9). Assays conducted under
the 'zero $CaCl_2$' condition included 0.5 mM DL-APB to suppress
residual APB-sensitive L-glutamate binding. Values are means ±
S.E.M. from 3 separate experiments (from Fagg et al., submitted).

examined only in the absence of $CaCl_2$ as earlier observations indicated it to be more effective under these conditions (8); however, its potency was low.
    A number of other analogues were tested as inhibitors of L-
glutamate binding at a concentration of 100 μM (8,13). Notably,
NMA displaced about 30% of L-glutamate binding in the absence of
Cl^- and Ca^{2+}, and was less effective in the presence of these
ions. Kainate and GABA were ineffective at both sites.
    The phosphonic acid analogues deserve further mention at this
point, since their relative potencies as antagonists of NMDA-
evoked excitation (6,7,26) provide a useful 'marker' for this
receptor type. Our initial investigations were conducted using
APP, APB and APV, although the recent availability of the longer
chain hexanoate (APHX) and heptanoate (APH) derivatives has allowed us to extend our observations. NMDA receptors are characterized by their preference for the 5-carbon (APV) and 7-carbon
(APH) members of this series, with maximal activity residing in
the D isomers (6,7,26), and this specificity is quite unlike that
observed at Cl^-/Ca^{2+}-dependent L-glutamate binding sites (Tables
1 and 2). However, when tested as inhibitors of L-glutamate
binding in the absence of $CaCl_2$, the relative potencies of these
compounds corresponded closely to that expected of an NMDA receptor (Table 1). Kinetic analyses showed that DL-APV and D-APH
were of similar potency (K_i's 7 ± 3 μM and 6 μM, respectively)
and maximally inhibited 50-60% of the Cl^-/Ca^{2+}-independent specific L-glutamate binding (Fagg et al., submitted).

CONCLUSIONS AND IMPLICATIONS

The observations presented in this chapter indicate that Na^+-independent binding sites for L-glutamate may be subdivided into two distinct populations on the basis of their Cl^- and Ca^{2+} requirements and their pharmacological characteristics. Both sites exhibit a number of properties indicative of roles as synaptic receptors. Both are enriched in SPMs (8,12), show differential distributions within the CNS (23; Whittemore et al., submitted), and are sensitive to inhibition by a number of compounds with agonist or antagonist activity at acidic amino acid receptor sites (this chapter). The Cl^-/Ca^{2+}-dependent (APB-sensitive) binding sites display a pharmacological specificity (assessed using the shorter chain phosphonic acid analogues) which closely corresponds to that determined electrophysiologically at the perforant path-granule cell synapse in the rat dentate gyrus (15) where glutamate is probably the neurotransmitter (3). Recent studies have demonstrated the existence of APB-sensitive sites both at the photoreceptor-ON bipolar cell synapse in the retina (29)(where the potencies of the phosphonic acid derivatives were shown to be similar to that reported here, ref. 24) and at the primary afferent-motoneuron synapse in the spinal cord (5,7). Hence, there is strong evidence for proposing that Cl^-/Ca^{2+}-dependent L-glutamate binding sites are of physiological significance at acidic amino acid-using synapses in the CNS.

The Cl^-/Ca^{2+}-independent population displays a number of properties which suggest that some of these sites function as NMDA-type receptors. Fundamental to this postulate is the characteristic pharmacological profile demonstrated amongst the phosphonic acid homologues, the high potencies of DL-APV and D-APH at these sites, and the finding that NMA is a more effective inhibitor of L-glutamate binding in the absence than in the presence of Cl^- and Ca^{2+} (8). These NMDA receptor-like sites probably represent a sub-population of Cl^-/Ca^{2+}-independent binding sites, since DL-APV, D-APH and the NMDA receptor agonists D-glutamate and D-aspartate maximally inhibited only 50-70% of L-glutamate binding. Although some anomalies are apparent (the similar potencies of quisqualate and ibotenate, and the low potency of $D_\alpha AA$ at these sites), these data provide the most compelling description to date of putative NMDA receptors in isolated membrane fractions, and additionally confirm the conclusions of electrophysiological studies, that L-glutamate is a 'mixed agonist' (32) acting at multiple acidic amino acid receptor sites.

A survey of the literature reveals that the K_i values for inhibition of L-glutamate binding presented here are in good agreement with those reported by other investigators, when the wide variations in assay methodology are taken into account. Binding assays for L-glutamate and L-aspartate have been conducted using Cl^--containing (Tris-Cl) and Ca^{2+}-chelating (Tris-citrate) buffers, and the present study helps to resolve a number of discrepancies between laboratories.

A question for the future concerns the precise function of

Cl^-/Ca^{2+}-dependent (APB-sensitive) L-glutamate binding sites. The anion specificity for stimulation of glutamate binding suggests, by analogy with the GABA-benzodiazepine system (25), that these sites may be linked to a membrane Cl^- channel, and therefore it is of interest that, at the retinal ON-bipolar cell, APB has been shown to mimic the hyperpolarizing actions of the natural transmitter (glutamate?)(29), possibly by decreasing Cl^- conductance (22). Cl^-/Ca^{2+}-dependent L-glutamate binding sites may be located postsynaptically, just as hyperpolarizing L-glutamate receptors are found on the locust muscle membrane (4), or presynaptically, to function as autoreceptors regulating the release of acidic amino acid neurotransmitters (18). The studies reported here will facilitate solution of this question, and hopefully will lead to greater understanding of the mechanisms of excitatory amino acid synaptic transmission in the CNS.

Acknowledgements

We should like to thank Drs. Alan Foster, Dan Monaghan, Tom Lanthorn, Eric Harris, Alan Ganong and Scott Whittemore for their participation in or valuable comment on this work, and Drs. J.C. Watkins, J.F. Collins, H. Shinozaki and C.H. Eugster for generous gifts of compounds. This work was supported by grant NS 08957 from the National Institutes of Health.

REFERENCES

1. Baudry, M. and Lynch, G. (1980): Proc. Natl. Acad. Sci. USA., 77: 2298-2302.
2. Baudry, M. and Lynch, G. (1981): J. Neurochem., 36: 811-820.
3. Cotman, C.W., Foster, A.C. and Lanthorn, T.H. (1981): Adv. Biochem. Psychopharmac., 27: 1-27.
4. Cull-Candy, S.G. and Usherwood, P.N.R. (1973): Nature, 246: 62-64.
5. Davies, J. and Watkins, J.C. (1982): Brain Res., 235: 378-386.
6. Davies, J., Francis, A.A., Jones, A.W. and Watkins, J.C. (1981): Neurosci. Lett., 21: 77-81.
7. Evans, R.H., Francis, A.A., Jones, A.W., Smith, D.A.S. and Watkins, J.C. (1982): Br. J. Pharmac., 75: 65-75.
8. Fagg, G.E., Foster, A.C., Mena, E.E. and Cotman, C.W. (1982): J. Neurosci., 2: 958-965.
9. Fagg, G.E., Foster, A.C., Harris, E.W., Lanthorn, T.H. and Cotman, C.W. (1982): Neurosci. Lett., in press.
10. Foster, A.C. and Roberts, P.J. (1978): J. Neurochem., 31: 1467-1477.
11. Foster, A.C., Fagg, G.E., Mena, E.E. and Cotman, C.W. (1981): Brain Res., 229: 246-250.
12. Foster, A.C., Mena, E.E., Fagg, G.E. and Cotman, C.W. (1981): J. Neurosci., 1: 620-625.
13. Foster, A.C., Fagg, G.E., Harris, E.W. and Cotman, C.W. (1982): Brain Res., 242: 374-377.

14. Hoffman, B.B. and Lefkowitz, R.J. (1980): Ann. Rev. Pharmac. Toxicol., 20: 581-608.
15. Koerner, J.F. and Cotman, C.W. (1981): Brain Res., 216: 192-198.
16. Lane, J.D., Smith, J.E. and Fagg, G.E. (1982): In: Neurobiology of Opiate Reward Mechanisms, edited by J.E. Smith and J.D. Lane. Elsevier, Amsterdam, in press.
17. London, E.D. and Coyle, J.T. (1979): Eur. J. Pharmac., 56: 287-290.
18. McBean, G.J. and Roberts, P.J. (1981): Nature, 291: 593-594.
19. Mena, E.E., Fagg, G.E. and Cotman, C.W. (1982): Brain Res., 243, 378-381.
20. Mena, E.E., Fagg, G.E., Monaghan, D.T. and Cotman, C.W. (1982): Soc. Neurosci. Abstr., 8, in press.
21. Michaelis, E.K., Michaelis, M.L. and Grubbs, R.D. (1980): FEBS Lett., 118: 55-57.
22. Miller, R.F. and Dacheux, R.F. (1976): J. Gen. Physiol., 67: 639-659.
23. Monaghan, D.T., Foster, A.C., Fagg, G.E., Mena, E.E. and Cotman, C.W. (1981): Soc. Neurosci. Abstr., 7: 503.
24. Neal, M.J., Cunningham, J.R., James, T.A., Josephs, M. and Collins, J.F. (1981): Neurosci. Lett., 26: 301-305.
25. Olsen, R.W. (1982): Ann. Rev. Pharmac. Toxicol., 22: 245-277.
26. Perkins, M.N., Stone, T.W., Collins, J.F. and Curry, K. (1981): Neurosci. Lett., 23, 333-336.
27. Roberts, P.J. (1981): Adv. Biochem. Psychopharmac., 28: 379-386.
28. Sharif, N.A. and Roberts, P.J. (1981): Brain Res., 211: 293-303.
29. Slaughter, M.M. and Miller, R.F. (1981): Science, 211: 182-185.
30. Snyder, S.H. and Childers, S.R. (1979): Ann. Rev. Neurosci., 2: 35-64.
31. Vargas, F., Greenbaum, L. and Costa, E. (1980): Neuropharmacology, 19: 791-794.
32. Watkins, J.C. and Evans, R.H. (1981): Ann. Rev. Pharmac. Toxicol., 21: 165-204.

CNS Receptors—From Molecular
Pharmacology to Behavior, edited by
P. Mandel and F. V. DeFeudis.
Raven Press, New York © 1983.

Cysteine Sulfinate Receptors in the Rat CNS

*M. Recasens, *F. Saadoun, **M. Maitre, *M. Baudry,
*G. Lynch, **P. Mandel, and *G. Vincendon

*Department of Psychobiology, University of California; and **Unite 44 de l'INSERM,
Université Louis Pasteur, 67084 Strasbourg Cedex, France

Increasing evidence, based mainly on the actions of a range
of selective antagonists, indicates the existence of several acidic
amino acid receptors (11,12, 23,24). On the basis of their agonist specificities, they have been termed N methyl-D-aspartate,
quisqualate and kainate and essentially related to the proposed
transmitter function of L-glutamate and L-Aspartate (5,6,22). We
recently suggested a neurotransmitter role for another excitatory compound: L-cysteine sulfinate (19,20): an endogenous
sulfur-containing acid amino acid, structurally related to
aspartate and glutamate, and this has been extended by other
laboratories (9,10).

This presentation discusses the properties of the cysteine
sulfinate (CSA) receptor binding site, its specificity, and its
possible physiological role in the mechanisms of synaptic transmission.

Properties of cysteine sulfinate receptor binding sites

The Na+ independent specific L-[3H] CSA binding to synaptic
membranes derived from rat brain was saturable and appeared to
occur by a single high affinity process with a Kd of about 100
nM (20). However, depending on the type of synaptic membranes
used (light, medium or high density membranes) the Kd varied
between 60 to 500 nM. The Na+-independent specific L-[3H] CSA
binding was maximal at pH 7.5 and decreased sharply at basic and
acidic values. It reaches the equilibrium after 40 min of incubation at 0°C, although this time was found variable according
again to the membrane preparation used (Recasens et al, unpub-

lished results). As could be expected for a putative neurotransmitter, the specific L-[^{3}H] CSA binding was enriched in
synaptic membranes as compared to whole brain homogenate (19).
Moreover, the density of L-[^{3}H]CSA binding sites was heterogeneous among the brain regions. The region displaying the
highest L-[^{3}H]CSA binding was the cerebellum (19,20). Although
the density of binding sites in a brain region may be related
usually to the "density of innervation" of that region by
neurons using the relevant neurotransmitter (the "density of
innervation" must be derived from independent studies of levels
of the neurotransmitter and of its synthetic enzymes, or
metabolites, of high affinity uptake sites and of other presynaptic markers), no obvious correlations between the density
of CSA binding sites and the "density of innervation" occurred,
as shown in Table I. This could be explained by: the differential localisations of the presynaptic markers to cell bodies
versus nerve terminals, which have been found for the CSA
synthesizing and degradative enzymes (18); the different size
and types of nerve terminals using the same transmitter; the
lack of proportionality between the number of terminals and
the number of neurons receiving these nerve terminals; the
fact that the CSA receptor sites represent a subpopulation of
sites and not all the sites responding to the given neurotransmitter (shown later in this chapter); finally, by the lack of
specificity of the high affinity uptake system, probably shared
by all the acid amino acids and at least by CSA, glutamate and
aspartate (20). High concentrations of monovalent cations
(K$^+$, Li$^+$) usually inhibited the L-[^{3}H]CSA binding. Only Na$^+$
ions produce an increase in the L-[^{3}H]CSA binding at concentrations of Na$^+$ above 30 mM. The divalent cations (Mn^{++}, Mg^{++},
Ca^{++}) first increased the L-[^{3}H]CSA binding to synaptic membranes and inhibited it at higher concentrations (19). In
sum, these data indicated that the "specific" L-[^{3}H]CSA binding
to synaptic membrane possessed many characteristics which
could be expected of an interaction with a physiological L-CSA
receptor.

Pharmacological specificity of the L-[^{3}H]CSA binding.
    *Substrate specificity of the Na$^+$-independent specific
L-[^{3}H] CSA binding
        The pharmacological specificity is particularly crucial in
evaluating the significance of the L-[^{3}H]CSA binding to synaptic membranes (Table II). L-CSA was the most potent inhibitor,
being threefold more potent than L-glutamate and eighty times
more potent than L-aspartate. Some other amino acids such as
taurine, glycine and GABA did not affect this binding. Kainic
acid and N-methyl-DL-aspartate, which are both considered as a
marker of one type of acid amino acid receptor site were also
ineffective in displacing L-[^{3}H]CSA binding. It should be
noted that the most potent inhibitors were α-amino acids with
an acidic group in position ω. Compounds containing ω-carboxyl
group (glutamate, aspartate) were more efficient than those

TABLE I: Regional distribution of CSA , of the activities of its metabolizing enzymes, of L-CSA uptake and binding

	CSA content (a) nmol/g wet wt	Synthesizing Enzyme (CO) (b) µmol/h/mg prot	Degradative Enzymes CSD(c)	CSA-T(d)	L-[³H] CSA uptake (e) pmol/30s/mg prot	L-[³H] CSA binding (f) pmol/mg prot
CEREBRAL CORTEX	287	0.42	3.16	11.4	839	1.04
CEREBELLUM	253	0.69	2.05	8.36	551	2.65
HYPOTHALAMUS	168	0.99	-	10.7	658	0.98
PONS MEDULLA	156	1.32	2.95	8.14	428	1.15
HIPPOCAMPUS	149	0.67	-	9.69	-	0.46
SPINAL CORD	132	0.86	-	-	-	-
STRIATUM	129	-	-	12.4	911	0.85
OLFACTORY BULBS	108	-	-	7.93	-	-
MIDBRAIN	68	-	3.26	-	-	-

a) Baba et al.: Anal. Biochem. 101(1980) 288-293. b) Misra and Olney: J. Neurochem. 35(1980) 1303-1308.
c) Agrawal et al.: Biochem. J. 122(1971) 759-763. d) Recasens et al.: BBRC 83(1978) 449-456.
e) Recasens et al.: Brain Res. 239(1982) 153-173. f) Recasens et al.: Neurochem Int. (1982) in press.

containing ω-sulfonic group (cysteic acid, homocysteic acid).
The fact that the displacement of L-[^{3}H] CSA by L-CSA was
found to be of similar potency to that produced by L-glutamate
and vice versa raises the question of the existence of distinct
receptor sites for CSA and for glutamate. Since N-methyl-DL-
aspartate and kainate are totally ineffective in displacing L-
[^{3}H]CSA binding under our assay conditions, CSA and glutamate may
share only the so-called "quisqualate" site, although each may
have other "specific" receptors.

TABLE II: Inhibition constants (IC$_{50}$) and displacement of [^{3}H]
cysteine sulfinate and L-[^{3}H] glutamate by various compounds

Compound	L-[^{3}H] CSA binding		L-[^{3}H] Glutamate binding	
	IC$_{50}$ (μ M)	displace-ment %	IC$_{50}$ (μ M)	displace-ment %
L-CSA	0.23	100	1.9	85
D-CSA	140	87	110	68
L-Glutamate	0.80	93	2.3	100
D-Glutamate	-	0	23	32
L-Aspartate	20	78	14	67
D-Aspartate	-	0	63	34
L-α Aminoadipate	-	47	-	-
DL Cysteate	16	29	71	68
DL Homocysteate	77	28	70	51
L Glutamate γ monoethylester	79	52	59	64
L Glutamate γ monomethylester	87	52	23	60
N-methyl-DL- Aspartate	-	0	-	13
Kainate	-	0	-	19
GABA	-	0	-	20
Taurine	-	0	-	0

Specific binding of L-[^{3}H] CSA and L-[^{3}H] Glutamate was determined as described (19) (final concentrations of radioactive

ligands CSA or glutamate 100nM). IC_{50} was defined as the concentration of substance which displaced 50% of the L-[^{3}H]CSA or L-[^{3}H]glutamate binding displaceable by this substance at a concentration of I mM. Displacing compounds were added at concentrations ranging from 10^{-8} M to 10^{-3} M. Log dose inhibitor concentration was plotted against L-[^{3}H] CSA or L-[^{3}H] glutamate binding values as a percentage of control. Percentages of displacement were calculated from the equation:

$$\frac{\text{displaceable binding by inhibitor (at a concentration of 1 mM)}}{\text{displaceable binding by CSA or glutamate (at a concentration of 1 mM)}} \times 100$$

All the results are the means of two or three experiments which varied by less than 10% (each experiment in triplicate). Each individual experiment was conducted so that L-[^{3}H] CSA and L-[^{3}H] glutamate binding were determined in parallel, under the same conditions, using the same membrane preparation.

Stereospecificity of the Na$^+$-independent specific L-[^{3}H]CSA binding
     The L-[^{3}H]CSA receptor site showed a high stereospecificity. D-CSA was 609 times less effective than L-CSA in displacing L-[^{3}H]CSA binding. D-glutamate and D-aspartate were ineffective with regard to L-[^{3}H]CSA binding. The high stereospecificity of the L-[^{3}H] CSA binding suggested also the existence of an interaction of L-CSA with its physiological receptor.

Comparison of the L-[^{3}H]CSA and L-[^{3}H]Glutamate binding.
     In order to determine whether the binding sites for CSA and glutamate belong to two distinct classes, we have systematically compared the subcellular (Table III) and regional distributions (Table IV), the ionic sensitivities and the pharmacological properties (Table II) of L-[^{3}H]CSA and L-[^{3}H]glutamate binding to synaptic membranes (19). In subcellular fractionation experiments, we observed a different pattern for L-[^{3}H]CSA and L-[^{3}H]-glutamate binding, suggesting the existence of distinct sites for both substances. The relative density of L-[^{3}H]CSA and L-[^{3}H]glutamate binding sites differed among brain regions although their regional distribution was correlated, indicating the possibility that some sites are shared by CSA and glutamate, and that some specific sites might exist for each substance. The complexity of the pharmacological results involves the existence of several binding sites. For example, D-L cysteate had a high apparent affinity for CSA sites but not for glutamate sites, although at high concentrations it did displace more L-[^{3}H]glutamate than L-[^{3}H]CSA binding. The reverse occurred for D-glutamate and L-glutamate γmonomethylester. Thus, the tested compounds displaced L-[^{3}H]CSA from a subpopulation of

sites with a high "affinity" (e.g. cysteate) or most of the sites with a relatively low "affinity" (e.g. D-CSA). Similar patterns of displacement were observed for L-[3H]glutamate binding with different compounds. Finally, L-[3H]glutamate and L-[3H]CSA binding exhibited roughly similar sensitivities to ion manipulation, but quantitative differences were evident.

Taken together, these data indicate that CSA and glutamate may have a common site, possibly the "quisqualate" site, although distinct membrane binding sites also exist. As CSA did not interfere with kainate and N-methyl-D-aspartate sites, this could represent the distinct site for L-glutamate, whereas there exists another specific site for CSA, probably different from the kainate, the quisqualate and the N-methyl-D-aspartate sites.

TABLE III: Subcellular distribution of L-[3H] CSA and

L-[3H] glutamate binding

	L-[3H] CSA binding pmol/mg protein	L-[3H] Glutamate binding pmol/mg protein
Homogenate	0.79 ± 0.16	0.57 ± 0.16
Mitochondrial synaptosomal membranes (P2)	1.49 ± 0.27	1.02 ± 0.20
A myelin	0.32 ± 0.08	0.59 ± 0.12
B synaptosomal membranes, membranes, myelin	0.43 ± 0.14	0.99 ± 0.12
C synaptosomal membranes	2.22 ± 0.51	0.84 ± 0.23
D synaptosomal membranes, mitochondria	2.39 ± 0.31	0.82 ± 0.17
E mitochondrial membranes	0.72 ± 0.19	0.36 ± 0.12

Subcellular fractionation has been performed as described (19). Final concentrations of L-[3H] cysteine sulfinate and L-[3H] glutamate were 100 nM. Results represent specific binding, as determined by the amount of radioactive ligand displaced in 1 mM unlabeled CSA or glutamate. Each value is the mean ± SD of five separate experiments. Triplicate determinations were performed for each experiment and differed by less than 5%. Each individual experiment of L-[3H] CSA and L-[3H] glutamate binding was undertaken the same day, on the same membrane preparation, under the same conditions.

TABLE IV: Regional distribution of L-[3H] CSA and L-[3H] Glutamate binding

REGIONS	L-[3H] CSA binding pmoles/mg protein	L-[3H]Glutamate binding pmoles/mg protein	L-[3H] CSA binding/ L-[3H] Glutamate binding
CEREBELLUM	2.65 ± 0.28	1.67 ± 0.21	1.58
FRONTAL CORTEX	1.25 ± 0.22	0.84 ± 0.14	1.49
PARIETAL CORTEX	1.02 ± 0.15	0.63 ± 0.11	1.62
OCCIPITAL CORTEX	0.84 ± 0.09	0.59 ± 0.08	1.42
PONS MEDULLA	1.15 ± 0.09	0.99 ± 0.19	1.16
OLFACTORY TUBERCLE	0.10 ± 0.03	0.25 ± 0.08	0.40
STRIATUM	0.85 ± 0.07	1.18 ± 0.10	0.72
SEPTUM	0.17 ± 0.03	0.29 ± 0.09	0.59
HIPPOCAMPUS	0.46 ± 0.07	0.48 ± 0.06	0.96
HYPOTHALAMUS	0.98 ± 0.08	1.01 ± 0.13	0.97

Specific binding of L-[3H] CSA and L-[3H] Glutamate was determined using crude synaptosomal fractions (P_2) as described (19). Results represent specific binding as determined by the amount of radioactive ligand displaced by 1 mM unlabelled CSA or Glutamate. The binding values are means ± SD of four different experiments (each in duplicate).

L-CSA and Neurotransmission

CSA exhibits potent neuroexcitatory activity in the spinal cord (7,8) and depolarizes the horizontal cells of the carp retina (25). The activities of the synthesizing enzyme (cysteine oxidase) and the degradative enzymes (cysteine sulfinate decarboxylase and cysteine sulfinate aminotransferase) are found in the nerve endings (1,11,14,15,16,17). The degradative enzymes have been located immunohistochemically in regions enriched in synaptic contacts (4,18). CSA is unevenly distributed in the rat brain (3). It increases the level of cyclic AMP and cyclic GMP in guinea pig cerebral cortex in vitro (21). It also induces an increase of cyclic AMP in other brain regions, and particularly in the hippocampus where taurine was reported to significantly reduce the CSA-induced cyclic AMP increase (2). CSA has been found to be released by rat brain slices (10). We, as well as others (10), recently reported the existence of a Na^+-dependent CSA uptake mechanism (20). We demonstrated that CSA binds to synaptic membranes in a Na^+-independent manner (19). Some L-CSA binding sites are specific and different from the glutamate binding sites (19). Thus L-CSA fulfills most of the criteria which define a neurotransmitter.

Conclusion

The neurochemical evidence strongly favours L-CSA as a transmitter. However, electrophysiological investigations have not yet been carried out systematically. It is hoped that such studies will lead to a clear confirmation of the physiological role of L-CSA in the mammalian central nervous system.

ACKNOWLEDGMENTS

M. Recasens is charge de Recherche a l"INSERM and was supported by an O.T.A.N. fellowship.

REFERENCES

1. Agrawal, H.C., Davison, A.N., and Kaczmarek, L.K. (1971): Biochem. J., 122:759-763.
2. Baba, A., Lee, E., Tatsuno, T.,and Iwata, H. (1982): J. Neurochem., 38:1280-1285.
3. Baba, A., Yamagami, S., Mizuo, H., and Iwata, H. (1980): Anal. Biocem., 101:288-293.
4. Chan-Palay, V., Lin, C.T., Palay, S.L., Yamamoto, H., and Wu, J.Y. (1982): Proc. Natl. Acad. Sci., 79:2695-2699.
5. Cotman, C.W. and Nadler, J.V. (1981): In: Glutamate: Transmitter in the Central Nervous System, edited by P.J. Roberts, J. Storm-Mathisen, and G.A.R. Johnston, pp. 117-154. John Wiley α Sons, Chichester.

6. Curtis, D.R. (1979): In: Advances in Biochemistry and Physiology, edited by L.J. Filer, S. Garatini, M.R. Kare, W.A. Reynolds, and R.J. Wurtman, pp. 163-175. Raven Press, New York.

7. Curtis, D.R., Duggan, A.W., Felix, D., Johnston, G.A.R., Tebecis, A.K., and Watkins, J.C. (1972): Brain Res., 41:283-301.

8. Curtis, D.R. and Watkins, J.C. (1960): J. Neurochem., 6:117-141.

9. Iwata, H., Yamagami, S., and Baba, A. (1982): J. Neurochem., 38:1275-1279.

10. Iwata, H., Yamagami, S., Mizuo, H., and Baba, A. (1982): J. Neurochem., 38:1268-1274.

11. McLennan, H. (1981): In: Advances in Biochemical Psychopharmacology, Volume 12, edited by G. Di Chiara and G.L. Gessa, pp. 253-262. Raven Press, New York.

12. McLennan, H., Hicks, T.P., and Hall, J.G. (1981): In: Amino Acid Neurotransmitters: Receptors for the Excitatory Amino Acids, edited by F.V. DeFeudis and P. Mandel, pp. 213-221. Raven Press, New York.

13. Misra, C.H. and Olney, J. (1975): Brain Res., 97:117-126.

14. Pasantes-Morales, H., Loriette, C., and Chatagner, F. (1977): Neurochem. Res., 2:671-680.

15. Rassin, D.K. and Gaull, G.E. (1975): J. Neurochem., 24: 969-978.

16. Recasens, M., Benezra, R., Basset, P., and Mandel, P. (1980): Biochemistry, 19:4583-4589.

17. Recasens, M. and Delaunoy, J.P. (1981): Brain Res., 205: 351-361.

18. Recasens, M., Gabellec, M.M., Austin, L., and Mandel, P. (1978): Biochem. Biophys. Res. Commun., 83:449-456.

19. Recasens, M., Saadoun, F., Varga, V., DeFeudis, F.V., Mandel, P., Lynch, G., and Vincendon, G. (1982): Neurochem. Internat., (in press).

20. Recasens, M., Varga, V., Nanopoulos, D., Saadoun, F., Vincendon, G., and Benavides, J. (1982): Brain Res., 239:153-173.

21. Shimizu, H. and Yamamura, Y. (1977): J. Neurochem., 28:383-388.

22. Usherwood, P.N.R. (1978): Adv. Comp. Physiol. Biochem., 7:227-309.

23. Watkins, J.C. (1981): In: Amino Acid Neurotransmitters, edited by F.V. DeFeudis and P. Mandel, pp. 205-212. Raven Press, New York.

24. Watkins, J.C., Davies, J., Evans, R.H., Francis, A.A., and Jones, A.W. (1981): In: Advances in Biochemical Psychopharmacology, Volume 27, edited by G. Di Chiara and G.L. Gessa, pp. 263-273. Raven Press, New York.

25. Wu, S.M. and Dowling, J.E. (1978): Proc Natl. Acad. Sci. (USA), 75:5205-5209.

CNS Receptors—From Molecular
Pharmacology to Behavior, edited by
P. Mandel and F. V. DeFeudis.
Raven Press, New York © 1983.

Block of Glutamate Receptors by a Spider Toxin

*Nobufumi Kawai, *Akiko Miwa, and **Takashi Abe

*Department of Neurobiology, Tokyo Metropolitan Institute for Neurosciences, Fuchu-City,
Tokyo 183 Japan; and **Laboratory of Insect Toxicology, Institute of Physical and Chemical
Research, Wako-City, Saitama 351 Japan

Abundant evidence has been accumulated which indicates that L-glutamate is the excitatory transmitter
in the neuromuscular junctions of crustacea and insects
(6,8,19,20). The amino acid is also a strong
candidate for the transmitter in various parts of CNS
(4,14). In search of neurotoxins derived from
biological sources, we have found that a spider venom
contains a specific blocker of the glutamate receptors
in lobster neuromuscular junctions (10,11). The toxin
was also effective in blocking the synaptic transmission in mammalian brain (12).

SPIDER TOXIN

Spiders (Nephila Clavata, Joro spider) were collected
at outskirts of Tokyo. Toxin (Joro Spider Toxin JSTX)
was separated after gel filtration using Sephadex G-50
and Sephadex G-15. The effective fractions were
further purified using high-performance liquid
chromatography. The toxin was found stable after
heating at 80°C for 15 min.

LOBSTER NEUROMUSCULAR TRANSMISSION

The lobster nerve-muscle preparation is suited for
investigation of aminergic transmission since the
excitatory and the inhibitory nerves are readily
accessible for independent stimulation (9,15). Fig. 1
shows the effect of JSTX on EPSPs and IPSPs evoked in
the stretcher muscle of walking leg of lobster
(Palinurus japonicus). JSTX selectively suppressed

221

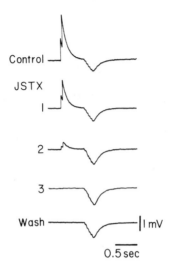

Fig. 1. Effect of the spider toxin (JSTX) on the postsynaptic potentials in the stretcher muscle of lobster walking leg. EPSPs and IPSPs were evoked successively by repetitive stimuli on the excitatory and inhibitory nerve, respectively. In this and all following Figures the numerals on each record indicate time in minutes after applying the toxin. Wash record was taken 90 min after application of the toxin.

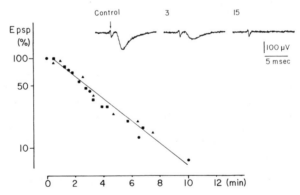

Fig 2. Inset records : effect of JSTX on the extra-cellularly recorded nerve terminal spike (arrow) followed by the excitatory postsynaptic potentials. Each beam shows averaged records of 20 consective sweeps. Graph shows time course of suppression of EPSPs. Ordinate: relative amplitude of the extra-cellularly recorded EPSPs in a logarithmic scale. Abscissa: time after applying the toxin at 0 min. Data are taken from three different preparations (indicated by different symbols) treated with the same concentration of the toxin.

EPSPs without altering IPSPs. The resting membrane potential and the input membrane resistance were unaffected by JSTX. When the extracellular recording was made from the synaptic region, stimuli on the excitatory nerve elicited the nerve terminal spike followed by extracellular EPSP which is proportional to the excitatory postsynaptic current at single synapse (5). JSTX suppressed the extracellularly recorded EPSPs without altering the nerve terminal spike. (Fig. 2) The amplitude of the extracellularly recorded EPSPs declined nearly exponentially with time after toxin application as shown in the graph of Fig. 2. Further study of the relation between dosage of the toxin and decline of EPSPs in various preparations showed that the rate constant of decline is linearly proportional to the toxin concentration.

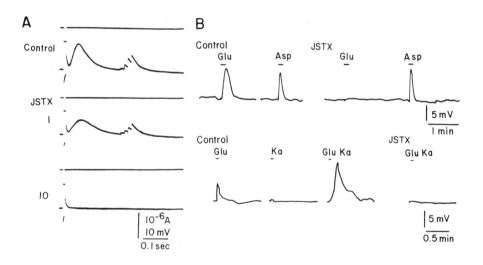

Fig. 3. Effect of JSTX on glutamate and its analogues (11). A. In each record, lower beam registered glutamate potentials by iontophoretic application of L-glutamate followed by EPSPs. Upper beam monitors applied current. B. Effects of the toxin on the depolarization evoked by bath application of glutamate and its analogues. In this experiment, the preparation was continuously perfused at a rate of 5 ml/min, and compounds were applied for the time indicated by bars. The concentrations were L-glutamate (0.1 mM), L-aspartate (1 mM) and kainic acid (0.1 mM).

GLUTAMATE AND ITS ANALOGUES

JSTX blocked depolarization of the postsynaptic membrane induced by L-glutamate. Both glutamate potentials and EPSPs evoked in the same muscle fiber were suppressed by the toxin (Fig. 3A). In contrast to L-glutamate, L-aspartate-induced depolarization was unaffected by JSTX (Fig. 3B). Kainic acid is known to potentiate the glutamate-induced depolarization in crustacean neuromuscular junction (2,17). In the presence of JSTX, however, no depolarization was found by applying kainate simultaneously with glutamate. The results suggest that the toxin blocked glutamate receptors irrespective of whether they are junctional or extra-junctional (16). On the other hand, depolarizaton induced by quisqualic acid was suppressed by JSTX, indicating that quisqualate is a potent glutamate-analogue like in the insect neuromuscular junction (1) and in various synapses of CNS (21).

MAMMALIAN BRAIN SYNAPSES

The effects of JSTX were further studied on CNS using brain slices. The preparation has an advantage in that the drug can be applied to the vicinity of the target receptors under direct visual control (13, 23). Slices were made from two parts of guinea-pig brain, hippocampus and olfactory cortex, where L-glutamate is a putative neurotransmitter (3,18). Hippocampal slices were made by transverse section and the field potentials were recorded from the pyramidal cell layer of CA3 in response to the stimulation on the granule cell layer. Paired stimuli on the granule cell layer elicited a marked facilitation in the postsynaptic component of the potentials of the pyramidal neurones (22) (Fig. 4B). JSTX suppressed postsynaptic potentials leaving the presynaptic volleys unaffected. Washing the preparation failed to restore the post-synaptic potentials. Fig. 4C shows the effect of JSTX on the field evoked potentials in the pyriform lobe by stimulation of the lateral olfactory tract. Post-synaptic potentials which showed a marked facilitation by paired stimuli, were suppressed almost completely by the toxin. As a control experiment, we made slices from the superior colliculus in connnection with the optic tract (13). The postsynaptic potentials in the superior colliculus evoked by optic tract stimulation were unchanged by JSTX even in high concentrations.

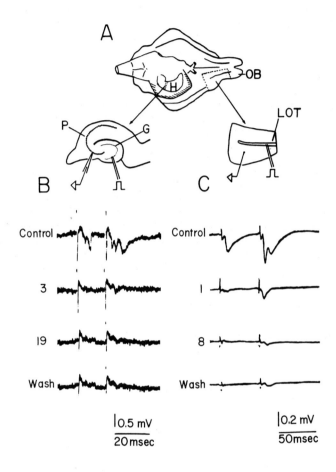

Fig. 4. Scheme of brain slice preparations and the effect of JSTX. A: ventral view of the guinea-pig brain. OB, olfactory bulb. H, Hippocampus. B: drawing of hippocampal slice. P, pyramidal cell layer. G, granule cell layer. Field potentials are taken from the pyramidal cells of CA3 in response to the paired stimuli on granular cells. C. drawing of slice of the olfactory cortex. LOT, lateral olfactory tract. Field potentials are recorded from the surface of pyriform lobe by paired stimuli on LOT.

The present study revealed that a neurotoxin purified from a spider (Nephila Clavata, Joro spider) has a specific blocking action on glutamate receptors in the crustacean neuromuscular junctions and also in the mammalian brain synapses. Investigations on the structure and physico-chemical properties of JSTX are now in progress. Based on profile of the chromatogram, molecular weight of JSTX can be assumed to be ca. 500. Rough estimate of the effective concentration of JSTX for suppressing EPSPs in lobster neuromuscular junction would then be in the range of 10-100 nM. This value is considerably lower than those of other glutamate antagonists that have been reported. In preliminary experiments, we have found that venoms of other spiders (Araneus ventricosus and Neoscone nautica) have similar effects on glutaminergic synapses (in preparation). Therefore, it may be inferred that a wide variety of spiders have the blocker of the glutamate receptor in their venoms. The specific and apparently irreversible action of spider toxin may serve as a useful tool for the study of the glutaminergic synapse.

ACKNOWLEDGEMENTS

This work was supported partly by grants from the Ministry of Education, Science and Culture, and from Nissan Science Foundation.

REFERENCES

1. Anderson, C.P., Cull-Candy, S.G., and Miledi, R. (1978): J. Physiol. (Lond.), 282:219-242.
2. Constanti, A., and Nistri, A. (1976): Brit. J. Pharmacol., 57:1-14.
3. Cotman, C.W., Foster, A., and Lanthorn, T. (1981): In: Glutamate as a Neurotransmitter, edited by C. Dichiara, and G.L.Gessa, pp.127. Raven Press, New York.
4. Curtis, D.R., and Johnston, G.A.R. (1974): Ergebn. Physiol., 69:97-188.
5. Dudel, J., and Kuffler, S.W. (1961): J. Physiol. (Lond.), 155:514-529.
6. Gerschenfeld, H.M. (1973): Physiol. Rev., 53: 1-119.
7. Johnson, J.L. (1972): Brain Res., 37:1-19.
8. Kawagoe, R., Onodera, K., and Takeuchi, A. (1981): J. Physiol. (Lond.), 312:225-236.

9. Kawai, N., and Niwa, A. (1980): J. Physiol. (Lond.), 305:73-85.
10. Kawai, N., Niwa, A., and Abe, T. (1982): Neurosci. Letters, suppl. 9:572.
11. Kawai, N., Niwa, A., and Abe, T. (1982): Brain Res., 247:169-171.
12. Kawai, N., Niwa, A., and Abe, T. (1982): Biomedical Res., 3:353-355.
13. Kawai, N., and Yamamoto, C. (1969): Int. J. Neuropharmacol., 8:437-449.
14. Krnjević, K. (1974): Physiol. Rev., 54:418-540.
15. Niwa, A., and Kawai, N. (1982): J. Neurophysiol., 47:353-361.
16. Onodera, K. and Takeuchi, A. (1980): J. Physiol. (Lond), 306:233-250.
17. Shinozaki, H., and Shibuya, I. (1974): Neuropharmacology, 13:1057-1065.
18. Storm-Mathisen, J. (1977): Prog. Neurobiol., 8:119-181.
19. Takeuchi, A., and Takeuchi, N. J. Physiol. (Lond.), 170:296-317.
20. Usherwood, P.N.R. (1972): Neurosci. Res. Prog. Bull., 10-2, 136-143.
21. Watkins, J.C. (1981): Advances in Biochemical Psychopharmacology: Amino Acid Neurotransmitters, edited by F.V. DeFeudis, and P. Mandel, pp. 205-212. Raven Press, New York.
22. Yamamoto, C. (1972): Exp. Brain Res., 14:423-435.
23. Yamamoto, C., and Kawai, N. (1969): Science, 155:341-342.

CNS Receptors—From Molecular
Pharmacology to Behavior, edited by
P. Mandel and F. V. DeFeudis.
Raven Press, New York © 1983.

Multiple Postsynaptic Responses Evoked by Glutamate on *In Vitro* Spinal Motoneurones

A. Nistri and M. S. Arenson

Department of Pharmacology, St. Bartholomew's Hospital Medical College, University of London, London EC1M 6BQ, England

L-glutamate, an endogenous amino acid, is thought to act as an excitatory transmitter in the central nervous system (10). Current studies which attempt to clarify the receptor pharmacology of this amino acid (5) indicate that spinal neurones possess different postsynaptic receptors for several structurally related analogues. Such studies have not, however, yet delineated whether these receptors mediate the same membrane response for the different compounds or whether one amino acid, acting through different receptors, can elicit several types of membrane response and therefore influence neuronal activity in a variety of ways. The reason why these questions have not been fully answered is that most investigations have been conducted either with extracellular recordings (which provide only indirect insight into neuronal membrane mechanisms) or with radioreceptor binding methods which of themselves cannot provide information on the physiological responsiveness of the neurone. Encouraged by reports of different modes of action of glutamate on unidentified neurones in tissue culture (6), the present study set out to examine, using intracellular recording techniques, the effects of glutamate on motoneurones of the frog *in vitro* spinal cord. Motoneurones are particularly suitable for this type of study because of their long-term stability and ease of identification. The *in vitro* slice preparation avoids the complications of anaesthesia and allows control of the amino acid concentrations and ionic composition of the bathing medium. Furthermore, rapid superfusion at low temperature ($7^\circ C$), while helping neuronal survival and depressing amino acid uptake, is not unphysiological for amphibia.

METHODS

Frogs (*Rana temporaria*) were used throughout. After dorsal laminectomy the spinal cord was longitudinally sliced into two

halves, one of which was placed in a perspex chamber (0.2 ml
volume) kept at 7°C. The preparation was constantly superfused
(5-10 ml/min) with oxygenated Ringer solution of the following
composition (mM): NaCl 111, KCl 2.5, NaHCO$_3$ 10, NaH$_2$PO$_4$.2H$_2$O
0.1, CaCl$_2$ 2; glucose 4. Several dorsal and ventral lumbar roots
were drawn into stimulating suction electrodes. Intracellular
recordings were usually obtained with 3 M KCl-filled glass microelectrodes (30-100 MΩDC resistance) connected to a high input
impedance amplifier with facilities for current injection, bridge
balancing and capacity neutralization. Recorded signals were
displayed on a storage oscilloscope and on a linear pen-recorder
and also stored on magnetic tape for subsequent analysis.

RESULTS

     Recordings were obtained from several tens of motoneurones,
immediately identified by their short-latency, all-or-none antidromic spike without a preceding EPSP. These cells had resting
membrane potentials between -50 and -80 mV, spikes over 50 mV
(always overshooting zero baseline) and input conductance of about
25 nS.
     Fig. 1 shows on a chart record that bath superfusion with
glutamate (1 mM) elicited a membrane depolarization associated
with a marked increase in input conductance at the peak of the
response (cf. much reduced size of downward deflections which
represent hyperpolarizing electrotonic potentials evoked by constant current pulses). During the glutamate-induced depolarization there was an intense synaptic bombardment of the motoneurone in Fig. 1 (cf. thick baseline at response peak) and
significant reduction in the latency and time-to-peak of the
antidromic spike (not shown). All these effects are indeed
typical of an excitatory response. In several other cells, the
depolarization produced by glutamate was however associated only
with modest increases in input conductance (on average 20%) and
such a phenomenon was indeed typical of cells receiving relatively small trans-synaptic discharges during glutamate superfusion.
This is in fact a well-documented finding of other authors (13,
14). Fig. 1 also shows (on the same cell) the action of glutamate
during superfusion with 1.5 mM Mn^{2+}/1 mM Ca^{2+} solution which
blocked chemical synaptic transmission. The depolarizing response
was largely reduced and there was little, if any, conductance
increase at plateau level. Moreover, the depolarization was
preceded by a membrane hyperpolarization (with conductance increase) large enough to block the antidromic spike generation.
Finally, during the glutamate washout phase, there was a transient
conductance decrease (cf. larger amplitude of hyperpolarizing
electrotonic potentials) with associated rise in neuronal excitability. Hence these findings indicated that a large proportion

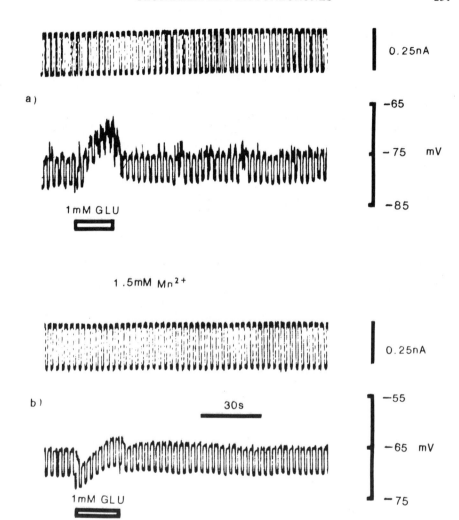

FIG. 1. Effect of 1 mM glutamate superfusion on frog motoneurone.
Chart record of membrane potential (bottom) and injected current
(top) in control Ringer (a) and in 1.5 Mn^{2+}/1 mM Ca^{2+} containing
solution (b). Downward deflections are hyperpolarizing electrotonic potentials elicited by 600 ms current pulses injected at
0.33 Hz and used to monitor input conductance. The motoneurone is
also stimulated antidromically (0.33 Hz) to fire action potentials
which are truncated by the frequency response of the pen recorder.
Note in b that the tracing is less "noisy" indicating the synaptic
transmission has been blocked and that the depolarizing effect of
glutamate is reduced and now clearly preceded by a hyperpolarizing
response.

of the depolarizing action of glutamate on motoneurones was indirect and that it was compounded with an early hyperpolarization
and a late conductance decrease.

The ionic mechanisms responsible for the direct depolarizing
effect of glutamate are not fully understood: increases in Na^+
permeability and/or decrease in K^+ permeability have been
suggested (4,14). In the present experiments the possible con-
tribution of K^+ channels to the glutamate action was investigated
using intracellular injections of Cs^+, a K^+ channel blocker (11).
Cs^+ was applied iontophoretically inside motoneurones by outward
1-3 nA currents delivered for up to 15 min to a 3 M CsCl containing electrode. Immediately after termination of the Cs^+
iontophoresis the motoneuronal membrane was depolarized by 5-8 mV,
its input conductance decreased by 20-40% and the spike after-
hyperpolarizations (believed to be due to K^+ currents) blocked.
Under these conditions, the depolarization evoked by glutamate
was reduced by over 50% and little or no conductance change was
noted at the peak of the response (1). The hyperpolarizing
effect of glutamate was however unaltered or even unmasked by
Cs^+, suggesting that K^+ was unlikely to play a role in this
particular response. Since an inhibitory compound such as GABA
(1-3 mM) which is thought to activate Cl^- conductances, was also
hyperpolarizing the same motoneurone, it seems likely that the
glutamate-induced hyperpolarization was caused by transmembrane
Cl^- influx (1).

The experiments described so far were mainly concerned with
multiple actions of relatively long (tens of seconds) administrations of glutamate on motoneurones. It was, nevertheless, of
interest to study the very initial response of these cells to
glutamate since one might expect that the endogenous transmitter
would act on a briefer timescale. It soon became apparent that
glutamate was acting on motoneurones before any measurable change
in their resting membrane potential or conductance. Fig. 2 shows
oscilloscope tracings of control antidromic spikes (left) and
within 3 s of 1 mM glutamate application (right). Although there
was no significant change in resting potential (see dashed line)
or early spike configuration, a late component of the spike, the
afterdepolarization (ADP), was enhanced, particularly in its rate
of rise (cf. arrow). A few seconds later, the glutamate depolarization developed and obscured this selective change. It is
conceivable that the ADP-enhancing effect of glutamate might have
been caused indirectly via presynaptic release of endogenous
substances. It was therefore necessary to examine the action of
glutamate in Mn^{2+}-containing media which fully blocked Ca^{2+}-
dependent synaptic transmission. Fig. 3 shows that in 2.5 mM
Mn^{2+} solution glutamate still enhanced the spike ADP and, in
particular, induced the appearance of small depolarizing waves
after the antidromic spike. It would therefore appear that the
earliest manifestation of glutamate effects on motoneurones was
a selective enhancement of the ADP.

Throughout this report it was stated that glutamate was an
excitatory agent on motoneurones. This point may not be

L-GLU(1mM)

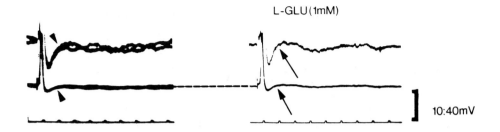

10:40mV

FIG. 2. Effect of 1 mM glutamate on frog motoneurone. Oscilloscope tracings of antidromic spikes in Ringer solution (left) and
in the presence of 1 mM glutamate (right). Each panel shows from
top to bottom: high gain AC trace, low gain DC trace and time
marks. Glutamate enhanced ADP (compare response marked by arrow
with control response marked by arrowhead) before changing resting
membrane potential (3 s application). Cell resting membrane potential was: -58 mV; resting input conductance: 29 nS. Time
marks: 10 ms.

Mn(2.5mM)   L-GLU(0.7mM)

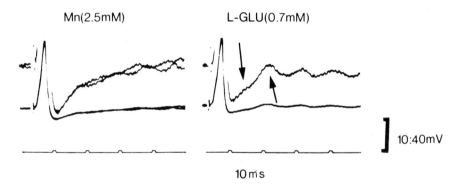

10:40mV

10ms

FIG. 3. Effect of 0.7 mM glutamate on frog motoneurone. Oscilloscope tracings of antidromic spikes in 2.5 mM Mn^{2+}/2 mM Ca^{2+}
solution (with complete block of chemical synaptic transmission).
Three seconds after start of glutamate superfusion and prior to
changes in membrane potential or conductance there is an enhancement of the ADP and the appearance of small depolarizing waves
(arrows). Other details as in Fig. 2. Resting membrane potential:
-65 mV, resting input conductance: 58 nS.

immediately obvious in view of the complex actions of this amino
acid on the neuronal membrane. It is however possible to demonstrate that, at the plateau of glutamate depolarization, incoming
orthodromic signals to motoneurones are more efficiently processed.
This is depicted in the oscilloscope tracings of Fig. 4 where

motoneuronal responses to dorsal root electrical stimulation
(0.33 Hz; 0.1 ms duration; fixed intensity) are represented at
fast (top row) and slow (bottom row) speed. On the left, superimposed control responses consist of polysynaptic EPSP with
spikes, spike due to direct current injection and, finally,
hyperpolarizing electrotonic potential. During glutamate superfusion the orthodromic spike latency was reduced and its rate
of rise increased (centre) and, in spite of the minimal conductance change, an anode break spike ("off response") was fired
(perhaps as a result of sudden removal of Na^+ channel inactivation). On the right, recovery responses are shown.

DISCUSSION

The present study offers an insight into the very complex,
multiple membrane responses elicited by glutamate on a single
central neurone. The first detectable response was a selective
enhancement of the spike ADP prior to changes in membrane potential or conductance. Since this effect was probably a direct
one on the motoneurone, it may represent a glutamate influence
on the mechanism(s) generating the ADP. Taking into account
current theories on the origin of the ADP which is believed to
be the expression of dendritic currents flowing to the cell soma
(12), it is possible that glutamate initially increased the
excitability of dendrites either through activation of their
ionic conductances (for example to Na^+; cf. appearance of small
waves in Fig. 3) or through blockade of some conductances (e.g.
to K^+). This mode of action might well make motoneurones more
responsive to afferent impulses and thus raise their excitability.
Secondly, the glutamate-induced depolarization was likely
caused partly by release of endogenous transmitter (note its
depression by Mn^{2+} solutions) and partly by increased Na^+ and
Ca^{2+} influx as reported by Sonnhof and Bührle (15). The relatively small associated conductance increase may have several
explanations: remote location of glutamate-sensitive sites, very
positive reversal potential for glutamate (7) and even the simultaneous deactivation of K^+ currents (as proposed by Engberg et al.
(4) and supported by present data on Cs^+ antagonism).
Thirdly, the depolarizing action of glutamate was usually
"contaminated" by a hyperpolarizing response (with conductance
increase) more easily attributed to Cl^- rather than K^+ fluxes
since it was resistant to Cs^+ injections. The presence of a
hyperpolarizing effect of glutamate is not entirely surprising as
this agent is known to have direct inhibitory effects on brain
neurones in vitro (8) and a chemical analogue of glutamate,
ibotenate, also has biphasic (inhibitory-excitatory) effects on
motoneurones (9). Fourthly, as previously noted on olfactory
cortex neurones (2) during the glutamate washout period there
was often a decrease in input conductance below the predrug
values and an associated rise in neuronal excitability. We have
at present no clear explanation for this phenomenon, though it is

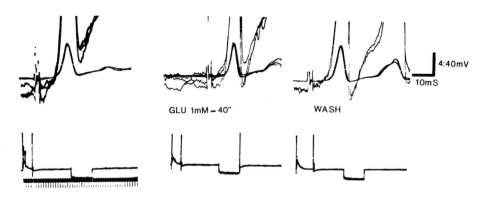

GLU 1mM – 40"   WASH   4:40mV   10mS

FIG. 4. Effect of 1 mM GLU on frog motoneurone. Oscilloscope tracing of response taken at fast (top row) and slow (bottom row) sweep. In top row from left to right: control orthodromic spike (with AC high gain and DC low gain), 40 s of glutamate superfusion (note faster rising phase of spike and shorter latency) and recovery a few min later. In bottom row from left to right: control orthodromic spikes riding on EPSP and followed by direct stimulation spike and hyperpolarizing electrotonic potential (bottom tracing shows 100 ms time marks), same sequence after 60 s of glutamate superfusion (note rather small change in amplitude of the electrotonic potential and appearance of anode break spike - i.e. an action potential at the end of the hyper-polarizing electrotonic response) and recovery a few min later. Orthodromic stimuli were applied at 0.33 Hz (0.1 ms duration) to a dorsal lumbar root. Resting membrane potential and conductance: -58 mV and 91 nS respectively.

of interest to note how a single application of glutamate may influence neuronal activity beyond the duration of its administration. It has previously been reported that invertebrate excitable membranes may display a degree of "memory" for the action of some excitatory amino acids (3).

Finally, one should be aware that other consequences of glutamate administration, namely electrogenic uptake (cf. 4) and post-application activity of Na^+/K^+ membrane pumps, might have been considerably reduced in our experiments owing to the low temperature used for recording. Using glutamate at higher temperature may well introduce these additional components to its overall effect on nerve cells.

In conclusion, although the present investigation was not designed to elucidate the receptor pharmacology of glutamate in the spinal cord and therefore does not carry stringent arguments in favour or against multiple receptor theories, it has demonstrated a variety of membrane responses to this amino acid. If it is accepted that glutamate may be a central transmitter, it becomes then feasible to suppose that one transmitter is employed to convey different kinds of neuronal signals. Admittedly, there is not much direct evidence to support this view except the fact that it would be "economical" for the nervous system and would reduce the level of biological noise and error in the network by avoiding the use of too many different chemicals.

ACKNOWLEDGEMENT

This work was supported by a grant from the Joint Research Board of St. Bartholomew's Hospital.

REFERENCES

1. Arenson, M.S. and Nistri, A. (1982): J. Physiol. (Lond.), in press.

2. Constanti, A., Connor, J.D., Galvan, M., and Nistri, A. (1980): Brain Res., 195: 403-420.

3. Constanti, A. and Nistri, A. (1979): Brit. J. Pharmacol., 65: 287-301.

4. Engberg, I., Flatman, J.A., and Lambert, J.D.C. (1979): J. Physiol. (Lond.), 288: 227-261.

5. Evans, R.H. and Watkins, J.C. (1981): Life Sci., 28: 1303-1308.

6. MacDonald, J.F. and Wojtowicz, J.M. (1982): Can. J. Physiol. Pharmacol., 60: 282-296.

7. Matthews, G. and Wickelgren, W.O. (1979): J. Physiol. (Lond), 293: 417-433.

8. Nicoll, R.A. and Alger, B.E. (1981): Science, 212: 957-959.

9. Nistri, A. (1981): Brain Res., 208: 397-408.

10. Puil, E. (1981): Brain Res. Revs., 3: 229-322.

11. Puil, E. and Werman, R. (1981): Can. J. Physiol. Pharmacol., 59: 1280-1284.

12. Schwindt, P.C. (1976): In: Frog Neurobiology, edited by R. Llinás and W. Precht, pp. 750-764. Springer, Berlin.

13. Shapovalov, A.I., Shiriaev, B.I., and Velumian, A.A. (1978): J. Physiol. (Lond.), 279: 437-455.

14. Sonnhof, V. and Bührle, Ch. Ph. (1980): Pflügers Arch., 388: 101-109.

15. Sonnhof, V. and Bührle, Ch. (1981): Adv. Biochem. Psychopharmacol., 27: 195-204.

CNS Receptors—From Molecular
Pharmacology to Behavior, edited by
P. Mandel and F. V. DeFeudis.
Raven Press, New York © 1983.

Benzodiazepine Receptor Ligands with Positive and Negative Efficacy[1]

*,†C. Braestrup, *M. Nielsen, and †T. Honoré

*Sct. Hans Mental Hospital, 4000 Roskilde, Denmark; and †A/S Ferrosan,
DK-2860 Soeborg, Denmark

There seems to exist at least three overlapping groups of benzodiazepine (BZ) receptor ligands (6), of which one group comprises
benzodiazepine-like ligands, in the following referred to as
agonists. Binding of this group of ligands to BZ receptors install
the classical anticonvulsant, sedative and anxiolytic effects of
minor tranquillizers. High affinity binding of benzodiazepine-like
ligands has been extensively studied (37, for review 3). GABA
agonists such as GABA and muscimol enhance the binding affinity of
benzodiazepine agonists; in some cases the affinity for BZ receptors
is about doubled by GABA agonists (5,21,38). A second group of BZ
receptor ligands are benzodiazepine receptor antagonists; these
ligands binds to BZ receptors and inhibit pharmacological and
other effects elicited via the BZ receptor recognition site.
Several benzodiazepine receptor antagonists are known, for example
β-CCE, PrCC, Ro 15-1788 and CGS 8216; these have all been investigated using high affinity binding techniques (12,26,28,31). The
pharmacological profile and the binding characteristics of these
four receptor antagonists are similar but clearly not identical.
Apparently, they all bind to the benzodiazepine recognition site,
but GABA agonists fail to substantially enhance the binding
affinity of the compounds (1,12,15,23,26,28,31). A third group of
BZ receptor ligands comprise convulsive (and/or anxiogenic)
ligands, tentatively called inverse agonists. Inverse agonists
bind to BZ receptors, but install exactly the opposite effects as
compared to benzodiazepine agonists. To our knowledge, no other
examples in pharmacology have been reported where receptors
respond in opposite directions depending on the nature of the
agonist. Two compounds of the inverse agonist type have recently
been described, methyl β-carboline-3-carboxylate (β-CCM) (1,20)
and methyl 6,7-dimethoxy-4-ethyl-β-carboline-3-carboxylate (DMCM)
(6).

---

[1] This paper was also presented at the Soc. Neuroscience,
Minneapolis, November 1982, and at the Nato Advance Study
Institute, Urbino, September 1982.

In this presentation we will discuss some of the distinct features of the binding of DMCM and β-CCM to BZ receptors; furthermore, the difference in binding properties of DMCM and β-CCM as compared to those of the benzodiazepines will be related to the difference in the pharmacology of these two groups of agents.

1.   β-CCM and DMCM bind   to BZ receptors

Several arguments support the idea that β-CCM and DMCM bind to BZ receptors: β-CCM and DMCM inhibit completely specific ^{3}H-flunitrazepam (^{3}H-FNM) binding in several brain regions, including hippocampus, cortex and cerebellum (7). Pharmacological effects of β-CCM and of DMCM can be inhibited by benzodiazepine receptor antagonists (6,33,40). The affinities for brain membranes of ^{3}H-β-CCM (K_D = 0.8 nM) (1) and of ^{3}H-DMCM (K_D = 0.5-6 nM) (4) are in accordance with IC_{50} values for β-CCM and DMCM, respectively, as inhibitors of ^{3}H-FNM binding to brain membranes (7). Specific binding of ^{3}H-β-CCM and ^{3}H-DMCM has   the same gross regional and subcellular distributions as specific binding of ^{3}H-FNM (1,4). Several compounds that are active on benzodiazepine receptors inhibit specific binding of ^{3}H-β-CCM and ^{3}H-DMCM in approximately the expected concentrations, as evaluated from inhibition of ^{3}H-FNM binding (1,4); conversely, several compounds that fail to inhibit ^{3}H-FNM binding also fail to inhibit ^{3}H-β-CCM and ^{3}H-DMCM binding. The total number of specific ^{3}H-β-CCM and ^{3}H-DMCM binding sites seems to equal the number of ^{3}H-FNM binding sites (1,4). The target size, found in radiation inactivation experiments (which is related to molecular weight) of ^{3}H-PrCC and ^{3}H-DMCM binding are equal to that of ^{3}H-FNM (27,32, E.A. Barnard unpublished). β-CCM and DMCM do not inhibit specific binding of several other brain receptor ligands (6 and unpublished). Specific binding of ^{3}H-β-CCM and ^{3}H-DMCM is affected by GABA agonists indicating that the binding sites are coupled to GABA receptors (1,4; for details see below). Photoshifts for BZ receptor ligands are similar regardless of whether ^{3}H-β-CCM (22), ^{3}H-DMCM (table 2) or other BZ receptor ligands are used as radioligand (see below).

2.   GABA effects

It has recently been proposed that the ability of GABA agonists to enhance or reduce the affinity of ligands for BZ receptors would reflect the pharmacological efficacy of BZ receptor ligands (1,6,13,15,26,35). These studies are exemplified in table 1, which shows the GABA-ratio for several benzodiazepine receptor ligands. A GABA-ratio above one, which means that GABA enhances the affinity of that ligand, is observed for benzodiazepine-like ligands, e.g. flunitrazepam. Ligands of this group are defined as having positive efficacy and are considered to be agonists to the BZ receptor. GABA-ratios of ca. 1 reflect that the compounds have grossly the same affinity in the presence and absence of GABA; thus, these compounds lack efficacy and are designated as receptor antagonists. A third group of ligands, comprising the anxiogenic (but not convulsive) ligand, FG 7142 (14) and the convulsive ligands β-CCM and DMCM have GABA-ratios below unity. These compounds have negative efficacy at the BZ receptors and may be named inverse agonists. As mentioned above, there seems to be a correlation between pharmacological efficacy and the GABA-ratio. Consequently, the GABA-ratio seems predictive of the pharmacological efficacies of new BZ receptor ligands.

TABLE 1. The effect of GABA receptor stimulation on the affinity of ligands for BZ receptors (from ref. 6)

Ligand	GABA ratio	N
Group 1		
Flunitrazepam	2.45 ± 0.2	4
Estazolam	2.43	2
Oxazepam	2.35	2
Diazepam	2.30 ± 0.3	4
Chlordiazepoxide	2.23 ± 0.1	3
Clonazepam	2.12 ± 0.2	3
CL 218872	1.98 ± 0.1	4
Lorazepam	1.75	2
Lormetazepam	1.71	2
Zopiclone	1.53 ± 0.1	3
Group 2		
Ro 15-1788	1.22 ± 0.1	3
PrCC	1.11	2
Group 3		
β-CCE	0.86 ± 0.1	4
FG 7142	0.87 ± 0.1	4
β-CCM	0.61	2
DMCM	0.46 ± 0.1	3

A GABA-ratio of 2 means that GABA (or muscimol) enhances the affinity of the ligand for BZ receptors twofold (see ref. 6).

3. Photoshift

Recently it has been suggested that BZ receptor agonists and antagonists can be distinguished in another biochemical model (22). In this model BZ receptors are inactivated by exposure to ultraviolet light in the presence of flunitrazepam (photoaffinity labelling). However, only 25% of the sites are labelled. A major part of the remaining receptors (unlabelled) lose their high affinity for benzodiazepines, whereas the affinity for some receptor antagonists is only slightly affected or unaltered (see fig. 1).

Thus, photoshifts for benzodiazepines are 0.02-0.04 (table 2) corresponding to 20-50 fold less affinity for UV/FNM exposed BZ receptors than for untreated receptors, whereas BZ receptor antagonists have photoshifts close to unity (table 2). These findings confirm several recent reports (9,16,25,39).

FIGURE 1.   Schematic representation of the postulated conformational
shift in BZ receptors upon UV/FNM exposure

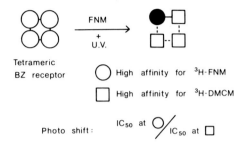

Tetrameric
BZ receptor   ○ High affinity for ³H-FNM

□ High affinity for ³H-DMCM

Photo shift : $\dfrac{IC_{50} \text{ at } ○}{IC_{50} \text{ at } □}$

TABLE 2.   Photoshift[a] for several BZ receptor ligands using
³H-DMCM as radioligand

Group	Compound	Photoshift
1, Agonist	Midazolam	0.02
	Flunitrazepam	0.03
	Lorazepam	0.03
	Triazolam	0.05
2, Receptor	Ro 15-1788	0.85
Antagonist	CGS 8216	0.93
3, Inverse	FG 7142	1.0
Agonist	β-CCM	1.4
	DMCM	2.6

a. The photolabelling procedure was done by preincubation of washed rat cortex membranes with
FNM (10 nM, final conc.) for 15 min followed by
exposure to long wave UV light for 10 min and
subsequent washing as previously described (4).
The assays were done in triplicate using ³H-DMCM
(0.1 nM) as a radioligand as described (4).
IC_{50} values in photolabelled and normal membranes
were obtained from a Hill analysis of the
inhibitory effect of at least three different
concentrations of the test substances.

From the above conjectures it is anticipated that DMCM would
have a particular high photoshift; this was confirmed because DMCM
exhibited the highest photoshift yet measured (table 2). There
exist, however, a few BZ receptor ligands, which do not fit well
into this scheme. Zopiclone (25), for example, has a intermediate
value for the photoshift albeit this compound possess pharmacological properties almost indistinguishable from those of the
benzodiazepines (22). Extended series of BZ receptor ligands,
ideally including several chemical types should be investigated

before the photoshift can be regarded as a reliable predictor of pharmacological efficacy.

4. Chloride channel related interactions

The affinity of BZ receptors for ^{3}H-diazepam is increased in the presence of anions that penetrate chloride ionophores (11,24). Likewise, some barbiturates and other agents believed to interact directly with chloride channels, enhance binding of ^{3}H-diazepam and ^{3}H-flunitrazepam to BZ-receptors (30). These findings point to a link between BZ receptors and the chloride ionophore related to GABA receptors. If the increase in binding in the presence of chloride ions reflects the pharmacological efficacy of BZ receptor ligands, we would expect that chloride ions would reduce binding affinity of inverse agonists, e.g. DMCM. This was not experimentally verified. Chloride ions, on the contrary, enhanced the binding of ^{3}H-DMCM to hippocampal membranes (unpublished).

DISCUSSION

It is generally accepted that benzodiazepines exert the majority of their pharmacological effects via the GABA-system (18); the molecular basis of this interaction is probably the GABA/BZ-receptor-chloride channel complex (fig. 2).

FIGURE 2.   A schematic representation of the GABA/BZ receptor chloride channel complex. Shown are drugs presumed to interact with the complex (from ref. 2)

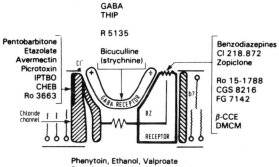

In this complex the BZ receptor might be functionally similar to allosteric sites in enzymes, which are sites distinct from the catalytic site (which could be likened to the GABA receptor/ chloride channel). The compound that binds to the allosteric site is named the effector. At constant enzyme and substrate concentrations, the binding of negative effectors reduces the reaction rate of enzymes (allosteric inhibition); the binding of positive effectors increases the reaction rate (allosteric activation). If the allosteric effector is the substrate molecule itself, the effector is said to be homotropic; if the effector is a molecule other than the substrate, the effector is said to by heterotropic. Thus, by analogy to enzyme biochemistry, benzodiazepines correspond to positive heterotropic effectors; they enhance GABA neurotransmission indirectly. Likewise, DMCM and β-CCM would correspond to negative heterotropic effectors. The concept of allosteric mechanism has previously been applied to pharmacological systems. For example the inhibitory effect of toxins on cholinergic transmission at the nicotinic receptor and also of local anesthetics have been described as negative heterotropic effectors (19). However, there were no examples of the existence of positive heterotropic effectors which act on the same allosteric site. To our knowledge BZ receptor is the first pharmacological example known where both positive and negative heterotropic effectors exist. The pharmacological term for a positive effector would be an agonist (agonist = drug that produce a response (8)). However, also the agents with negative efficacy (negative effectors, i.e. DMCM) produce a response and are therefore agonists. The term inverse agonist would signify that the reponse is opposite to that of already known agonists. Partial agonists and partial inverse agonists fit nicely into this scheme. Receptor antagonists inhibit responses both to partial and full agonists and to inverse agonists by occupying the receptors.

An alternative to the existense of inverse agonists would be the presence of a tonically active endogenous substance which interacts with the BZ receptor. In that case the above-mentioned receptor antagonist might represent partial agonists and the inverse agonists (or the agonists!) might be described as antagonists to the endogenous ligand and thereby produce a response without having any efficacy. However, several findings support the existence of agonist, inverse agonist and receptor antagonist. Firstly, the GABA-ratio is unity for receptor antagonists, that means, the washed membrane receptor preparation equilibrates in the middle position corresponding to agents having no efficacy, and not in one of the extremes, which would be expected if a soluble endogenous ligand was removed. Secondly, in well-washed cultured neurones, where no tonic release of endogenous ligand is likely to occur, the GABA response is enhanced by benzodiazepine agonists and reduced by inverse agonist (10,29,36,41). This again suggest that the equilibrium without endogenous ligand is in the middle position. A spectrum of BZ receptor ligands with partial and full positive and negative efficacies is exemplified in fig. 3. Note that PrCC and Ro 15-1788 have weak positive efficacy whereas CGS 8216, FG 7142 and β-CCE have weak negative efficacy.

There has been some uncertainty as to how the GABA-ratio relates to pharmacological efficacy in terms of mechanisms. The biochemical observation is that GABA enhances the affinity of benzodiazepine agonist, while the fact to be explained is that benzodiazepine agonists enhance the effects of GABA. Benzodiazepine agonists do enhance GABA receptor affinity, but only slightly and only in certain conditions (17,34). These two sets of results can be explained by adapting the two state concept of

FIGURE 3. A continuum of BZ receptor ligands in relation to their efficacy (agonists, receptor antagonists and inverse agonists)

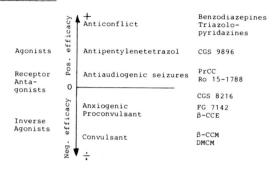

receptor function, which is visualized in fig. 4. The BZ receptor is assumed to occur in two forms, the active form (fig. 4, right) and the inactive form (fig. 4, left), these forms are in equilibrium under normal conditions, with both forms being present in appreciable amounts even without endogenous or exogenous ligands being present at the BZ recognition site. The presence of benzodiazepine agonists, which have high affinity for the active form,

FIGURE 4. A two state model for BZ receptors, relative to GABA-receptors and chloride channels (this model reflects fig. 5 in ref. 7; see Discussion for further details)

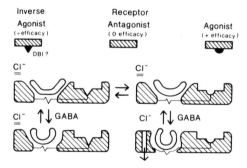

will change the equilibrium to the right, which is the active state for the GABA/chloride channel to be operative in GABAergic transmission; GABA itself will shift the equilibrium to the right. BZ receptor antagonists will not affect the equilibrium, because they have similar affinity to both forms of the BZ receptor and consequently they will not change GABAergic transmission. Inverse agonists have the opposite selectivity as compared to benzodiazepines and will shift the equilibrium to the left reducing GABAergic transmission. This scheme (figs. 2 and 4) is consistent with the above-mentioned experiments with cultured neurones. It is not known at present how a tetrameric BZ receptor complex might be incorporated into a GABA/BZ receptor chloride channel complex. Furthermore, there is at present no simple way to incorporate the results found in photoshift experiments (table 2) into a theoretical model that describes how the photoshift might relate to pharmacological efficacy.

REFERENCES

1. Braestrup, C., and Nielsen, M. (1981): Nature 294: 472-474.
2. Braestrup, C., and Nielsen, M. (1982): Lancet 1030-1034.
3. Braestrup, C., and Nielsen, M. (1982): In: Handbook of Psychopharmacology vol. 17, edited by L.L. Iversen, S.D. Iversen, and S.H. Snyder, pp. 285-384. Plenum Press, New York.
4. Braestrup, C., Nielsen, M., and Honoré, T. (1983): J. Neurochem. submitted.
5. Braestrup, C., Nielsen, M., Krogsgaard-Larsen, P., and Falch, E. (1979): Nature 280:331-333.
6. Braestrup, C., Schmiechen, R., Neef, G., Nielsen, M., and Petersen, E.N. (1982): Science, 21 6:1241-1243.
7. Braestrup, C., Schmiechen, R., Nielsen, M., and Petersen, E.N. (1982): In: Pharmacology of Benzodiazepines, edited by S.M. Paul et al., in press, McMillan Press.
8. Bowman, W.C., and Rand, M.J. (1980): Textbook of Pharmacology 2nd edition, Blackwell Scientific Publications, Oxford.
9. Brown, C.L., and Martin, I.L. (1982): Brit. J. Pharmacol. 77:312P.
10. Chan, C.Y., Gibbs, T.T., and Farb, D.H. (1982): Soc. Neurosci. 12th annual meeting abstract no. 158.6.
11. Costa, E., Robard, D., and Pert, C.B. (1979): Nature 277:315-316.
12. Czernik, A.J., Petrack, B., Kalinsky, H.J., Psychoyos, S., Cash, W.D., Tsai, C., Rinehart, R.K., Granat, F.R., Lovell, R.A., Brundish, D.E., and Wade, R. (1982): Life Sci. 30:363-372.
13. Doble, A., Martin, I.L., and Richards, D.A. (1982): Brit. J. Pharmacol. 76:238P.
14. Dorow, R. 13th C.I.N.P. congress (1982).
15. Ehlert, F.J. Roeske, W.R., Braestrup, C., Yamamura, S.H., and Yamamura, H.I. (1981): Eur. J. Pharmacol. 70:593-596.
16. Gee, R.W., and Yamamura, H.I. (1982): Eur. J. Pharmacol. 82:239-241.
17. Guidotti, A., Toffano, G., Baraldi, M., Schwartz, J.P., and Costa, E. (1979): In: Gaba-Neurotransmitters, edited by P. Krogsgaard-Larsen, J. Scheel-Krüger and H. Kofoed, pp. 406-415, Munksgaard, Copenhagen.
18. Haefely, W., Polc, P., Schaffner, R., Keller, H.H., Pieri, L., and Möhler, H. (1979): In: Gaba-Neurotransmitters, edited by P. Krogsgaard-Larsen, J. Scheel-Krüger and H. Kofoed, pp. 357-375, Munksgaard, Copenhagen.

19. Heidmann, T., and Changeux, J.P. (1979): Eur. J. Biochem. 94:281-296.
20. Jones, B.J., and Oakley, N.R. (1981): Brit. J. Pharmacol. 74:884P-885P.
21. Karobath, M., and Sperk, G. (1979): Proc. nat. Acad. Sci. 76:1004-1006.
22. Karobath, M., and Supavilai, P. (1982): Neurosci. lett. 31:65-69.
23. Marangos, P.J., and Patel, J. (1981): Life Sci. 29:1705-1714.
24. Martin, I.L., and Candy, J.M. (1978): Neuropharmacol. 17:993-998.
25. Möhler, H. (1982): Eur. J. Pharmacol. 80:435-436.
26. Möhler, H., and Richards, J.G. (1981): Nature 294:753-765.
27. Nielsen, M., Honoré, T., and Braestrup, C. (1982): Biochem. Pharmacol. in press.
28. Nielsen, M., Schou, H., and Braestrup, C. (1981): J. Neuro-chem. 36:276-285.
29. O'Brian, R.A., Schlosser, W., Spirt, N.M., Franco, S., Horst, W.D., Polc, P., and Bonetti, E.P. (1981): Life Sci. 29:75-81.
30. Olsen, R.W. (1982): Ann. Rev. Pharmacol. 22:245-277.
31. Patel, J., Marangos, P., and Goodwin, F. (1981): Eur. J. Pharmacol. 72:419-422.
32. Chang, L.R., Barnard, E.A., Lo, M.M.S., and Dolly, J.O. (1981): FEBS LETT. 126:309-312.
33. Schweri, M., Cain, M., Cook, J., Paul, S., and Skolnick, P. (1982): Pharmac. Biochem. Behav. 17: in press.
34. Skerrit, J.H., Willow, M. and Johnston, G.A.R. (1982): Neurosci. lett. 29:63-66.
35. Skolnick, P., Schweri, M.M., Williams, E.F., Moncada, V.Y., and Paul, S.M. (1982): Eur. J. Pharmacol. 78:133-136.
36. Study, R.E., and Barker, J.L. (1982): JAMA 247:2147-2151.
37. Squires, R.F., and Braestrup, C. (1977): Nature 266:732-734.
38. Tallmann, J.F., Thomas, J.W., and Gallager, D.W. (1978): Nature 274:383-385.
39. Thomas, J.W., and Tallman, J.F. (1982): Soc. Neurosci. 12th annual meeting abstract no. 111.1.
40. Vallin, A., Dodd, R.H., Liston, D.R., Potier, P., and Rossier, J. (1982): Eur. J. Pharmacol. 85:93-99.
41. White, W.F., Dichter, M.A., and Snodgrass, S.R. (1981): Brain Res. 215:162-176.

CNS Receptors—From Molecular
Pharmacology to Behavior, edited by
P. Mandel and F. V. Defeudis.
Raven Press, New York © 1983.

Benzodiazepine Receptors: Mode of Interaction of Agonists and Antagonists

H. Möhler

*Pharmaceutical Research Department, F. Hoffmann-La Roche & Co., Ltd.,
CH-4002 Basel, Switzerland*

It is well established that the main central actions of tranquillizing benzodiazepines such as their anxiolytic, hypnotic,
muscle relaxant and anticonvulsant actions are based on the enhancement of GABAergic synaptic transmission (12, 13). The initial event in this process is the activation of benzodiazepine
receptors (25, 38). These receptors could be localized, at least
in part, in GABAergic synapses (28), where they appear to be part
of a supramolecular complex consisting of the GABA-receptor, the
chloride-ionophore, the benzodiazepine receptor and probably
other proteins (22, 27). The GABA-dependent activation of the
chloride ionophore is modulated in the presence of benzodiazepines
in such a way that the frequency of chloride channel opening is
increased (39).

The recent development of novel benzodiazepine receptor ligands
has led to a new concept: opposite pharmacological effects can be
mediated via the same receptors· Depending on the type of
ligand, not only anxiolytic, muscle relaxant and anticonvulsant
actions but also anxiogenic and convulsant actions can be mediated via benzodiazepine receptors. This view is based mainly on
studies of the pharmacology and biochemistry of the imidazobenzo-
diazepine Ro 15-1788 and some β-carboline-3-carboxylates. This
paper describes the mode of interactions of various types of
ligands with benzodiazepine receptors.

BENZODIAZEPINE ANTAGONISTS

Compounds which antagonize the effects of tranquillizing benzodiazepines at the level of the benzodiazepine receptor have only
recently been discovered (11). They were found among imidazodiazepines, β-carboline-3-carboxylates and pyrazoloquinolines. Among
the imidazodiazepines, Ro 15-1788 was found to selectively an-

tagonize all major central actions of benzodiazepines by competitive high affinity interaction with benzodiazepine receptors in the central nervous system. Ro 15-1788 per se, in doses sufficient to antagonize benzodiazepine actions, has no major pharmacological actions in most animal test systems and in man (3, 9, 14, 19, 24, 34). Ro 15-1788 can be used clinically to alleviate benzodiazepine effects,e.g. in case of intoxication or overdosage (G. Scollo-Lavizzari, personal communication).

Among β-carboline-3-carboxylate derivatives, the methyl-, ethyl- and propylesters (βCCM, βCCE, βCCP), the methylamide (βCCMA) and 6,7-dimethoxy-4-ethyl-β-carboline-3-carboxylate (DMCM) are high affinity ligands for benzodiazepine receptors (4, 5, 6, 7, 29, 30) and antagonize benzodiazepine effects in vivo (8, 10, 20, 31, 32, 33, 35, 37, 41). However, in contrast to Ro 15-1788, some of these compounds show major pharmacological actions per se. βCCE shows proconvulsant activity, DMCM and βCCM are convulsants and βCCMA induces anxiety attacks in man (7, 8, 15, 31, 32). Thus, the pharmacological effects of these β-carbolines are opposite to those of tranquillizing benzodiazepines. Correspondingly, their mechanism of action was found to be the reverse of that of benzodiazepines. While GABAergic synaptic transmission is enhanced by tranquillizing benzodiazepines, it is reduced by βCCE and βCCM (33, 35, 36). Although tranquillizing benzodiazepines and the above-mentioned β-carbolines show opposite pharmacological effects,they appear to interact with the same receptor sites in the CNS. This view is based on the finding that Ro 15-1788 antagonizes not only the effects of tranquillizing benzodiazepines but also those of β-carbolines, as shown for βCCE and βCCM (31, 33, 36). Furthermore, in vitro, the ligand specificity and maximum number of binding sites for ^{3}H-Ro 15-1788 were the same as those for ^{3}H-clonazepam (26) and largely similar to those of ^{3}H-βCCE, ^{3}H-βCCP and ^{3}H-βCCM (5, 6, 29, 30).

NOMENCLATURE OF RECEPTOR LIGANDS

In order to differentiate the various groups of benzodiazepine receptor ligands the term agonist is used for ligands with tranquillizing and anticonvulsant actions. This group of ligands includes the classical benzodiazepines and chemically unrelated compounds with similar pharmacological characteristics such as zopiclone (2) and CL 218 872 (18). In contrast, compounds which exert proconvulsant, convulsant and anxiogenic actions may be termed "inverse agonists" (36). This group of compounds is so far restricted to β-carboline-3-carboxylates such as βCCE, βCCM, βCCMA and DMCM. Obviously, when both an agonist and an inverse agonist are administered, the pharmacological effects of the agonist are alleviated by the inverse agonist and vice versa.

The third category of receptor ligands comprises compounds which lack major pharmacological actions per se, but antagonize the effects of other receptor ligands. Classically, this group of compounds is termed antagonists. Their representative is Ro 15-1788. The effect of both agonists and inverse agonists are antagonized by Ro 15-1788.

In the future, compounds may be found with properties of both agonists and antagonists contained in the same molecule (mixed agonist/antagonists) and those with properties of antagonists and inverse agonists (mixed inverse agonists/antagonists).

MODE OF LIGAND RECEPTOR INTERACTIONS

Although agonists, inverse agonists and antagonists appear to interact with the same sites in the CNS, their mode of receptor interaction must be different, since these groups of compounds elicit different pharmacological effects. Experimental evidence for a differential mode of receptor interaction is provided by two types of in vitro receptor binding studies:

1) Measurement of receptor affinity in the presence and absence of GABA:
Since the affinity of benzodiazepine receptor agonists is known to be enhanced in the presence of GABA (16, 40), an attempt was made to determine whether the affinity of other receptor ligands would also be altered in the presence of GABA. Their IC_{50} values were determined in the absence and presence of GABA on ^3H-Ro 15-1788 binding (Tab. 1). It was found that the IC_{50} ratio (-GABA/+GABA) was greater than 1.0 for receptor agonists (Group A), while the IC_{50} ratio of inverse agonists (Group C) was less than 1.0. Thus, compounds with opposite pharmacological profile showed opposite changes in the GABA-dependent IC_{50} ratio. However, receptor ligands which lack major pharmacological activity per se, such as Ro 15-1788 and its desfluoroanalogue Ro 14-7437 (Group B), showed the same IC_{50} value in the presence and absence of GABA (26). Thus, the GABA-dependent affinity shift (IC_{50} ratio) may be useful to predict the pharmacological profile of a receptor ligand. For example, the pharmacological spectrum of the pyrazoloquinoline CGS 8216 (1) is expected to be similar to that of βCCE and βCCMA (Tab. 1). Results similar to those in Tab. 1 were found with ^3H-diazepam as radioligand (7).

2) Receptor affinity after photoaffinity labelling.
In brain synaptic membranes, four benzodiazepine binding sites appear to occur in close spatial association (23). After photo-labeling maximally with flunitrazepam only one of the sites becomes irreversibly blocked. The binding characteristics of the remaining sites were investigated in reversible binding studies

TABLE 1. Effect of GABA on the inhibitory potency of various benzodiazepine receptor ligands[a]

Ligands		IC_{50} Ratio (-GABA/+GABA)
Group A	Flunitrazepam	3.3 ± 0.4
	Diazepam	2.9 ± 0.1
	Oxazepam	2.7 ± 0.4
	Zopiclone	1.6 ± 0.1
	CL 218 872	1.6 ± 0.2
	PK 9084	1.5 ± 0.1
Group B	Ro 15-1788	1.1 ± 0.05
	Ro 14-7437	0.9 ± 0.1
	βCCP	1.0 ± 0.05
Group C	CGS 8216	0.7 ± 0.1
	βCCE	0.7 ± 0.1
	βCCMA	0.7 ± 0.1
	βCCM	0.6 ± 0.05
	DMCM	0.5 ± 0.1

[a]IC_{50} values were determined in ^3H-Ro 15-1788 binding in the absence and presence of 100 $\mu mol \cdot 1^{-1}$ GABA at 35 °C. The ratio of the IC_{50}-value $\pm$ SEM (-GABA/+GABA) (n=3) is given (26). For the structure of PK 9084 and CGS 8216 see ref. 17 and 1, respectively.

using ^3H-Ro 15-1788 as radioligand (Tab. 2) (21). Compared to non-photolabeled membranes the displacing potency of various receptor agonists was reduced (Group A), while that of Ro 15-1788 remained unchanged (Group B). Among inverse agonists only βCCM and DMCM showed a reduction in inhibitory potency after photolabeling (Group C). Apparently this assay is less sensitive as a predictor of the pharmacological profile of inverse agonists than the test of the GABA shift described above. However, if βCCM and DMCM are considered as representatives for inverse agonists, the results of both assays are compatible. When the affinity of agonists is either increased or decreased under the assay conditions, the affinity of inverse agonists was altered in the opposite direction. This result may reflect the property of agonists and inverse agonists to induce different conformational changes of the benzodiazepine receptor protein which result in opposite pharmacological effects.

In contrast, Ro 15-1788 seems to interact with a part of the benzodiazepine binding site which is not affected by the conformational changes induced by either GABA or the photolabeling reaction with flunitrazepam. This lack of susceptibility to conformational changes may reflect the inability of Ro 15-1788 to induce a conformational change of the receptor. The analysis of the thermodynamics of the ligand binding reaction supports this view.

TABLE 2. Effect of photoaffinity-labeling on the inhibitory
potency of various benzodiazepine receptor ligands[a]

	Ligands	IC_{50} ratio
Group A	Diazepam	48
	Oxazepam	37
	Flunitrazepam	30
	Clonazepam	20
	Zopiclone	2.5
	CL 218 872	2.7
Group B	Ro 15-1788	1.1
	βCCP	1.0
Group C	CGS 8216	1.0
	βCCE	0.9
	βCCMA	1.0
	βCCM	0.7
	DMCM	0.4

[a] IC_{50} values were determined on ^{3}H-Ro 15-1788 binding using
photolabeled and control membranes from rat cerebral cortex. The
IC_{50} ratios (photolabeled/control) are the means of two determinations (21).

THERMODYNAMICS OF THE LIGAND–RECEPTOR INTERACTION

Differences in the type of ligand-receptor interaction can be
detected by an analysis of the thermodynamics of the binding reaction. The changes in free energy (ΔG^0) and free enthalpy
(ΔH^0) have previously been shown to be different for the binding
reaction of agonists and antagonists, e.g. at the β-adrenergic receptor (42). In the case of benzodiazepines, the ligand receptor
interaction of the agonist clonazepam was found to be mainly an enthalpy driven process, while that of the antagonist Ro 15-1788
was enthalpy as well as entropy (ΔS^0) driven at 37 ^{0}C (Tab. 3)
(26). This result is in line with a differential mode of interaction of agonists and antagonists with benzodiazepine receptors.
The difference in the thermodynamics of the binding reaction
of clonazepam and Ro 15-1788 was apparent only at temperatures
> 21 ^{0}C. Below that temperature, where phase transitions of lipids
are known to occur, clonazepam and Ro 15-1788 binding showed the
same thermodynamic parameters (26). Possibly the agonist-dependent
change in benzodiazepine receptor conformation can only be induced
at temperatures > 21 ^{0}C.

TABLE 3. Thermodynamic parameters of the binding reaction of
          clonazepam and Ro 15-1788 to benzodiazepine
          receptors[a]

	ΔG^0 (kcal·mol^{-1})	ΔH^0 (kcal·mol^{-1})	ΔS^0 (EU)
Clonazepam	- 11.2	- 15.0	- 12.2
Ro 15-1788	- 11.5	- 9.9	+ 5.1

[a]Binding assays were performed at 37 °C with membranes from
rat cerebral cortex (26).

MODEL OF LIGAND-RECEPTOR INTERACTION

The electrophysiological, pharmacological and biochemical evidence concerninq the mode of receptor interaction of various types
of benzodiazepine receptor ligands can be summarized in a simple
model: Receptor agonists induce a conformational change of the receptor which results in an increased frequency of the opening of
the GABA-dependent chloride channel. This effect is the basis of
the tranquillizing, anticonvulsant and muscle relaxant action of
this group of compounds. By contrast, inverse agonists which show
proconvulsant, convulsant and anxiogenic activity induce a different conformational change of the receptor, resulting in a reduction of GABAergic synaptic transmission. It is not known whether
this effect is based on a decrease of the mean channel open time
or a decrease of the frequency of chloride channel opening. Finally, antagonists of the type of Ro 15-1788 interact with the
receptor protein without inducing a conformational change, which
explains the lack of major pharmacological activity of such compounds per se. They antagonize,however, the effects of agonists as
well as of inverse agonists by competitive interaction at the
binding site.
    The manipulation of the efficiency of a synaptic process in op-
posite directions via one receptor site is a novelty in the field
of pharmacology. Possibly, a continuous spectrum of receptor ligands exists ranging from pure agonists to pure inverse agonists
by which the GABAergic synaptic transmission may be enhanced or
reduced to various degrees. The pharmacological properties and
mechanisms of action of such compounds will be of great interest.

Acknowledgment
I thank Dr. W. Haefely for critical reading of the manuscript.

REFERENCES

1. Bernard,P., Bergen, K., Sobiski, R. and Robson, R.D. (1981): Pharmacologist, 23: 150.
2. Blanchard, J.C., Boireau, A., Garret, C. and Joulou,L. (1979): Life Sci., 24: 2417-2420.
3. Bonetti, E.P., Pieri, L., Cumin, R., Schaffner, R., Pieri, M., Gamzu, E.R., Müller, R.K.M. and Haefely, W. (1982): Psychopharmacology, 78: 8-18.
4. Braestrup, C., Nielsen, M. and Olsen, C.E. (1980): Proc. Natl. Acad. Sci. USA, 77: 2288-2292.
5. Braestrup, C. and Nielsen, M. (1981): Nature, 294: 472-474.
6. Braestrup, C. and Nielsen, M. (1981): J. Neurochem., 37: 334-341.
7. Braestrup, C., Schmiechen, R., Neff, G., Nielsen, M. and Petersen, E.N. (1982): Science, 216: 1241-1243.
8. Cowen, P.J., Green, A.R., Nutt, D.J. and Martin, I.L. (1981): Nature, 290: 54-55.
9. Darragh, A., Scully, M., Lambe, R., Brick, I., O'Boyle, C. and Downie, W.W. (1981): Lancet, 2: 8-10.
10. Fujimoto, M., Kawasaki, K., Tatsushita, A. and Okabayashi, T. (1982): Eur. J. Pharmacol., 80: 259-262.
11. Haefely, W., Bonetti, E.P., Burkard, W.P., Cumin, R., Laurent, J.-P., Möhler, H., Pieri, L., Polc, P., Richards, J.G., Schaffner, R. and Scherschlicht, R. (1983): Benzodiazepines: Molecular Biology to Clinical Practice, edited by E. Costa, R. Amrein, W. Haefely, and J. Ward, (in press). Raven Press, New York.
12. Haefely, W., Pieri, L., Polc, P. and Schaffner, R. (1981): In: Handbook of Experimental Pharmacology, Vol. 55, Psychotropic Agents, Part 2, edited by F. Hoffmeister and G. Stille, pp. 13-262. Springer, New York.
13. Haefely, W., Polc, P., Pieri, L., Schaffner, R. and Laurent, J.-P. (1983): In: Benzodiazepines: Molecular Biology to Clinical Practice, edited by E.Costa, R.Amrein, W.Haefely and J. Ward, (in press). Raven Press, New York.
14. Hunkeler, W., Möhler, H., Pieri, L., Polc, P., Bonetti, E.P., Cumin, R., Schaffner, R. and Haefely, W. (1981): Nature, 290: 514-516.
15. Jones, B.J. and Oakley, N.R. (1981): Br. J. Pharmacol., 74: 223P.
16. Karobath, M. and Sperk, G. (1979): Proc. Natl. Acad. Sci. USA, 76: 1004-1006.
17. Lefur, G., Mizoule, J., Burgevin, M.C., Ferris, O., Heaulme, M., Gauthier, A., Gueremy, C. and Uzan, A. (1981): Life Sci., 28: 1439-1448.
18. Lippa, A.S., Coupet, E.N., Greenblatt, C.A., Klepner, C.A. and Beer, B. (1979): Pharmac. Biochem. Behav., 11: 99-106.

19. Lotz, W. (1982): Neuroendocrinology, 35: 32-36.
20. Mitchell, R. and Martin, I. (1980): Eur. J. Pharmacol., 68: 513-514.
21. Möhler, H. (1982): Europ. J. Pharmac., 80: 435-436.
22. Möhler, H. (1983): In: Benzodiazepines: Molecular Biology to Clinical Practice, edited by E. Costa, R. Amrein, W. Haefely and J. Ward, (in press). Raven Press, New York.
23. Möhler, H., Battersby, M.K. and Richards, J.G. (1980): Proc. Natl. Acad. Sci. USA, 77: 1666-1670.
24. Möhler, H., Burkard, W.P., Keller, H.H., Richards, J.G. and Haefely, W. (1981): J. Neurochem., 37: 714-722.
25. Möhler, H. and Okada, T. (1977): Science, 198: 849-851.
26. Möhler, H. and Richards, J.G. (1981): Nature, 294: 763-765.
27. Möhler, H. and Richards, J.G. (1983): In: Anxiolytics: Neurochemical, Behavioral and Clinical Perspectives, edited by J.B. Malick, S.J. Enna and H.I. Yamamura, (in press). Raven Press, New York.
28. Möhler, H., Richards, J.G. and Wu, J.-Y. (1981): Proc. Natl. Acad. Sci. USA, 78: 1935-1938.
29. Nielsen, M. and Braestrup, C. (1980): Nature, 286: 606-607.
30. Nielsen, M., Schou, H. and Braestrup, C. (1981): J. Neurochem., 36: 276-285.
31. Nutt, D.J., Cowen, P.J. and Little, H.J. (1982): Nature, 295: 436-438.
32. Oakley, N.R. and Jones, B.J. (1980): Eur. J. Pharmacol., 68: 381-382.
33. O'Brien, R.A., Schlosser, W., Spirt, N.M., Franco, S., Horst, W.D., Polc, P. and Bonetti, E.P. (1981): Life Sci., 29: 75-82.
34. Polc, P., Laurent, J.-P., Scherschlicht, R. and Haefely, W. (1981): Naunyn-Schmiedeberg's Arch. Pharmacol. 316: 317-325.
35. Polc, P., Ropert, N. and Wright, D.M. (1981): Brain Res., 217: 218-220.
36. Polc, P., Bonetti, E.P., Schaffner, R., and Haefely, W. (1983): Naunyn-Schmiedeberg's Arch. Pharmacol., (in press).
37. Prado de Carvalho, L., Grecksch, G., Chaponthier, G. and Rossier, J. (1983): Nature, (in press).
38. Squires, R.F. and Braestrup, C. (1977): Nature, 266: 732-734.
39. Study, R.E. and Barker, J.L. (1981): Proc. Natl. Acad. Sci. USA, 78: 7180-7184.
40. Tallman, J.F., Thomas, J.W. and Gallager, D.W. (1978): Nature, 274: 384-385.
41. Tenen, S. and Hirsch, J.D. (1980): Nature, 288: 609-610.
42. Weiland, G.A., Minneman, K.P. and Molinoff, P.B. (1979): Nature, 281: 114-117.

CNS Receptors—From Molecular
Pharmacology to Behavior, edited by
P. Mandel and F. V. Defeudis.
Raven Press, New York © 1983.

Classification of Dopamine Receptors

Ian Creese, David R. Sibley, and Stuart Leff

*Department of Neurosciences, School of Medicine, University of California, San Diego,
La Jolla, California 92093*

Rapid progress has been made during the past two years in the classification of dopamine receptor subtypes (3,27). Although direct biochemical studies of dopamine receptor interactions were initiated in 1972 with the identification of a dopamine-stimulated adenylate cyclase in both brain and peripheral nervous tissue (15), it was not until radioligand binding experiments were conducted in 1975 (6) that it first became apparent that dopamine receptor subtypes existed. It is now clear from both pharmacological and radioligand binding experiments that dopamine receptors can be classified into at least two broad categories (17). D-1 dopamine receptors have been associated with stimulation of adenylate cyclase, whereas D-2 dopamine receptors are associated with inhibition of adenylate cyclase activity. Radioligand binding experiments have been able to delineate these two receptor subtypes. Radioligand binding experiments have also identified additional sites whose relationship to the D-1 and D-2 dopamine receptors remains unclear, but which have been suggested to identify dopamine autoreceptors found on dopamine neurons and terminals (21,24,31). This chapter will review the recent radioligand binding experiments investigating each putative receptor subtype.

D-1 Dopamine Receptors

A dopamine-stimulated adenylate cyclase was first identified in mammalian superior cervical ganglion and subsequently in the retina and striatum (2,11,16). Briefly, phenothiazine antagonists have nanomolar potency, butyrophenone antagonists have micromolar potency and dopamine agonists stimulate activity at micromolar concentrations. The dopaminergic ergots are partial agonists or antagonists at this receptor having sub-micromolar to micromolar potency, and the benzamide antipsychotics show no antagonist activity.

D-1 receptors can be directly studied with radioligand binding experiments using [^{3}H]flupenthixol or [^{3}H]piflutixol, thioxanthene antagonists which label sites in striatum with nanmolar affinity and have structures similar to the phenothiazines (9,13,14). The potencies of dopaminergic antagonists in inhibiting dopamine-stimulated adenylate cyclase$_3$ activity correlates well with their potencies in competing for [^{3}H]flupenthixol binding. These sites are present in striatum at approximately three fold the density seen for D-2 binding sites. However, thioxanthene antagonists are not selective D-1 antagonists. Detailed competition studies have revealed that a proportion (about 20%) of [^{3}H]flupenthixol binding is to D-2 receptors (9). However, the D-1 receptor can be selectively labeled with [^{3}H]flupenthixol by including an appropriate "masking" drug, i.e., a low concentration of an unlabeled butyrophenone, in the assay to saturate D-2 receptors (29).

D-1 receptors in the striatum appear to be located exclusively on intrinsic neurons. Kainic acid-induced lesions of striatal neurons almost completely eliminate striatal dopamine-stimulated adenylate cyclase activity (10,21). The localization of D-1 receptors to striatal neurons is further supported by our findings that [^{3}H]flupenthixol binding shows a similarly large loss after kainic acid lesions (19).

Labeled dopamine agonists such as [^{3}H]dopamine, [^{3}H]apomorphine, and [^{3}H]n-propylnorapomorphine (NPA) label a population of divalent cation-dependent, guanine nucleotide-sensitive sites in striatum which display high affinity for thioxanthene and phenothiazine antagonists and low affinity for butyrophenone antagonists (12). These characteristics suggest that these sites may be a high affinity, agonist specific binding state of the D-1 receptor. Recent studies have demonstrated that, similar to the D-2 receptor found in brain and anterior pituitary (see below), agonist binding to D-1 receptors appears to involve heterogeneous receptor states showing high and low affinity for agonists (29). As seen in agonist/[^{3}H]flupenthixol competition experiments, the addition of guanine nucleotides can cause the conversion of a high affinity agonist binding state of the receptor to a low affinity agonist-receptor state. Likewise, guanine nucleotides reduce the amount of [^{3}H]agonist binding, some of which may represent the high affinity$_3$ agonist state of the D-1 receptor (12). This high affinity [^{3}H]aporphine binding is also substantially reduced by striatal kainic acid lesion (19).

D-2 Dopamine Receptors

Butyrophenone antagonists such as haloperidol and spiperone labeled to a high specific activity, have been utilized to label D-2 dopaminergic receptor sites. These binding sites are not only found in dopamine innervated areas of the brain but also in the pituitary where dopamine inhibits prolactin release with nanomolar affinity. The pharmacological and biochemical characteristics of this receptor are markedly different from those of the D-1 dopamine receptor. In the pituitary dopamine inhibits adenylate cyclase activity stimulated by either beta-adrenergic receptor activation [intermediate lobe] (23) or vasoactive intestinal peptide [anterior lobe] (25). Butyrophenone and phenothiazine antagonists, as well as dopamine agonists, demonstrate nanomolar potencies, while the dopaminergic ergots are potent agonists and the substituted benzamides are active as antagonists at these dopamine receptors.

We have conducted detailed studies of radioligand binding experiments to D-2 dopamine receptors in the pituitary using computer assisted data analysis (28) and found that the binding of antagonists to the D-2 receptor exhibits mass-action characteristics consistent with a simple bimolecular reaction. In contrast, agonist binding displays heterogeneous properties indicative of two separate classes of agonist binding sites. These phenomena are demonstrated in Figure 1. Shown here is the experimental data and the resulting computer-modeled competition curve for a (+)butaclamol/[^{3}H]spiperone experiment. The computer analysis employed is a nonlinear least squares curve fitting program which can analyze the data in terms of one or more classes of binding sites. The (+)butaclamol curve models best to a single homogeneous receptor state with a K_D of 1.1nM. Also shown in Figure 1 are agonist/[^{3}H]spiperone competition experiments employing the agonist apomorphine. In membrane preparations in the absence of guanine nucleotides, the apomorphine curve is shallow (pseudo-Hill coefficient=0.58) with computer analysis indicating that the data is best explained by a two-state binding model. The dissociation constants for the high and the low affinity binding states (R_H and R_L) have been designated K_H and K_L respectively. Interestingly, the two states are present in about equal proportions in the membranes. In the presence of a saturating concentration of GppNHp, a nonmetabolizable analogue of GTP, the apomorphine curve is shifted to the right and is steepened (pseudo-Hill coefficient=0.94). Moreover, computer analysis of the data now indicates a single homogeneous population of binding sites in the membranes whose affinity for apomorphine is not significantly different from the K_L value of the control curve (Fig. 1) suggesting a conversion from the R_H receptor state to the R_L receptor state.

Recently, we also investigated the dopamine receptor radioligand binding characteristics in intact, viable bovine anterior pituitary cells (30). In these experiments, bovine anterior pituitaries were first dispersed into single whole cells via collagenase treatment and then used directly in the binding experiments. Strikingly, agonist/[^{3}H]spiperone competition

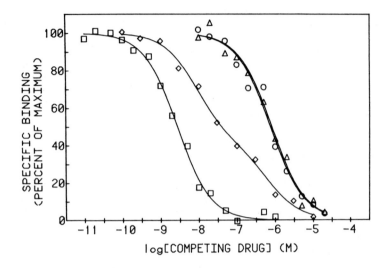

FIG. 1. Computer-modeled competition curves for [³H]spiperone binding to anterior pituitary preparations. The experimentally determined data points are shown by the open symbols while the solid lines are computer generated curves fitting the observed data points. The (+)butaclamol curve (□), performed using membranes, models best to a single binding site. The apomorphine curve (◇) fits best to two binding states of high (K_H=5nM) and low (K_L=350nM) affinity in about equal proportions (R_H=55%, R_L=45%) in the membranes. With the addition of 0.1mM GppNHp to the membranes (Δ), the apomorphine curve fits best to a single receptor state (K=360nM). Using whole cells (○), the apomorphine curve also models best to a single binding component (K=330nM).

curves are homogeneous with pseudo-Hill coefficients of about 1 (Fig. 1). Moreover, in Fig. 1, one can see that the apomorphine/[³H]spiperone curve in the cells is superimposable with the apomorphine/[³H]spiperone + GppNHp curve in membrane preparations. Additionally, exogenously added guanine nucleotides no longer affect the apomorphine/[^{3}H]spiperone curve. This suggests that in intact cells endogenous GTP regulates agonist binding in a fashion identical to that of exogenously added GTP in membrane preparations.

We have also characterized the binding of the radiolabeled agonist [^{3}H]NPA to dopamine receptors in bovine anterior pituitary membrane preparations (28). One of the more striking findings with this radioligand is that its Bmax is approximately 50% of that of [^{3}H]spiperone's suggesting that it labels only the high affinity agonist state (R_H) seen in agonist/[^{3}H]spiperone curves. This is also suggested by the finding that agonist/[^{3}H]NPA competition curves are homogeneous with the single affinities that are not significantly different from the K_H values obtained from the corresponding agonist/[^{3}H]spiperone curve. Furthermore, saturating concentrations of guanine nucleotides completely abolish the specific [^{3}H]NPA binding to pituitary membrane preparations without affecting the binding of [^{3}H]spiperone directly.

We have proposed that a two-step, three component ternary complex model can explain these unique properties of agonist binding to the D-2 dopamine receptor (28). This model proposes that agonist binding to the receptor takes place in two steps which involves the interaction of the agonist and receptor with an additional membrane effector unit (presumably a guanine nucleotide binding protein) to yield a high affinity ternary complex. It is this complex that is responsible for the high affinity agonist binding state. Guanine nucleotides exert their effects through inhibiting the formation and/or promoting destabilization of this high affinity ternary complex.

For the most part, D-2 receptors in brain appear to be identical to those of pituitary. Agonist/[^{3}H]spiperone competition experiments conducted in caudate membrane preparations indicate the presence of heterogeneous agonist states of the receptor which are regulated by guanine nucleotides. However, many investigators have observed that agonist/[^{3}H]spiperone competition curves conducted in these preparations show pseudo-Hill coefficients significantly less than 1, in the presence of maximally effective concentrations of guanine nucleotides. Several reasons for this should be considered. Firstly, [^{3}H]spiperone has high affinity for 5-HT$_2$ serotonin receptors which are present in the striatum (4). Thus, the heterogeneity still observed in the presence of guanine nucleotides could be due to labeling both 5-HT$_2$ and D-2 receptors. Consequently, D-2 receptor binding of [^{3}H]spiperone should be studied in the presence of a selective serotonergic antagonist such as ketanserin (29). Secondly, according to a two-step, three component ternary complex model, the proportion of the high affinity agonist binding state should be dependent upon the ratio of receptor and guanine nucleotide binding protein and the dissociation constant for their association (22). Consequently, full agonists at the D-2 receptor in brain may still show some high affinity binding in the presence of maximally effective concentrations of guanine nucleotides if the affinity of the guanine nucleotide binding protein for the receptor is only moderately decreased in the presence of guanine nucleotides. It should be considered that a population of high affinity butyrophenone sites may exist on cortico-striate terminals which are not GTP regulated (8). Following kainate lesion these sites may be studied in isolation (20). However, the lack of guanine nucleotide regulation of agonist binding at these sites may be an artifact of the kainate lesion.

We have recently obtained more direct evidence that D-2 receptor-agonist interactions in caudate nucleus may involve a GTP binding protein. When canine caudate membranes are solubilized with digitonin, agonist/[³H]spiperone competition curves are best described by a one-site model in which agonists show uniformly low affinity for D-2 [³H]spiperone binding sites (Fig. 2). Furthermore, guanine nucleotides have no additional effect on the agonist/[³H]spiperone competition curves, and we are unable to obtain any D-2 specific [³H]agonist binding in the solubilized receptor preparation (18). These findings suggested that solubilization of the receptor in digitonin inhibits or prevents the coupling of receptor with a GTP binding protein. However, if the membranes are preincubated with either labeled or unlabeled agonist, a GTP sensitive, high affinity agonist state of the D-2 receptor can be solubilized. If the membranes are preincubated with labeled [³H]agonists, reversible specific binding can be solubilized whose dissociation is enhanced by the addition of GTP but not ATP. When membranes are preincubated with unlabeled dopamine and subsequently solubilized, the addition of guanine nucleotides can reverse the prebound dopamine's inhibition of [³H]spiperone binding in the solubilized preparation, presumably by reducing agonist affinity for the solubilized D-2 receptor and enhancing its dissociation (5).

D-3 Binding Sites

We have seen that agonists can label D-2 dopamine receptors with nanomolar affinity, and that these sites show nanomolar affinity for butyrophenones as well. However, another site has been identified in the striatum which is labeled with nanomolar affinity by [³H]agonists but which demonstrates micromolar affinity for butyrophenones. It therefore cannot be a D-2 dopamine receptor. These sites have been designated as D-3 sites (32). [³H]Agonist binding to both D-2 and D-3 sites can be studied simultaneously. Competition curves between butyrophenone antagonists such as spiperone and labeled agonists such as [³H]dopamine (Fig. 3), [³H]apomorphine or [³H]NPA appear biphasic (Fig. 3). Computer analysis of this curve indicates that

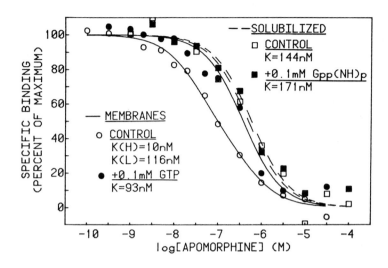

FIG. 2. Computer-modeled competition curves showing apomorphine inhibition of [³H]spiperone binding to canine caudate preparations. Data points are shown by symbols while the lines are computer generated curves fitting these points. Experiments using membrane homogenates (circles, solid lines) or extracts of digitonin solubilized membranes (squares, dashed lines) were conducted at 0-4°C. The control curve conducted in membranes fits best to two binding states of high $(K_H=10nM)$ and low $(K_L=116nM)$ affinity in about equal proportions $(R_H=59\%, R_L=41\%)$. With the addition of GTP to the membranes the curve fits best to a single receptor state (K=93nM). While agonist/[³H]spiperone competition curves from experiments on rat striatal membranes conducted in the presence of guanine nucleotides often do not fit best to a single receptor state, similar experiments conducted with several agonists in canine caudate membrane at this temperature always produce curves which fit best to one binding state. Using extracts of digitonin solubilized membranes, curves from competition experiments conducted in the presence or absence of guanine nucleotides models best to a single binding state (K=171nM and 144nM respectively).

[³H]dopamine labels two sites having nanomolar and micromolar affinity for spiperone respectively, and the respective density of these two sites in the striatum can be estimated by this

analysis. The portion of the curve showing nanomolar affinity
for spiperone represents binding to the D-2 receptor, while the
portion showing lower affinity for spiperone represents binding
to the D-3 site. As shown in Figure 3, binding to both sites can
be studied in striata after 6-hydroxydopamine denervation of the
nigrostriatal tract.

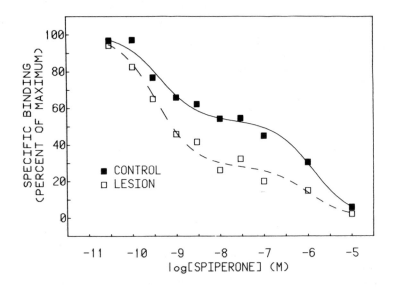

FIG. 3. Unilateral 6-OHDA lesions: representive fitted
curves for [³H]DA/spiperone competition in contralateral (■) and lesion (□₃) striata. Representative
spiperone competition for [³H]DA binding experiments in
control striatum were analyzed showing a best fit curve
modeling to two sites. The K_i's for spiperone for the
two sites were estimated to be 213pM and 0.65μM for the
high affinity (D-2) and low affinity (D-3) sites
respectively. D-3 sites comprised 53% of the total at
this [³H]DA concentration (1.3nM) in the non-lesioned
striatum. On the lesioned side D-3 sites comprised
only 28% of the total [³H]DA binding, or 47% of the
concentration of D-3 sites observed in the contralateral side. Final parameter estimates for curves shown
were; CONTRALATERAL: K#$_{D-2}$=213pM, R$_{D-2}$=9.1 fmol/mg tissue, K$_{D-3}$=0.65μM, R$_{D-3}$=10.2 fmol/mg tissue; LESION:
K$_{D-2}$=176pM, R$_{D-2}$=12.6 fmol/mg tissue; K$_{D-3}$=0.50μM, R$_{D-3}$=4.8 fmol/mg tissue. #K=affinity, R=receptor concentration.

6-OHDA-induced denervation of the nigrostriatal pathways leads to

Table 1. Characteristics of dopaminergic binding sites

	D-1	D-2 $R_H \rightleftharpoons R_L$		D-3
Usable radioligands				
[³H]thioxanthenes	+	+	+	?[1]
[³H]butyrophenones	-[2]	+	+	-
[³H]agonists	+[2]	+	-	+
Agonist affinity	μM[2]	nM	μM	nM
Butyrophenone affinity	μM	nM	nM	μM
Adenylate cyclase association	Stimulatory	Inhibitory or unassociated		?[3]
Guanine nucleotide sensitivity	++	++	-	+
Function	A) Parathyroid hormone release B) Striatum: unknown	A) Inhibition of pituitary hormone release B) DA mediated behavioral responses and their antagonism by neuroleptics		A) Autoregulation of DA neurones?
Striatal location	A) Intrinsic neurons	A) Intrinsic neurons B) Cortico-striate afferents?[4]		A) Intrinsic neurons B) Nigro-striatal terminals[5]
Pituitary location	-	+		-

1 [³H]flupentixol binding to D-3 receptors has yet to be investigated.

2 [³H]agonists may label a high affinity state of D-1 receptors in membrane preparations although stimulation of adenylate cyclase requires μM dopamine.

3 D-3 autoreceptors are definitely not linked to stimulation of adenylate cyclase. However their association with inhibition of adenylate cyclase has not been studied. Postsynaptic D-3 binding sites may be a high agonist-affinity state of D-1 receptors.

4 [³H]butyrophenone binding sites on cortico-striate terminals may be a distinct receptor subtype as they have low agonist affinity and no guanine nucleotide sensitivity. Alternatively, their lack of guanine nucleotide regulation may be an artifact of the kainic acid lesion used to isolate them.

5 D-3 binding sites appear to be found only postsynaptic to dopamine terminals in the striatum in our latest studies.

a 50% decrease in D-3 binding sites in rat striatum, which has suggested that they may identify dopamine autoreceptors on the presynaptic nigrostriatal terminals (24,31). D-2 receptors are increased by 10-40% due to degeneration-induced supersensitivity (7).

However, a 6-OHDA lesion not only removes the dopamine terminals from the striatum but also leads to a rapid depletion of dopamine. Recently, we and others (1,20) have seen that acute reserpine injections produce decreases in D-3 binding similar to that produced by 6-OHDA denervation. 6-Hydroxydopamine denervation produces a decrease of $64+4\%$ of D-3 [^{3}H]agonist binding which was observed to be due to a decrease in Bmax for these sites. Twenty hours after an injection of reserpine (4 mg/kg s.c.) D-3 binding decreases $42+6\%$. Preincubating membranes from reserpine-treated animals with either dopamine (100nM) or the supernatant from a membrane preparation of a normal striatum reverses the loss in D-3 [^{3}H]agonist binding. Similarly, preincubating striatal membranes from 6-OHDA denervated striata with dopamine also reverses the "lesion-induced" loss in D-3 [^{3}H]agonist binding (20). Thus the loss in D-3 binding seen after these two treatments appears to be an artefact of the depletion of striatal dopamine. Furthermore D-3 binding appears to be located on either striatal neurons and/or glia since the addition of dopamine to 6-OHDA lesioned striata produced normal levels of D-3 binding. Our studies of binding in striata after kainic acid lesion support the hypothesis that D-3 binding is localized largely on striatal neurons since D-3 binding is decreased by 75% after this treatment. We are therefore currently investigating the possibility that D-3 binding identifies a high affinity agonist state of the D-1 receptor.

CONCLUSION

Table 1 summarizes our present classification of dopamine receptors from radioligand binding experiments. Future studies investigating the properties of solubilized receptors will determine if they are one or the same gene products, or distinct molecular entities.

ACKNOWLEDGEMENTS

We wish to thank K. Tatsukawa for technical assistance and D. Taitano for manuscript typing. This work was supported by PHS grant #MH32990.

REFERENCES

1. Bacopolous, N.G. (1981): Life Sci., 29:2407-2414.
2. Brown, J.H., and Makman, M.H. (1972): Proc. Natl. Acad. Sci. USA, 69:539-543.
3. Creese, I. (1982): Trends in Neurosci., 5:40-43.
4. Creese, I., and Snyder, S.H. (1978): Eur. J. Pharmacol., 49:201-202.
5. Creese, I., and Leff, S.E. (1982): Soc. Neurosci. Abstr., (in press).
6. Creese, I., Burt, D.R., and Snyder, S.H. (1975): Life Sci., 17:993-1002.
7. Creese, I., Burt, D.R., and Snyder, S.H. (1977): Science 197:596-598.
8. Creese, I., Usdin, T., and Snyder, S.H. (1979): Nature, 278:577-578.
9. Cross, A.J., and Owen, F. (1980): Eur. J. Pharmacol., 65:341-347.
10. Govoni, S., Olgiati, V.R., Trabucchi, M., Garau, L., Stefanini, E., and Spano, P.F. (1978): Neurosci. Lett., 8:207-210.
11. Greengard, P. (1976) Nature, 260:101-108.
12. Hamblin, M.W., and Creese, I. (1982): Life Sci., 30:1587-1595.
13. Hyttel, J. (1978): Prog. Neuro-Psychopharmacol., 2:329-335.
14. Hyttel, J. (1978): Life Sci., 23:551-556.
15. Iversen, L.L. (1975): Science, 188:1084-1089.
16. Kebabian, J.W., Petzold, G.L., and Greengard, P. (1972): Proc. Natl. Acad. Sci. USA, 79:2145-2149.
17. Kebabian, J.W., and Calne, D.B. (1979): Nature, 277:93-96.
18. Leff, S.E., and Creese, I. (1982): Fed. Proc. 41:1633.
19. Leff, S., Adams, L., Hyttel, J., and Creese, I. (1981): Eur. J. Pharmacol. 70:71-75.
20. Leff, S.E., Hamblin, M.W., and Creese, I. (1982): Soc. Neurosci. Abstr., (in press).
21. List, S., Titeler, M., and Seeman, P. (1980): Biochem. Pharmacol., 29:1621-1622.
22. Molinoff, P.B., Wolfe, B.B., and Weiland, G.A. (1981): Life Sci., 29:427-443.
23. Munemura, M., Eskay, R.L., and Kebabian, J.W. (1980): Endocrinology, 106:1795-1803.
24. Nagy, J.I., Lee, T., Seeman, P., and Fibiger, H.C. (1978): Nature, 274:278-281.
25. Onali, P., Schwartz, J.P., Costa, E. (1981): Proc. Natl. Acad. Sci. USA, 78:6531-6534.
26. Schwarcz, R., Creese, I., Coyle, J.T., and Snyder, S.H. (1978): Nature, 271:766-768.
27. Seeman, P. (1980): Pharm. Rev., 32:229-313.
28. Sibley, D.R., De Lean, A., and Creese, I. (1982): J. Biol. Chem., 257:6351-6361.

29. Sibley, D.R., Leff, S.E., and Creese, I. (1982): Life Sci., 31:637-645.
30. Sibley, D.R., Mahan, L.C., Creese, I. (1981): Soc. Neurosci. Abstr., 7:126.
31. Sokoloff, P., Martres, M.-P., and Schwartz, J.-C. (1980): Nature, 288:283-286.
32. Titeler, M., List, S., and Seeman, P. (1979): Comm. Psychopharmacol., 3:411-420.

CNS Receptors—From Molecular
Pharmacology to Behavior, edited by
P. Mandel and F. V. Defeudis.
Raven Press, New York © 1983.

Solubilization of Brain Dopamine Receptors

Philip G. Strange, Patricia A. Frankham, Jean M. Hall,
and Mark Wheatley

*Department of Biochemistry, The Medical School, Queen's Medical Centre,
Nottingham NG7 2UH, England*

Of the several dopaminergic binding sites described
using in vitro assays, at present only the D_2 sites
show clearly the properties expected of a receptor
site (8,9). The D_2 receptor is involved in many
important dopaminergic functions and good correlations
are observed between potencies for substances in
in vitro D_2 receptor assays and in vivo dopaminergic
tests (8,9). We have initiated a programme aimed at
isolating and characterising the D_2 receptor protein
in brain and some of our studies are described below.

CHARACTERISATION OF MEMBRANE-BOUND D_2 RECEPTORS

We have characterised membrane-bound D_2 receptors
in bovine caudate nucleus using [^{3}H]spiperone binding
(13). Spiperone is a potent neuroleptic that has been
shown to interact strongly with dopaminergic D_2
receptors (5) but it has also been shown to interact
with serotonergic S_2 receptors (6) and this must be
taken into account in its use especially in tissues
like caudate nucleus that receive serotonergic
innervation in addition to dopaminergic innervation
(1,11). [^{3}H]Spiperone binding in bovine caudate
nucleus could be resolved into dopaminergic D_2 and
serotonergic S_2 contributions and the binding
properties of the dopaminergic D_2 sites could be
determined by using [^{3}H]spiperone binding in the
presence of a low concentration (0.3µM) of the
selective serotonergic antagonist mianserin to block
the serotonergic S_2 sites. Under the conditions used
antagonist binding to the D_2 sites was generally
homogeneous and characterised by slope factors (n)
close to one whereas agonist binding was heterogeneous

267

(n<1). We and others have resolved the agonist binding data into contributions from two classes of sites with equal antagonist affinities but differing agonist affinities which have been termed R_H (higher) and R_L (lower) (2,13). Good correlations were observed between antagonist affinities in these experiments and physiological measures of dopaminergic antagonist activity (9) and extensive examples of such correlations have been obtained by others (see for example 8).

ISOLATION AND CHARACTERISATION OF D_2 RECEPTOR PROTEIN

Initially we fractionated a bovine caudate nucleus homogenate by differential centrifugation and sucrose density gradient centrifugation in order to obtain a fraction enriched in D_2 receptor bearing membrane fragments (14). Enrichments of roughly six fold could be obtained by this approach but muscarinic acetylcholine receptors were also enriched in the preparation so that the technique is unlikely to be suitable for D_2 receptor purification. Therefore we have used the alternative approach of solubilisation of receptors using detergents as a preliminary to purification.

A series of detergents (non-ionic, zwitterionic and ionic) was tested for solubilisation of D_2 receptors from bovine caudate nucleus and good results were obtained with CHAPS (3 -[(3-cholamidopropyl)dimethyl-ammonio]-1-propane sulphonate), cholate (in the presence of sodium chloride), digitonin and lysophosphatidylcholine (LPC) (9,10,12,15). Solubilised receptors were assayed by [3H]spiperone binding using a charcoal adsorption technique to separate bound and free radioligand and defining specific receptor associated binding of [3H]spiperone as the difference in binding in parallel assays containing 1μM (+) and (-)-butaclamol. As this definition of specific binding does not distinguish dopaminergic and serotonergic sites it was necessary to characterise the solubilised preparations more fully. This was also necessary in order to determine that the preparations were truly solubilised and in order to gain some information on the physical characteristics of the solubilised receptors. This characterisation will be considered below for the LPC and cholate/sodium chloride solubilised preparations.

Solubilised preparation obtained with LPC

In using LPC for solubilisation it was found

(9,10,12) that unless proteinase inhibitors were present during solubilisation the pharmacological profile of the solubilised preparation was rather different from that seen for the membrane bound receptors and was dominated by the presence of [³H] spiperone binding sites that showed little or no ability to discriminate the isomers of the drug butaclamol (non-stereospecific sites or spirodecanone sites (3,4)). If solubilisation was carried out in the presence of proteinase inhibitors these non-stereospecific sites were less important, specific [³H] spiperone binding to receptors could easily be detected and a good correlation was observed between the binding of ligands to the solubilised sites and the membrane-bound D_2 receptors (9) so that the LPC solubilised preparation contains solubilised D_2 receptors with no major serotonergic component detectable under these conditions. Thus inhibition of receptor proteolysis during solubilisation may be important in obtaining a useful preparation of solubilised D_2 receptors. This effect of proteinase inhibitors in these experiments is largely due to benzethonium, a compound reported to be an inhibitor of cysteine proteinases (7). However, other specific inhibitors of cysteine proteinases do not exert the same effect so alternative explanations for the action of benzethonium must be considered. For example the combination of LPC and benzethonium could be solubilising a different combination of proteins or the same proteins in a different state, or benzethonium could be inhibiting [³H]spiperone binding to the non-stereospecific sites (9).

The LPC/benzethonium preparation can be passed through a 200nm filter without loss of specific [³H] spiperone binding and if the preparation is examined in the electron microscope (after fixation) no membranous elements are observed. Sucrose density gradient centrifugation in the presence of soluble marker enzymes gives a sedimentation coefficient (not corrected for detergent binding) of 11.9S. Thus the preparation appears to be truly solubilised. We have also shown the receptors to be glycoproteins by mannoside sensitive adsorption to concanavalin A-sepharose. The adsorbed receptors may be eluted from concanavalin A-sepharose by α-methyl mannoside with a five fold enrichment. These are preliminary experiments and should be amenable to improvement for use as a purification procedure.

The LPC/benzethonium solubilised preparation therefore offers a useful preparation of solubilised D_2 receptors. Even in this preparation, however, non-specific binding of [³H]spiperone is high, representing about 50% of the total [³H]spiperone binding. We have managed to reduce this non-specific binding considerably by running the ligand-binding assays at 25°C (30 mins.) as opposed to 4°C (4 hrs.) which was used for the other studies. At the higher temperature specific [³H]spiperone binding constituted 80% of the total binding (10). Some pharmacological data are given in Fig. 1: the selective dopaminergic antagonist domperidone shows evidence of binding to two classes of sites and the selective serotonergic antagonist mianserin inhibits a portion of the binding with high affinity. This is probably due to the presence of major dopaminergic D_2 and minor serotonergic S_2 components of [³H]spiperone binding. It is not clear why the S_2 component was not observed when the assays were carried out at 4°C. One possibility is that the

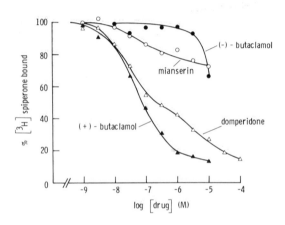

FIG. 1. Pharmacological profile of LPC (0.1%)-solubilised preparation assayed at 25°C. [³H)Spiperone binding was determined in the presence of varying concentrations of competing ligands.

affinity of the serotonergic sites for [³H]spiperone increases as the temperature is raised so that at the concentration of [³H]spiperone used for the assays the S_2 component is detected only at the higher temperature.

Solubilised preparation obtained with cholate/sodium chloride

The solubilised preparation obtained using cholate (0.2%)/sodium chloride (1M) and assayed at 4°C showed a high (80% approx.) proportion of specific [³H]

spiperone binding, the remainder consisting of minor
non-specific and non-stereospecific components. Some
pharmacological data are given in Fig. 2: the
selective dopaminergic antagonist domperidone and the

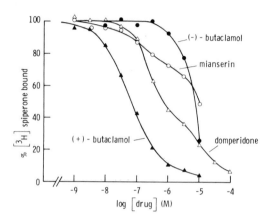

FIG. 2. Pharmacological profile of cholate/salt-
solubilised preparation. [³H]Spiperone binding was
determined in the presence of varying concentrations
of competing ligands.

selective serotonergic antagonist mianserin showed
evidence of binding to high and low affinity sites.
This may be due to the presence of D_2 and S_2
components of [³H]spiperone binding as described above
for the LPC-solubilised preparation.
    The solubilised [³H]spiperone binding sites pass
readily through a 200nm filter. Electron microscopy
of the cholate/sodium chloride solubilised preparation
did not reveal the presence of membranous elements.
Sucrose density gradient centrifugation gave a
sedimentation coefficient of 7.3S (not corrected for
detergent binding) and gel filtration on a calibrated
sepharose 4B column gave a Stokes Radius for the
solubilised preparation of 5nm. These data are
entirely consistent with the presence of truly
solubilised sites.

CONCLUSION

    In conclusion these studies show that either LPC
(in the presence of benzethonium) or cholate/sodium
chloride may be used for solubilisation of brain D_2
receptors. The yield of solubilised sites is much

greater with cholate/sodium chloride (10) and the
easily dialysable nature of the detergent may be useful
in receptor reconstitution studies. On the other hand
the presence of an ionic detergent may cause problems
in some future purification steps so that the
availability of the two detergent systems for receptor
solubilisation may be very important. The presence of
serotonergic components in the solubilised preparations
is to be expected given the properties of the starting
tissue and should be viewed favourably as it may enable
studies on solubilised S_2 receptors to be carried out.
As in the case of studies on membrane bound receptors,
serotonergic components of [^{3}H]spiperone binding may be
eliminated using an appropriate concentration of a
selective serotonergic antagonist such as mianserin.

ACKNOWLEDGEMENTS

We thank the Wellcome Trust and the M.R.C. for
financial support and Mrs. M. Spooner for help with
manuscript preparation.

REFERENCES

1. Anden, N., Fuxe, K., Hamberger, B. and Hokfelt, T.
    (1966): Acta. Physiol. Scand., 67:306-312.
2. Creese, I. (1982) Trends in Neurosciences, 5: 40-43.
3. Gorissen, H., Ilien, B., Aerts, G. and Laduron, P.
    (1980) FEBS Letts. 121:133-138.
4. Howlett, D.R., Morris, H. and Nahorski, S.R.
    (1979): Mol. Pharmacol., 15: 506-514.
5. Leysen, J.E., Gommeren, W. and Laduron, P.M.
    (1978): Biochem. Pharmacol., 27: 307-316.
6. Leysen, J.E., Niemegeers, C.J.E., Tollenaere, J.P.
    and Laduron, P.M. (1978): Nature (London) 272:
    168-171.
7. Otto, K. (1971): In: Tissue Proteinases: edited
    by A. J. Barrett and J. T. Dingle, pp. 1-25,
    North Holland Publishing Co., Amsterdam.
8. Seeman, P. (1980): Pharmacol. Rev. 32:229-313.
9. Strange, P.G. (1983): In: Cell Surface Receptors,
    edited by P.G. Strange, Ellis Horwood,
    Chichester, U.K. in press.
10. Strange, P.G., Frankham, P.A., Hall, J.M.,
    Lancaster, S., Wheatley, M. and Withy, R.M.
    (1983): In: Investigation of membrane-located
    receptors, edited by E. Reid, G.M.W. Cook and
    D.J. Morre, Plenum Press, New York, in press.
11. Van der Kooy, D. and Hattori, T. (1980): Brain
    Res. 186:1-7.
12. Wheatley, M., Frankham, P.A., Hall, J.M. and
    Strange, P.G. (1982): Biochem. Soc. Trans.
    10:373.

13. Withy, R.M., Mayer, R.J. and Strange, P.G. (1981):
    J. Neurochem. 37:1144-1154.
14. Withy, R.M., Mayer, R.J. and Strange, P.G. (1982):
    J. Neurochem. 38:1348-1355.
15. Withy, R.M., Wheatley, M., Frankham, P.A. and
    Strange, P.G. (1981): Biochem. Soc. Trans. 9:416.

CNS Receptors—From Molecular
Pharmacology to Behavior, edited by
P. Mandel and F. V. Defeudis.
Raven Press, New York © 1983.

Modulation of Dopamine Receptor Binding by Ascorbic Acid

Bertha K. Madras and Betty Chan

Psychopharmacology Section, Clarke Institute of Psychiatry; and Department of Pharmacology, University of Toronto, Toronto, Ontario, M5T 1R8 Canada

Brain dopamine/neuroleptic receptors (D_2-type) are the most probable site of action of neuroleptic drugs (28). Neuroleptic binding to the receptor correlates with neuroleptic doses which elicit clinical and behavioural responses (27,28).

Increased density of D_2 receptors is detectable in post-mortem schizophrenic brains (13). These excess receptors may be a characteristic of a subtype of schizophrenia, although a component of the increase is probably drug-induced (13,18,25). Tardive dyskinesia, a partly irreversible neurological disorder, develops after chronic neuroleptic treatment and elevated dopamine receptor density has been proposed as the cause (12). Thus, an understanding of dopamine receptor regulation is of obvious clinical importance. Regulation of dopamine receptor density, binding affinity, and activity is not well understood and may be exerted through proximal or distal (1,10) influences. Possible regulatory mechanisms include turnover (internalization, synthesis, degradation); receptor binding may also be modified by membrane constituents such as GTP (5), or membrane lipids (3,9,20). D_2 receptor regulation by these systems is currently under investigation in our laboratory. The present report outlines the evidence for membrane lipid modulation of dopamine receptors in vitro.

Recently, the binding of several neurotransmitter receptors dopamine D_1 (11,31), D_2

(3,9,11,16,20), opiate (16), $\propto$-adrenergic (16), serotonin S_1 (24,32) and S_2 (24) were reportedly decreased by inclusion of ascorbic acid in the assay medium. In the present report ascorbic acid reduced ^{3}H-spiperone binding to membrane, but not to solubilized receptors. Both EDTA and manganese prevented the ascorbate-induced decline of membrane receptors. Solubilized dopamine receptors retain the binding characteristics (Kd, I.C.$_{50}$'s, rank order of potencies) of membrane receptors (20) yet binding was not affected by ascorbate, EDTA, or manganese. The results indicate that ascorbic and/or manganese modulate dopamine receptors indirectly, possibly by modifying the membrane matrix of the receptor. Ascorbic acid may reduce D_2 receptor binding by catalyzing lipid peroxidation (3,9,20). In brain this reaction is catalyzed by ascorbate and Fe++ (26) and inhibited by EDTA.

MATERIALS AND METHODS

[3H]-Spiperone (26-51Ci/mmol) was obtained from New England Corp. (+)-Butaclamol was a gift from Ayerst Research Laboratories, Montreal. Digitonin (Fisher) and polyethylene glycol (6000) were obtained from commercial sources. Either fresh or frozen (Pelfreeze, AK) canine striata were used. The main difference between the two preparations is that dopamine displacement of ^{3}H-spiperone binding is less in the frozen (I.C.$_{50}$:15-25 μM) than the fresh (I.C.$_{50}$:5 μM) preparation.

Tissue Preparation

Membrane bound and solubilized receptors were prepared as described (19,21). Following homogenization (sucrose, 0.25 M, 10 vol.) and centrifugation, 1100 x g), the pellet was rehomogenized. The suspension was then centrifuged at 105,000 x g for 60 min. The pellet was resuspended in various buffers by homogenization (TEAN: 50 mM Tris HCl pH 7.4 at 0^0 C; 5 mM Na$_2$ EDTA; 0.01% ascorbic acid, 10 μM nialamide. TN: Tris, nialamide, TAN: tris, ascorbate, nialamide).

The membrane suspension was solubilized by exposure to digitonin (1% final concentration) in one of three buffers described above (19,21). After 30 min, the suspension was centrifuged at 105,000 x

g for 1 h and was used as soluble receptor
preparation.   Electron microscopy of the soluble
preparation revealed no membrane fragments (19,21).

Receptor Binding Assays

Membrane Assay:

Receptor preparations (when indicated) were
preincubated prior to the binding assay
(incubation).   Membranes prepared in various
buffers were preincubated for various time periods
(0, 2 h, 3 h, 24 h) at 22^0 C or 37^0 C.   The
preincubation medium was removed by dialysis of the
membrane preparation against at least 1000-fold
dilution with TN buffer.   Then binding assays were
performed with the following incubation
constituents: ^{3}H-spiperone (0.2 ml, 1 nM final)
and buffer for total binding, or ^{3}H-spiperone (0.2
ml, (+)-butaclamol: 1 M final) for non-specific
binding measurement.   A 3 h incubation at 0^0 C was
followed by filtration of 0.5 ml aliquot on Whatman
GF/B filters.   Radioactivity on the filter was
eluted with aquasol and measured by liquid
scintillation spectrometry (42% efficiency).   Each
experiment was repeated 3 times using a different
brain.

Soluble Assay:

The incubation medium was the same as
described earlier (19,21).   The soluble receptor
(0.1 ml, 1 mg/ml protein) and 0.05 ml of ion
solutions were preincubated for the indicated time
period.   Then 0.2 ml of either [^{3}H]-spiperone in
buffer or 0.2 ml of [^{3}H]-spiperone and (+)-
butaclamol (1 μM) were added.   Additional
incubation for 16 h at 0^0 C was followed by assay
using a modified (6), polyethylene glycol
precipitation assay (2).   The association time was
longer for the soluble preparation (5 h) and 16 h
was chosen for convenience.   At 0^0 C the receptor
was stable if ^{3}H-spiperone was present.   Bovine
gamma globulin (0.3 w/v, 100 μl) was added,
followed immediately with polyethylene glycol 6000
(30% w/v, 200 μl) final concentration, 10% in TEAN
or Tris-nialamide buffer at 4^0 C.   After stirring
and standing on ice for 10-15 mins, an aliquot (0.5
ml) was then filtered slowly through Whatman GF/B
glass fibre filters.   The filters were washed twice
with 7 ml of polyethylene glycol (10% in TEAN at 4^0

C) and incubated for 10 h at 4^0 C as described
above. Soluble receptors prepared in Tris-
nialamide buffer were used for the EDTA/ascorbate
experiments. Statistical analysis of each group
was done by the two-tailed Student's t-test
(multiple comparison procedure).

RESULTS

Preincubation of Receptors

Preparation Buffer,   TAN

    Preincubation of membrane receptors prepared
in tris-ascorbate-nialamide buffer (TAN) resulted
in an 80% loss of ^{3}H-spiperone binding (Fig. I).

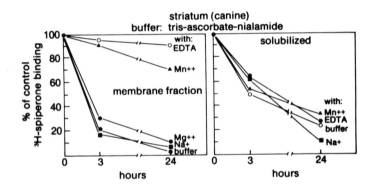

Fig. I   Effects of ions and Na₂EDTA on the
stability of [^{3}H]spiperone binding. Receptor
preparations were preincubated with ions NaCl (100
mM), MgCl₂ (1mM) MnCl₂ (1mM), EDTA (5mM) or no
additions (buffer), for various times (0,3,24h).
(The CaCl₂ curve is omitted but is almost identical
to that of MgCl₂). Then [^{3}H]spiperone (1nM) or
[^{3}H]spiperone and (+)-butaclamol (1 M) were added
to measure total and non-specific binding. Each
point is a mean of three experiments done in
triplicate. The y-axis: specific binding at 0 time
(in presence of individual ions) is the denominator
for the percentage calculations. The x-axis, hours
refers to preincubation time. At 3 h and 24 h
binding to the EDTA and Mn^{2+} treated membranes are
significantly different from controls (P < 0.005).

After 24 h only 5% of the binding remained. Both EDTA (5 mM) and Mn^{++} (5 mM), but not Ca^{++}, Mg^{++} or Na^+, prevented significant losses of receptor binding. Solubilized receptors also declined during preincubation. However, binding decreased to a lesser extent than membrane receptors at 3 h. Solubilized receptors were not affected by ascorbate, manganese, or EDTA. More recently, we have found that preincubation at 37^0 C for 2 h is sufficient to demonstrate the ascorbate effect.

Preparation buffer: TN

^{3}H-Spiperone binding to membrane receptors exposed to ascorbate alone for 3 h (not shown) or 24 h decreased significantly (Fig. II). EDTA prevented the decline. Solubilized receptor binding was reduced irrespective of buffer constituents.

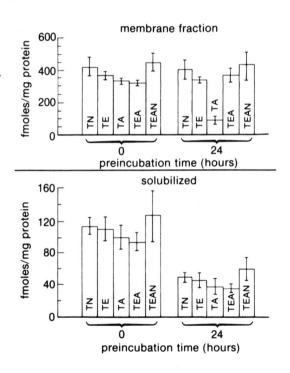

Fig. II   Influence of ascorbate and Na_2EDTA [^{3}H] spiperone binding to membrane and soluble fractions prepared in tris-nialamide buffer. Assays were done as described (legend fig. 1). TN

(Tris-nialamide), TE (Tris-Na$_2$EDTA), TA (Trs-ascorbate), TEA (Tris-Na$_2$EDTA, ascorbate), TEAN (tissue prepared in TEAN buffer). All values are mean $\pm$ S.E.M. of three experiments done in triplicate using individual canine brains.

Ascorbate and manganese modification of dopamine and neuroleptic displacement curves.

Receptors were prepared in various buffers and preincubated for 3 h at 22^0 C. Both dopamine and (+)-butaclamol displacement of ^{3}H-spiperone binding were reduced by ascorbate (TAN buffer, Fig. III). The IC$_{50}$ values for (+)-butaclamol increased 8-fold and dopamine 2-fold. Inclusion of manganese in the preincubation buffer prevented ascorbate-induced receptor binding decline.

Receptors preincubated in TEAN (not shown) or TN buffers showed similar displacement curves whether manganese was present or not (Fig. IV).

Preincubation of membranes with Ascorbate in the presence of Dopaminergic Drugs.

Membranes (prepared in TN or TAN buffer) were preincubated at 37^0 C for 2 h with dopamine (100 μM), apomorphine (50 μM) or haloperidol (100 nM). The concentrations selected were based on 5 x I.C.$_{50}$ values. Following dialysis to remove the drugs, specific ^{3}H-spiperone binding was measured. Haloperidol was minimally effective in preventing the ascorbic acid response. In contrast, in the presence of dopamine or apomorphine ^{3}H-spiperone binding was retained at 96 and 72% (resp.) of control (TN) values (Table 1). Glutathione failed to reverse the ascorbate effect.

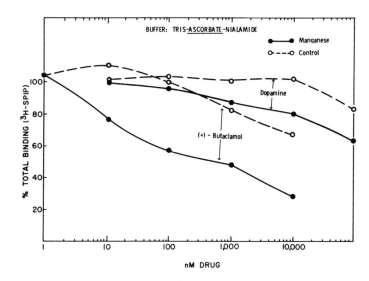

Fig. III and IV   Influence of manganese on ³H-spiperone binding to membranes preincubated either with or without ascorbic acid.

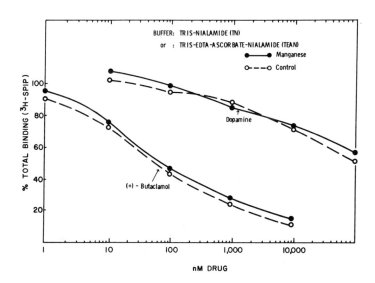

Table 1. Preincubation of membranes with ascorbate and dopaminergic drugs.

% OF CONTROL (TN) BINDING

		TN	TAN
Control		100	4
Haloperidol	(100 nM)	100	13
Dopamine	(100 μM)	80	96
Apomorphine	(50 μM)	81	72
GSH	(100 μM)	100	5

Ascorbate and neurotransmitter receptors

Recent reports on ascorbic acid modulation of CNS receptors are summarized in the following table (II).

Table II   Neurotransmitter Receptor binding in the presence of Ascorbic Acid.

RECEPTOR	%DECREASE	^{3}H-LIGAND		REF
Dopamine D_1 a	50	^{3}H-dopamine,	cAMP	11,31
Dopamine D_2 b	15-95,91	^{3}H-spip,	^{3}H-halo	3,16,20
Dopamine D_3 c		^{3}H-NPA		14
Serotonin S_1d	30,30	^{3}H-serotonin		24,32
Serotonin S_2	43	^{3}H-spiperone		24
Opiate	85	^{3}H-etorphine		16
α-Adrenergic	70,33	^{3}H-clonidine		16
Muscarinic- e	19	^{3}H-QNB		16

a ^{3}H-dopamine (11) does not necessarily label D_1 sites specifically or exclusively.
b   Decrease depends on exposure time, temperature, ascorbate concentration.
c   Ascorbate enables reversible dopamine agonist binding (N-propylnorapomorphine:NPA).
d   Binding not characterized.
e   Muscarinic-cholinergic, quinuclidinylbenzilate.

Manganese administration and dopamine receptor density

MnCl$_2$ (1.5 mg/ml) was administered to rats

(150-175 g) in drinking water. Controls received tap water. Both groups drank equal amounts of water and showed similar weight gain. After 1 and 2 weeks dopamine receptor density increased by 10% and 17% resp. The results were not statistically significant. After one month both control and experimental values were the same. (Fig.V).

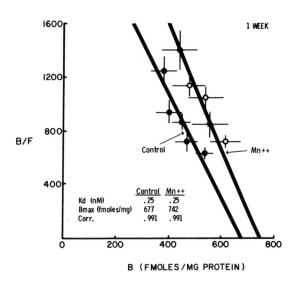

B (FMOLES/MG PROTEIN)

Fig. V MnCl₂ administration and ³H-spiperone binding (N=15)

DISCUSSION

Ascorbic acid produces a profound time-dependent decrease in specific ³H-spiperone binding to striatal membranes. The effect is irreversible because removal of ascorbate from the buffer did not restore binding. Heikilla et al. showed that the loss was due to a reduction in Bmax (12). Both EDTA and Mn⁺⁺ prevented the reduction in binding, although Mn⁺⁺ was not as effective. Dopamine and (+)-butaclamol displacement of ³H-spiperone showed loss in both affinity (increased I.C.₅₀) and sites. Inclusion of dopamine or apomorphine during ascorbate exposure (concentration 5-fold greater than I.C.₅₀ values) prevented the ascorbate-induced decline. Haloperidol (100 nM) however did not. Agonist occupancy of the receptor may induce a conformational change in the receptor which prevents the ascorbate effect; antagonist occupancy presumably involves no change in receptor conformation. Alternatively, catechols, as reducing agents, may specifically inhibit lipid peroxidation. The binding of ^{3}H-spiperone to solubilized receptors was lost during preincubation whether or not ascorbate was included in the buffer. Thus, it would appear that the binding changes induced by ascorbate may be indirect and not related to the binding site. To further this point, both EDTA and Mn^{++} which reversed the ascorbate-induced decline of binding, had no effect on the solubilized receptors.

The mechanism of ascorbic injury is unknown but increasingly thought to be related to lipid peroxidation. Lipid peroxidase is catalyzed by ascorbic acid and Fe^{++} (26). It is possible that EDTA chelates the Fe^{++}, and Mn^{++} (another transition state metal) is a competitive inhibitor of the reaction. Manganese has been shown to inhibit brain lipid peroxidase (29).

Direct evidence was provided by Heikilla et al. who recently demonstrated that inhibitors of lipid peroxidase also prevented ascorbate-induced loss of ^{3}H-spiperone binding to membranes (8,9). These observations, combined with the susceptibility of membrane but not solubilized receptors to ascorbic acid injury are strongly suggestive of lipid modulation of dopamine receptors in vitro.

Does lipid peroxidation modulate dopamine receptors in vivo? The scanty evidence is indirect. Ascorbic acid administered to rats or mice blocks amphetamine-induced turning behaviour or locomotion (8,30).

Although the brain has very high concentrations of ascorbic acid its function remains unknown. Ascorbic acid efflux from synaptic receptors is coupled to depolarization in vivo and in vitro (23). It is also released together with catecholamines from adrenal chromaffin cells upon stimulation (7). Whether the released ascorbate modulates dopamine receptors, either directly or by catalysis of lipid peroxidation is unknown.

Manganese toxicity in humans is characterized by an initial phase of psychosis followed by onset of Parkinsonism. Manganese inhibits brain lipid peroxide formation in rats (29).

In these studies manganese elevated dopamine receptor density but not significantly. It is possible that oral ingestion of manganese does not result in comparable levels of brain Mn^{++} as manganese absorbed through the lungs. Manganese toxicity in humans is characterized by an initial phase of psychosis followed by onset of Parkinsonism. Manganese inhibits brain lipid per-oxide formation in rats (29).

ACKNOWLEDGEMENTS

The authors thank Karen Scully for excellent technical assistance. The work was funded in part by the Banting Institute, the Bickell Foundation and the Ontario Mental Health Foundation.

REFERENCES

1. Baume, S., Patey, G., Marchais, H., Protais, P., Constentin, J., and Schwartz, J.-C. (1979): Life Sci. 24:2333-2342.

2. Chan,, B., Madras, B.K., Davis, A. and Seeman, P. (1981): Eur. J. Pharmacol. 74:53-59.

3. Chan, B., Seeman, P., Davis, A. and Madras, B.K. (1982): Eur. J. Pharmacol. 81:111-116.

4. Constentin, J., Marchais, H., Protais, P., Baudry, M., LaBaume, S., Martres, M.-P. and Schwartz, J.-C. (1977): Life Sci. 21:307-314.

5. Creese, I., Usdin, T. and Snyder, S.H. (1979). Mol. Pharmacol. 16:69-76.

6. Cuatrecasas, P. (1972): Proc. Nat. Acad. Sci. Sci 69:318.

7. Daniels, A.J., Dean, G., Viveros, O.H., and Diliberto, E.J. (1982): Science, 216:737-739.

8.   Heilkilla, R.E., Cabbat, F.S., and Manzino, L.
     (1981):   Res. Commun. Chem. Path. and
     Pharmacol. 34:409-421.

9.   Heilkilla, R.E., Cabbat, F.S., and Manzino, L.
     (1982): J. Neurochem. in press.

10. Hruska, R.E., Silbergeld, E.K. (1980): Eur. J.
     Pharmacol. 61:397-400.

11. Kayaalp, S.O., Rubenstein, J.S., and Neff, N.H.
     (1981): Neuropharmacology 20:409-410.

12. Klawans, H.L. (1973). Amer. J. Psychiatry
     130:82-86.

13. Lee, T., and Seeman, P. (1980):   Amer. J.
     Psychiat. 137:191-197.

14. Leff, S., Sibley, D.R., Hamblin, M. and Creese,
     I. (1982): Life Sci. 29:2081-2090.

15. Lieber, D., Harbon, S. (1982): Mol. Pharmacol.
     121:654-663.

16. Leslie, F.M., Dunlop, C.E. and Cox, B.M.
     (1980): J. Neurochem. 34:219-221.

17. Lowry, O.H., Rosebrough, N.H., Farr, A.L. and
     Randall, R.J. (1951):   J. Biol. Chem.
     193:265-275.

18. MacKay, A.V.P., Bird, E.D., Spokes, E.G.,
     Rosser, N., Iversen, L.L., Creese, I. and
     Snyder, S.H. (1980): Lancet:915-916.

19. Madras, B.K., Davis, A., Junashko, P. and
     Seeman, P. (1980): Psychopharmacology and
     Biochemistry of Neurotransmitter Receptors.
     Yamamura, H., Olsen, R.W. and Usdin E. eds.
     Elsevier North Holland, p. 411-419.

20. Madras, B.K., Davis, A., Chan, B. and Seeman,
     P. (1981): Prog. Neuropsychopharmacol.
     5:543-548.

21. Madras, B.K., Davis, A. and Seeman, P. (1982):
     Eur. J. Pharmacol. 78:431-438.

22. Markwell, M.A.K., Hass, S.M., Bieber, L.L. and
     Tolbert N.E. (1978): Anal. Biochem. 87:206.

23. Milby, K.H., Mefford, I.N., Chey, W. and Adams, R.N. (1981): Brain Res. Bull. 7:237-242.

24. Muakkassay-Kelly, S.F., Andresen, J.W., Shih, J.C. and Hochstein, P. (1982): Biochem. Biophys. Res. Commun. 104:1003-1010.

25. Owen, F., Crow, J.J., Poulter, M., Cross, A.J., Longden, A. and Riley, G.J. (1978): Lancet 2:223-226.

26. Rehncrona, S., Smith, D.S., Akesson, B., Westerberg, E., and Siesjo, B.K. (1980). J. Neurochem. 34:1630.

27. Seeman, P., Lee, T., Chau-Wong, M. and Wong, K. (1976): Nature 261:717-719.

28. Seeman, P. (1980): Pharmacol. Revs. 32:229-313.

29. Shukla, G.S. and Chandra, S.V. (1981): Acta. Pharmacol. Toxicol. 48:95.

30. Tolbert, A.C. Thomas, T.N., Middaugh, L.D., and Zemp, J.W. (1979): Brain Res. Bull. 4:43-48.

31. Thomas, T.N. and Zemp, J.W. (1977): J. Neurochem. 28:663-665.

32. Weiner, N., Arold, N. and Wesemann, W. (1982): J. Neurosci. Methods 5:41-45.

CNS Receptors—From Molecular
Pharmacology to Behavior, edited by
P. Mandel and F. V. DeFeudis.
Raven Press, New York © 1983.

Behavioural Data Suggesting the Plurality of Central Dopamine Receptors

Jean Costentin, Isabelle Dubuc, and Philippe Protais

Laboratoire de Pharmacodynamie et de Physiologie, U.E.R. de Médecine et de Pharmacie de Rouen, St. Etienne du Rouvray, France

The emerging concept of the plurality of receptors for a given neurotransmitter now extends to most of the known neurotransmitters or neuromodulators. The development of new in vivo or in vitro tests (and especially binding studies) as well as the advent of new ligands has played a prominent part in this classification into receptor subtypes.

The dopamine receptors are also concerned by such a classification. As a matter of fact, the binding studies conducted by Sokoloff et al. (12) as well as Titeler et al. (13) have led to the identification (in addition to the dopamine receptor subtype linked to an adenylate cyclase which was termed D1 by Kebabian and Calne, 5) of three subtypes of dopamine binding sites:
. The D2 sites are, especially in the striatum, postsynaptically located, and are characterized by a high affinity for both the dopamine agonists (especially apomorphine) and the neuroleptic agents (except for some benzamide derivatives, such as sulpiride).
. The D3 sites seem to correspond, at least in the striatum, to dopamine autoreceptors; they display a high affinity (nM) for apomorphine and a low relative affinity for neuroleptic agents (μM).
. The D4 sites (for Sokoloff et al., 12, that Seeman, 10, termed D2 and reciprocally) display a lower affinity for apomorphine than D2; they have a high affinity for neuroleptics, including benzamide derivatives such as sulpiride.

This classification is founded upon binding studies and therefore could correspond either only to binding sites without functional implications or, on the contrary, to true receptors in the pharmacological sense.

The present experiments were designed to try and correlate these in vitro data with behavioural effects produced by apomorphine. This drug is, indeed, the reference dopamine agonist (3) which is operative on each of the above mentioned subtypes of binding sites. The following is an account of a series of studies about, particularly, the polyphasic modulations of various behaviours elicited by increasing doses of apomorphine with the aim to emphasize their dependence on different subtypes of dopamine receptors.

I - POLYPHASIC MODULATION OF LOCOMOTOR ACTIVITY IN MICE
BY INCREASING DOSES OF APOMORPHINE.

Male Swiss albino mice (CD1 Charles River, 22-24g) were injected s.c. with increasing doses of apomorphine. Immediately after, they were introduced singly into activity cages fitted with two photoelectric units (1). The number of beams crossed by the animals was recorded by electromechanical counters between the 5th and the 20th min following the introduction of mice into the actimeter.

Apomorphine, as a function of the test doses, induces polyphasic modifications in the locomotor activity of mice. They consist in (i) a hypokinesia observed for low doses of apomorphine, maximal at 25 ug/kg (ii) an apparent restoration of the locomotor activity for higher doses centered on 75 µg/kg (iii) another hypokinesia, somewhat more marked than that induced by 25 µg/kg apomorphine, which occurred for still higher doses and was maximal at 150 µg/kg (iv) and finally another restoration of the locomotor activity taking place from an apomorphine dose of about 250 µg/kg (Fig. 1). These observations were based, in fact, upon a dose-response curve established from many apomorphine test doses at very short intervals and many animals were used for each one.

These data prompted us to investigate the interactions of some neuroleptic and non-neuroleptic agents with these various effects of apomorphine. The hypokinesia produced by 25 µg/kg apomorphine was modified neither by 50 µg/kg haloperidol nor by 20 mg/kg sulpiride (Fig. 1) nor again by various other dopamine antagonists such as flupenthixol, levomepromazine, droperidol, pimozide, thioridazine and mezilamine (submited for publication). All these neuroleptics were used at the highest dose which, by itself, did not decrease significantly the spontaneous locomotor activity. When the tonic dopaminergic component exerting a stimulating influence on the locomotor activity was suppressed (either by the catecholaminergic denervation caused by an i.c.v. injection of the neurotoxin 6-hydroxy-dopamine, or by the administration of high doses of neuroleptics), the spontaneous locomotor activity of mice was decreased and the hypokinetic effect of 25 µg/kg apomorphine was no longer observed.

Taken together and considered with previous studies (2) these data are compatible with the involvement of dopamine autoreceptors in the hypokinetic effect of 25 µg/kg apomorphine. These autoreceptors, sensitive to low doses of apomorphine and with an apparently low sensitivity to neuroleptics present some similar characteristics with the D3 subtype of binding sites described by Sokoloff et al. (11) and by Titeler et al. (13). The antagonism induced by a low dose of yohimbine (Fig. 1) could be inconsistent with this hypothesis. However the involvement of an α2-adrenergic receptor could be only indirect (on the efferent pathway mediating the locomotor response to this low dose of apomorphine) or else yohimbine could directly interact with D3 receptors.

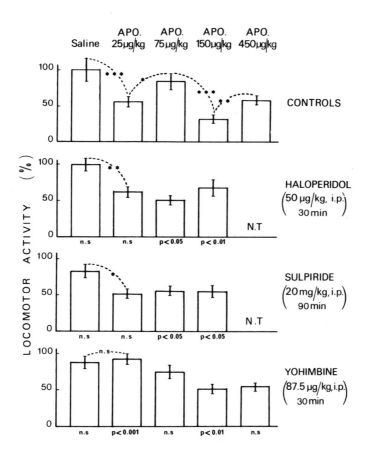

Fig. 1 - Effects of increasing doses of apomorphine on the locomotor activity in mice and interactions with haloperidol, sulpiride and yohimbine.

The locomotor activity in saline-treated controls corresponded to 297 ± 44 beams crossed. The time indicated between brackets corresponds to the interval between the pretreatment and the s.c. injection of the apomorphine test doses.

The statistical comparisons to respective controls are indicated under the columns.

n.s = non significant; * = p < 0.05; ** = p < 0.01; *** = p < 0.001

M ± S.E.M. of 22-43 animals per group.

N.T. = not tested

The interaction of neuroleptics and yohimbine with the effects of 75 and 150 µg/kg apomorphine was also studied. Haloperidol and sulpiride antagonized these two effects at doses which did not modify the hypokinesia produced by 25 µg/kg apomorphine (Fig. 1). Investigating the relative sensitivity to sulpiride of the locomotor effects elicited by 75 and 150 µg/kg apomorphine, it appeared that the hypokinesia produced by 150 µg/kg apomorphine was more sensitive to the neuroleptic than the restoration of the locomotor activity induced by 75 µg/kg apomorphine. As a matter of fact, whereas from 2 mg/kg sulpiride on, there was a significant antagonism of the hypokinesia elicited by 150 µg/kg apomorphine, it was necessary to reach a 20 mg/kg dose to significantly antagonize the effect of 75 µg/kg apomorphine. This could support the involvement, in these two effects, of dopamine receptors differing at least by their relative sensitivity to sulpiride. Furthermore, yohimbine was without effect on the restoration of the locomotor activity elicited by 75 µg/kg apomorphine but partly antagonized the hypokinesia induced by 150 µg/kg apomorphine.

II - BIPHASIC EFFECT OF INCREASING DOSES OF DOPAMINE AGONISTS ON YAWNING BEHAVIOUR AND PENILE ERECTIONS IN RATS

Male Wistar rats (150-200 g, IFFA CREDO) were injected with increasing doses of various dopamine agonists. They were put into individual wire netting cages (l = 25 cm; w = 20 cm; h = 30 cm) and the yawns and penile erections they presented were counted during the next hour.

All the tested dopamine agonists induced yawns and some penile erections whose frequency waxed then waned when the test doses were increased. The following indicates the approximate doses (mg/kg) of these drugs which induced about the maximum number of yawns/penile erections: N-propyl-nor-apomorphine = 0.0015/0.003; apomorphine = 0.1/0.1; lisuride = 0.012/0.025; lergotrile = 0.5/0.5; bromocriptine = 5/5; piribedil = 1.5/3; S 584 = 10/20; L-DOPA associated with benserazide (25 mg/kg) = 50/100. It was for an apomorphine dose of about 100 µg/kg that the yawns and penile erections had the highest frequency (Fig. 2, inset). The apomorphine-induced yawning was antagonized by all the neuroleptics tested up to now whether they be "classical" (4,8,14) or "atypical" (submitted for publication). For the few neuroleptics tested on the apomorphine-induced penile erections, it appeared that their ID 50 values were roughly similar to that determined on the apomorphine-induced yawning (Table 1).

The yawns' and penile erections' frequency decreased beyond 100 µg/kg apomorphine and cancelled out at about the 600 µg/kg dose level (Fig. 2, inset). When increasing doses of neuroleptics were opposed to this 600 µg/kg apomorphine test dose, it was observed that, like haloperidol (Fig. 2), most of the tested agents made the yawns and the penile erections reappear. On the contrary, sulpiride, tested at doses up to 150 mg/kg, did not (Fig. 2 and Table 1).

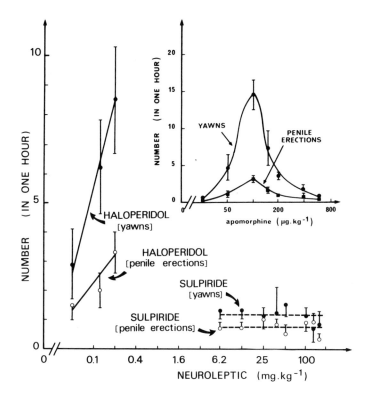

Fig. 2 - Dose-response curves of apomorphine-induced yawning behaviour and penile erections (inset) and effects of increasing doses of haloperidol and sulpiride on the disappearance of yawns and penile erections elicited by a high
apomorphine dose.

Apomorphine (0.6 mg/kg) was injected s.c. either 30 min after
haloperidol or 90 min after sulpiride i.p. administrations.
M ± S.E.M. of 6-13 animals per group.

III - COMPARATIVE ANTAGONIST EFFICACY OF VARIOUS NEUROLEPTICS
TOWARDS SNIFFING, LICKING AND CLIMBING BEHAVIOURS ELICI-
TED BY APOMORPHINE IN RATS.

We examined in Wistar rats the apomorphine-induced climbing
behaviour (submitted for publication) previously described in mice
(6, 9). Simultaneously with the verticalisation of the rats along
the wire netting walls of their cages, two other stereotyped behaviours, sniffing and licking, were evaluated. The relative effica-

Neuroleptics	YAWNING BEHAVIOUR		PENILE ERECTIONS	
	APPEARANCE ID 50 (mg/kg)	DISAPPEARANCE ID 50 (mg/kg)	APPEARANCE ID 50 (mg/kg)	DISAPPEARANCE ID 50 (mg/kg)
Haloperidol	0.11 ± 0.01	0.11 ± 0.01	0.09 ± 0.03	0.08 ± 0.01
Pimozide	0.18 ± 0.03	0.23 ± 0.03	0.23 ± 0.07	0.17 ± 0.02
Sulpiride	21 ± 8	> 150	24 ± 8	> 150
Metoclopramide	1.35 ± 0.64	1.38 ± 0.11	1.86 ± 0.39	1.17 ± 0.09
Mezilamine	0.97 ± 0.07	0.69 ± 0.07	1.26 ± 0.20	0.83 ± 0.07

Table 1 : Comparative efficacy of various neuroleptics on the apomorphine-induced appearance and disappearance of yawns and penile erections in rats.

Neuroleptics were injected i.p. 30 min or 90 min (benzamide derivatives) before the s.c. injections of apomorphine. Rats were injected with a 100 μg/kg apomorphine test dose for the determination of ID 50 on the appearance of behaviours and with a 600 μg/kg apomorphine test dose for the determination of ID 50 on the disappearance of behaviours.

The ID 50 and their standard errors were calculated according to the method of Miller and Tainter (7). For each drug at least 6 dose levels were tested ; 6 to 13 rats per dose.

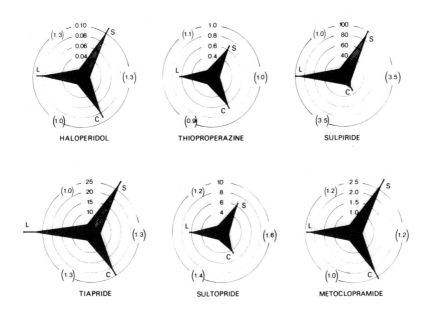

Fig. 3 - Comparative potencies of various neuroleptics for antagonism of three apomorphine-induced behaviours in rats.

Each branch of the stars corresponds to the ID 50 + S.E.M. (mg/
kg) on the sniffing (S), the licking (L) and the climbing (C) behaviours.

The numbers indicated between brackets correspond to the ratio
of the ID 50: S/C, L/C and S/L.

6-13 determinations for each result.

cy of some neuroleptics was compared on these three apomorphine
effects occurring simultaneously. Neuroleptics were administered
i.p. 90 min (benzamide derivatives) or 30 min (others) before the
s.c. injection of 0.6 mg/kg apomorphine. From the 5th to the 65th
min following this later injection, the sniffing, licking and climbing behaviours were simultaneously scored every two minutes in an
all or none manner. The final score for each animal was obtained
by summing up the scores (0 or 1) attributed at each observation.
For each experiment an ID 50 was calculated according to the graphic method of Miller and Tainter (7). The means + S.E.M. were
obtained by averaging the individual ID 50 values.

For most of the neuroleptics tested, considered individually,
ID 50s were roughly similar on the three apomorphine effects studied
whilst for some benzamide derivatives there was a more or less dissociated efficacy. As a matter of fact, the individual efficacy of
haloperidol, thioproperazine, tiapride, sultopride and metoclopramide with regard to sniffing, licking and climbing were roughly

similar. On the contrary, sulpiride antagonized relatively easily the climbing behaviour but only with difficulty the sniffing and licking behaviours (Fig. 3).

From the data of the second and third section of this paper, it is tempting to suggest the involvement of two dopamine receptor subtypes in each experiment. In the appearance of yawns and penile erections, then in their disappearance, there seem to be involved dopamine receptors differing in their relative sensitivity to apomorphine (and other dopamine agonists) and to neuroleptics. The appearance of yawns and penile erections could depend on the stimulation of a dopamine receptor subtype with a high sensitivity to both apomorphine and neuroleptics; the disappearance of these two behaviours could depend on the stimulation of a dopamine receptor subtype with a lower sensitivity to apomorphine than the preceding one and with a similar apparent sensitivity to neuroleptics except sulpiride. Since this latter drug does not make the yawns and penile erections reappear, one may suggest that the dopamine receptor subtype involved in the disappearance of these behaviours is less sensitive to sulpiride than those involved in their appearance.

A similar disparity in sensitivity to sulpiride is also observed in the third group of experiments since, whereas the apomorphine-induced climbing is easily antagonized by sulpiride, the apomorphine-induced sniffing or licking behaviours are antagonized only at very high doses close to the toxic doses. Other studies on these tests are in progress which indicate that some new benzamide derivatives display a still more discriminant property than sulpiride.

These results are apparently well correlated with the recent data of J.C. Schwartz et al. (personal communication) resulting from binding studies on the D2 and D4 dopamine receptor subtypes. The ratio of the Ki determined for various neuroleptics on the D2 and D4 binding sites are, indeed, very similar to the ratio of the ID 50 of these neuroleptics on the sniffing and climbing or on the licking and climbing. These ratio are more generally equal or close to 1 except for sulpiride for which it was 3.9 in binding studies and 3.5 in behavioural studies both in the sniffing/climbing ratio and in the licking/climbing ratio.

When attempting to interpret the present behavioral data in terms of the discriminative properties of sulpiride and some other new benzamide derivatives (to be published) with regard to the D4 and D2 dopamine receptor subtypes, as revealed by the binding studies of Schwartz and co-workers, it is attractive to suggest that the dopamine receptors involved in the apomorphine-induced appearance of yawns and penile erections, as well as in apomoprhine-induced climbing behavior, could correspond to the D4 subtype, whereas those involved in the apomorphine-induced disappearance of yawns and penile erection as well as in the apomorphine-induced sniffing and licking behaviors, could correspond to the D2 subtype. Such an interpretation can also be extended to the data presented in the first section of this paper. The dopamine receptors involved in the hypokinetic effect of 150 µg/kg apomorphine, easily blocked by sulpiride, could correspond to the D4 subtype, whereas those involved in the restoration of locomotor activity induced by 75 µg/kg apomorphine could correspond to the D2 subtype.

It is obvious that this demonstration would greatly profit by the advent of new agents more discriminative than sulpiride. The tests presented in this paper could perhaps be useful for their selection.

This work was supported in part by grant (ATP 4176) from the Centre National de la Recherche Scientifique.

REFERENCES

1. Boissier, J.R., and Simon, P. (1965) : Arch. Int. Pharmacodyn., 158 : 212-225.

2. Carlsson, A. (1975) : in Pre- and Post synaptic receptors, edited by E. Usdin and W.E. Bunney Jr, pp 49-63. Marcel Dekker, N.Y.

3. Ernst, A. (1967) : Psychopharmacologia, 10 : 316-323.

4. Holmgren, B., and Urbà-Holmgren, R. (1980) : Acta Neurobiol. Exp., 40 : 633-642.

5. Kebabian, J.W., and Calne, D.B. (1979) : Nature (London), 277: 93-96.

6. Marçais, H., Protais, P., Costentin, J., and Schwartz, J.C. (1978) : Psychopharmacology, 56 : 233-234.

7. Miller, L.C., and Tainter, M.L. (1944) : Proc. Soc. Exp. Biol. Med., 57 : 261-264.

8. Mogilnicka, E., and Klimek, V. (1977) : Pharmacol. Biochem. and Behav., 7 : 303-305.

9. Protais, P., Costentin, J., and Schwartz, J.C. (1976) : Psychopharmacology, 50 : 1-6.

10. Seeman, P. (1980) : Pharmacological Reviews, 32, 3 : 229-313.

11. Sokoloff, P., Martres, M.P., and Schwartz, J.C. (1980) : Nature (London), 288 : 283-286.

12. Sokoloff, P., Martres, M.P., and Schwartz, J.C. (1980) : Naunyn Schmiedeberg's Arch. Pharmacol., 315 : 89-102.

13. Titeler, M., List, S., and Seeman, P. (1979) : Commun. Psychopharmacol., 3 : 411-420.

14. Yamada, K., and Furukawa, T. (1980) : Psychopharmacology, 67 : 39-35.

CNS Receptors—From Molecular
Pharmacology to Behavior, edited by
P. Mandel and F. V. DeFeudis.
Raven Press, New York © 1983.

Dopamine Receptor Function and Spontaneous Orofacial Dyskinesia in Rats During 6-Month Neuroleptic Treatments

[1]John L. Waddington, Alan J. Cross, Stephen J. Gamble, and Rachel C. Bourne

Division of Psychiatry, MRC Clinical Research Centre, Northwick Park Hospital, Harrow HA1 3UJ, England

Supersensitivity of forebrain dopamine (DA) receptors after repeated neuroleptic treatments in animals has been widely investigated. Increased behavioural responsivity to DA agonists and elevated binding of ^{3}H-neuroleptic ligands are usually studied several days after withdrawal from neuroleptic treatments lasting a few weeks, and appear to be reliable and consistent effects (17). In considering the clinical implications of such phenomena, particularly relating to enduring anti-psychotic activity and emergence of tardive dyskinesia, wide discrepancies between the duration of treatment in animal studies (a few weeks) and in the clinic (up to several years, or more) are usually ignored. Only a few studies have investigated neuroleptic treatments constituting a significant proportion of an animal's adult life span (1, 26-29). We here describe and discuss some consequences of 6-month treatments with a wide range of typical and atypical neuroleptics.

MATERIALS AND METHODS

Typical phenothiazine (fluphenazine, FPZ; trifluoperazine, TPZ), butyrophenone (haloperidol, HAL), thioxanthene (piflutixol, PTX) and atypical substituted benzamide (metoclopramide, MET; 4-chloro-5-amino-2 (N-4- (1-benzylpiperidinyl)) - carboxamido anisole, BRL 20596, ref. 9) neuroleptics were given to male Sprague-Dawley rats via drinking water (26). Fluphenazine decanoate (FPZ-d) was given by i.m. depot injection, in oil, at 2-3 week intervals (27). Neuroleptics were given continuously for 6 months at doses in proportion with clinical neuroleptic potency (5, 20; data courtesy of Lundbeck, PTX, and Beecham,

---

[1]Present address: Royal College of Surgeons in Ireland, St. Stephen's Green, Dublin 2, Ireland.

BRL) as detailed in Fig. 1.   Age-matched control animals were
maintained drug-free under otherwise identical conditions.

At the 6 month point, while neuroleptic administration
continued, their spontaneous behaviour was assessed by direct
visual observation; they were then challenged s.c. with the
DA agonist apomorphine (APOM) and resultant stereotypy responses

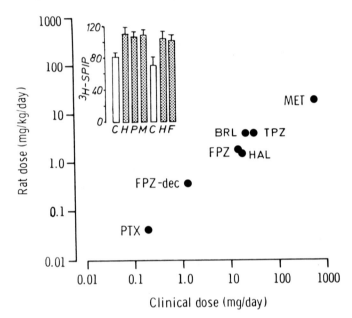

FIG. 1. Relationship between doses of neuroleptics in rats and
clinical neuroleptic dose in man.   Insert: striatal binding
of ^{3}H-SPIP (fmol/mg) in controls (C) and neuroleptic groups.
Means ± SEM (N = 5-9).

assessed by conventional rating scale (26).   After these
behavioural studies, neuroleptics were withdrawn.   At various
times thereafter further behavioural observations were made
and/or animals taken for assay of the binding of ^{3}H-spiperone
(^{3}H-SPIP) and ^{3}H-cis (Z)-flupenthixol (^{3}H-FPT) (2,29).

RESULTS

At the 6 month point, stereotypy to 0.15 mg/kg APOM was
antagonised (P < 0.05) in animals receiving typical phenothiazine, butyrophenone and thioxanthene neuroleptics; there
was no spontaneous stereotypy prior to APOM (Fig. 2).   In
separate colonies given HAL for 3, 6 or 9 months, responses to
0.15 mg/kg APOM were antagonised (P < 0.05) at each time point
(Fig. 3).   Log dose-response curves for induction of gnawing
by APOM (0.075-2.5 mg/kg) showed a uniform shift in curve to
the right in animals given HAL for 6 months (Fig. 4).   At 8
days after withdrawal from 6 months HAL, the incidence of
gnawing induced by 0.15 mg/kg APOM was raised (controls, 13%;

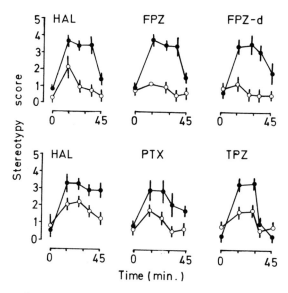

FIG. 2. Stereotypy responses at 6 months, before and after challenge with 0.15 mg/kg APOM at time zero for control (•) and typical neuroleptic (o) groups (N = 5-10).

HAL-withdrawn, 75%, P < 0.05, N = 8-23); APOM-induced gnawing was similarly enhanced at 9 days after withdrawal from TPZ (controls, 0%; TPZ-withdrawn, 80%, P < 0.05, N = 5-6). This supersensitive response to 0.15 mg/kg APOM had declined by 45 days after TPZ withdrawal (controls, 18%; TPZ-withdrawn, 43%; NS, N = 7-11). In animals given the substituted benzamides MET and BRL, stereotypy induced by 0.15 mg/kg APOM was not antagonised at the 6-month point (Fig. 5).

Following behavioural studies, striatal binding of ^{3}H-SPIP (0.8 nM) was assayed 7-11 days after withdrawal for a representative of each class of neuroleptic, and was similarly and significantly (P < 0.05) elevated in each case (Fig. 1 insert; FPZ, HAL, PTX, MET).

Direct visual observation prior to APOM challenge revealed a syndrome of spontaneous orofacial dyskinesia in certain animals. Its characteristics were principally jaw movements, bearing some similarity to abortive chewing but not directed onto physical material. Jaw movements in the lateral plane caused a characteristic "grating" sound as the teeth were drawn across one another and the presence or absence of this auditory sign, as assessed by a 'blind' investigator over a 10-min period, was used as the most reliable estimate of prevalence. The syndrome was present in each of 4 control colonies and occurred to excess in animals given all classes of neuroleptic except the butyrophenone HAL, when assessed at the 6-month point (Fig. 6). For each offending neuroleptic,

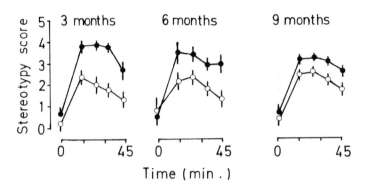

FIG. 3. Stereotypy responses to 0.15 mg/kg APOM in controls (●) and animals given HAL (o) for 3, 6 or 9 months (N = 5-18).

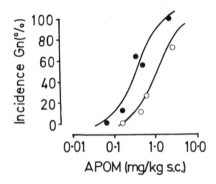

FIG. 4. Incidence of gnawing (Gn, %) to increasing doses of APOM in controls (●) and animals given HAL (o)   for 6 months (N = 6-23).

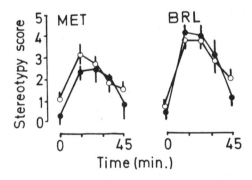

Fig. 5. Stereotypy responses to 0.15 mg/kg APOM in controls (●) and animals given substituted benzamides (o) for 6 months (N=5-10).

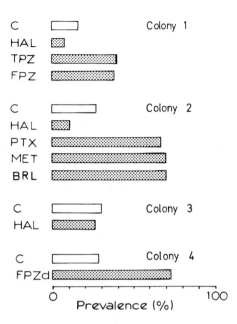

FIG. 6. Prevalence of spontaneous orofacial dyskinesia in
controls (C) and animals given neuroleptics for 6 months
(N = 8-32).

the prevalence was 2-3 x that of controls (overall prevalence:
controls, 21%; neuroleptic, 53%, N = 55-62; P < 0.01). For
HAL, no such effect was seen in each of 3 colonies (overall
prevalence: controls, 23%; HAL, 18%, N = 45-70, NS). The
syndrome was followed long into withdrawal in animals for whom
TPZ and PTX treatment had been terminated at 6 months. In
neither group did the excess of spontaneous orofacial dyskinesia
decline after withdrawal. Rather, a trend towards a greater
excess was noted over periods of 1 and 2.5 months for PTX- and
TPZ-withdrawn animals, respectively (Fig. 7 upper). Immediately
after final behavioural assessments at these withdrawal points
animals were taken for binding studies. While prevalences of
the syndrome were significantly increased (P < 0.05), they were
not associated with any changes in the binding of 0.8 nM
[3]H-SPIP or 2nM ^{3}H-FPT in either group (Fig. 7 lower).

DISCUSSION

In animals given typical phenothiazine, butyrophenone and
thioxanthene neuroleptics, functional DA receptor blockade,
assessed by antagonism of responsivity to 0.15 mg/kg APOM,
endured over 6 months of treatment. On the basis of poten-

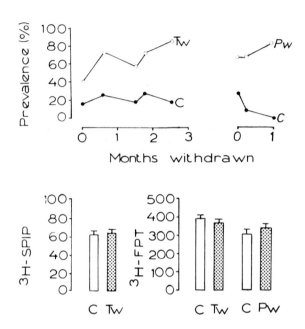

FIG. 7. Upper: Prevalence of spontaneous orofacial dyskinesia
during (o) withdrawal from trifluoperazine (Tw) and piflutixol
(Pw) after 6 months treatment, and in controls (C,●). Lower:
striatal binding of ^{3}H-SPIP and ^{3}H-FPT (fmol/mg) immediately
following final behavioural assessments (N = 3-10).

tiated gnawing responses to higher APOM doses (0.5-2.0 mg/kg)
it has been proposed (1) that after a crucial 6-month period
of phenothiazine treatment, DA receptor blockade has been
replaced by overt supersensitivity while on neuroleptics.   We
have found some potentiation of certain specific responses to
high APOM doses after 6 months of phenothiazine and thioxanthene
treatment (28,29) but argue that lower APOM doses are more
relevant for the detection of functional, competitive DA
receptor blockade.   HAL appears different from these other
typical neuroleptics, with dose-response curves for APOM-induced
gnawing being shifted to the right (competitive antagonism).
Also, while HAL can enduringly antagonise responses to 0.15
mg/kg APOM over 6 months, it fails to inhibit stereotypy to
1.0 mg/kg APOM after 1 week or 6 months of treatment at this
dose.   Scores 15 min after APOM were: 1 week, controls 3.7 ±
0.2, HAL 3.6 ± 0.3; 6 months, controls 3.4 ± 0.2, HAL 3.9 ± 0.3,
N = 7-8).   We can find no special functional significance for
the 6-month point, responses to 0.15 mg/kg APOM being antagonised

after 3, 6 or 9 months of HAL with only a trend towards tolerance.

In animals given atypical substituted benzamides, functional DA receptor blockade was not demonstrable at 6 months. However, MET has a very short $t\frac{1}{2}$ in the rat (21). Therefore, the interval between denial of access to water containing benzamide and administering APOM challenge may be confounding. Enhanced responsivity to 1.0 mg/kg APOM indicated DA receptor blockade had endured to maintain covert supersensitivity (stereotypy scores 15 min after APOM: controls, 2.6 ± 0.4; MET, 3.9 ± 0.2, N = 5-9, P < 0.05).

Representatives of each neuroleptic class given over a 500-fold dosage range (PTX, 0.04 mg/kg up to MET, 18 mg/kg/day) induced very similar increases in the striatal binding of ^{3}H-SPIP. At the given doses these drugs appear to be having a common action at those DA receptors (D$_2$) exemplified by striatal binding sites for ^{3}H-SPIP (17) and further suggest that DA receptor blockade had been present during continuous benzamide treatment. These data indicate induction of DA receptor supersensitivity that remains functionally 'masked' prior to withdrawal of neuroleptics. This is in agreement with enhanced gnawing responses to 0.15 mg/kg APOM after but not before withdrawal from HAL or TPZ at 6 months.

The syndrome of spontaneous orofacial dyskinesia did not appear to be related to these DAergic processes. It occurred independent of state of functional DA receptor blockade and degree of masked DA receptor supersensitivity. It endured and even increased long after neuroleptic withdrawal, beyond decline in DA supersensitivity. It was not associated with changes in striatal binding of two ligands preferentially labelling proposed subclasses of DAergic site (^{3}H-FPT, D$_1$; ^{3}H-SPIP, D$_2$; Refs. 2, 17, 29). This syndrome may therefore have an as yet unspecified non-DAergic basis; it is notable that neuroleptics interact to varying extents with a wide range of non-DAergic processes (16).

Clinical Antipsychotic Activity

Functional DA receptor blockade over 6-9 months of neuroleptic treatment is consistent with propositions that (i) blockade of at least some forebrain DA receptors is necessary for their antipsychotic action (12) and (ii) that antipsychotic efficacy is enduring with little evidence for tolerance in the absence of precipitating adverse psychosocial events (7). We have recently reported (28) stereospecific antagonism of such DAergic responses over 6 months treatment with cis (Z) - but not trans (E)-flupenthixol, paralleling corresponding stereospecific antipsychotic activity (12). As representatives of each neuroleptic class had very similar effects on striatal ^{3}H-SPIP binding sites when given at doses in proportion with clinical antipsychotic potency, this apparent uniformity of action at the D_2 receptor mirrors the correlation between affinity for ^{3}H-SPIP binding sites and antipsychotic potency (17). These data are consistent with the proposition that in schizophrenia there may be some hyperfunction of D_2 DAergic processes and that this may be equilibrated by neuroleptic-induced D_2 blockade, at least when the clinical profile is characterised by positive symptoms (12).

Tardive Dyskinesia

It is tempting to seek parallels between the observed spontaneous orofacial dyskinesia and clinical tardive orobuccolingual dyskinesia. The rodent syndrome was promoted only during very prolonged neuroleptic treatment and occurred in the presence of functional DA receptor blockade, paralleling the emergence of late-onset dyskinesia in the presence of enduring antipsychotic activity; it endured and increased for up to $2\frac{1}{2}$ months beyond cessation of 6 months neuroleptic treatment, paralleling exacerbation of tardive dyskinesia on neuroleptic withdrawal and equivocal evidence that in some patients the condition may be persistent (13). In offending neuroleptic groups the prevalence was between 2-3 x that in controls, and recent estimates put the prevalence of dyskinesia in neuroleptic-treated patients at approximately 3 x that in drug-free patients (11). Therefore, in both animals and man a neuroleptic-associated tardive component appears to be superimposed on a baseline prevalence that may reflect a combination of predisposing ageing and disease factors (3, 24) with which neuroleptics may interact.

As the rodent syndrome appeared to have a non-DAergic basis, this would be consistent with recent arguments (23) that DA receptor supersensitivity, the prevailing hypothesis for the pathophysiology of the disorder, may be too short-lived to account for persistent forms of tardive dyskinesia; no specific role for abnormal DA receptor function need follow from the sensitivity of dyskinetic features to modulation by drugs influencing DAergic function. A recent direct test of this DA supersensitivity hypothesis has involved binding studies with ^{3}H-SPIP and ^{3}H-FPT in striatal tissue from post-mortem brains of schizophrenics rated in life for the presence or absence of abnormal movements (3); the lack of increase in binding values in movement-disordered over non-movement-disordered patients agrees strikingly with the animal syndrome.

In querying the DA supersensitivity hypothesis of tardive dyskinesia it is possible to consider that tardive dyskinesia might be differentially associated with distinct neuroleptic drugs. Our finding that the rodent syndrome is most prominently promoted by FPZ-decanoate is notably consistent with statistical associations reported in studies of tardive dyskinesia (4, 6, 19). While HAL failed to promote the rodent syndrome, dyskinesia in HAL-treated patients need not be contradictory because of almost invariable polypharmacy. Data are required from patients who have received HAL alone (25), with no previous or concurrent treatment with other neuroleptics or anticholinergics. In the rodent studies, the lack of effect of HAL dissociates the syndrome from dystonic reaction, akathisia or parkinsonian tremor. In primates, tardive dyskinetic movements associated with chronic HAL may reflect a species sensitivity and are more reliably promoted by phenothiazines (8, 14, 15), as noted here. Associations between clinical tardive dyskinesia and HAL have been described as not common (18) or infrequent (22), and reports of such have been noted to be nearly non-existent in the medical literature (10). Thus, some current concepts of tardive dyskinesia may require re-evaluation.

ACKNOWLEDGMENTS

We thank Beecham, Janssen, Lundbeck, SKF & Squibb for facilitating these studies.

REFERENCES

1. Clow, A., Jenner, P., and Marsden, C.D. (1979): Eur. J. Pharmacol., 57: 365-375.
2. Cross, A.J. and Waddington, J.L. (1981): Eur. J. Pharmacol., 71: 327-332.
3. Crow, T.J., Cross, A.J., Johnstone, E.C., Owen, F., Owens, D.G.C., and Waddington, J.L. (1981): In: Biological Psychiatry 1981, edited by C. Perris, G. Struwe, and B. Jonsson. Elsevier, Amsterdam.
4. Csernansky, J.G., Grabowski, K., Cervantes, J., Kaplan, J., and Yesavage, J. (1981): Am. J. Psychiat., 138: 1362-1365.
5. Davis, J.M. (1975): Arch. Gen. Psychiat., 33: 858-861.
6. Ezrin-Waters, C., Seeman, M.V., and Seeman, P. (1981): J. Clin. Psychiat., 42: 16-22.
7. Falloon, I.R., Boyd, J.L., McGill, C.W., Razani, J., Moss, H.B., and Gilderman, A.M. (1982): New Eng. J. Med., 306: 1437-1440.
8. Gunne, L., and Barany, S. (1976): Psychopharmacol., 50: 237-240.
9. Hadley, M.S. (1982): In: Chemical Regulation of Biological Mechanisms, Royal Society of Chemistry (in press).
10. Jacobson, G., Baldessarini, R.J., and Manschreck, T. (1974): Am. J. Psychiat., 131: 910-913.
11. Jeste, D., and Wyatt, R.J. (1981): Am. J. Psychiat., 131: 910-913.

12. Johnstone, E.C., Crow, T.J., Frith, C.D., Carney, M.W.P., and Price, J.S. (1978): Lancet, i: 848-851.
13. Klawans, H.L., Goetz, C.G., and Perlik, S. (1981): Am. J. Psychiat., 138: 900-908.
14. McKinney, W.T., Moran, E.C., Kraemer, G.W., and Prange, A.J. (1980): Psychopharmacol., 72: 35-39.
15. Paulson, G.W. (1973): Adv. Neurol., 1: 647-650.
16. Peroutka, S., and Snyder, S.H. (1980): Am. J. Psychiat., 137: 1518-1522.
17. Seeman, P. (1980): Pharm. Rev., 32: 229-313.
18. Shader, R.I. (1972): In: Butyrophenones in Psychiatry, edited by A. DiMascio and R.I. Shader, pp. 97-114. Raven Press, New York.
19. Smith, R.C., Strizich, M., and Klass, D. (1978): Am. J. Psychiat., 135: 1402-1403.
20. Stanley, M., Lautin, A., Rotrosen, J., Gershon, S., and Kleinberg, D. (1980): Psychopharmacol., 71: 219-225.
21. Tam, Y.K., Axelson, J.E., McErlane, B., Ongley, R., and Price, J.D. (1981): J. Pharmacol. Exp. Ther., 217: 764-769.
22. Tarsy, D., and Baldessarini, R.J. (1976): In: Clinical Neuropharmacology, Vol. 1., edited by H. Klawans, pp. 27-61. Raven Press, New York.
23. Tarsy, D., and Baldessarini, R.J. (1977): Biol. Psychiat., 12: 431-450.
24. Varga, E., Sugerman, A., Varga, V., Zomorodi, A., Zomorodi, W., and Menken, W. (1982): Am. J. Psychiat., 139: 329-331.
25. Waddington, J.L. (1982): Am. J. Psychiat., 139: 703-704.
26. Waddington, J.L., and Gamble, S.J. (1980): Eur. J. Pharmacol., 67: 363-369.
27. Waddington, J.L., and Gamble, S.J. (1980): Eur. J. Pharmacol., 68: 387-388.
28. Waddington, J.L., Gamble, S.J., and Bourne, R.C. (1981): Eur. J. Pharmacol., 69: 511-513.
29. Waddington, J.L., Cross, A.J., Gamble, S.J., and Bourne, R.C. (1982): In: Advances in Dopamine Research, edited by M. Kohsaka, pp. 143-146. Pergamon Press, Oxford.

CNS Receptors—From Molecular
Pharmacology to Behavior, edited by
P. Mandel and F. V. Defeudis.
Raven Press, New York © 1983.

Brain Iron and Dopamine Receptor Function

*M. B. H. Youdim, *D. Ben-Shachar, *R. Ashkenazi,
and †S. Yehuda

*Rappaport Medical Research Center, Department of Pharmacology, Haifa, Israel;
and †Department of Psychology, Bar Elan University, Ramat Gan, Israel

Iron-deficiency, the most prevalent nutritional disorder in
man, is thought to affect behaviour in children and adults (19-27,
30) and also in the rat as shown by Youdim and Green (37). The
distribution of iron in the brain regions parallels that of DA
(37,42). However, the function of the large amounts of iron
found in these areas is not known. We have, therefore, investigated the effect of iron-deficiency on the binding sites of
several neurotransmitters in the rat brain and correlated them
with the behavioural response to apomorphine (3,40,41).
Youdim and Green (37) have shown that the serotonin (5-HT) and
the dopamine (DA) mediated behavioural responses induced by centrally acting drugs (amphetamine and apomorphine) were significantly diminished in rats fed an iron-deficient diet for 5 weeks.
By this procedure a reduction of 40% in brain levels of non-haem
iron was noted. The altered behavioural responses could not be
attributed to changes in monoamine metabolism, since the activities of the iron-dependent enzymes tryptophan hydroxylase,
tyrosine hydroxylase and monoamine oxidase were unchanged.
Furthermore, the turnover and brain levels of 5-HT, DA or
noradrenaline (NA) in the iron-deficient rats were similar to the
control groups (39).
It was suggested that the reduction in the functional activity
of monoaminergic pathways induced by nutritional iron-deficiency

might be due to post-synaptic changes, possibly at or beyond the DA receptor site (39). Supporting evidence for this concept has come from studies of nucleus accumbens DA-mediated hypothermia induced by d-amphetamine in rats kept at $4^{\circ}C$ (33-36). Iron-deficiency in rats greatly diminishes the hypothermic effect of d-amphetamine (40), a property shared by the action of neuroleptics (33,35).

METHODS

Preparation of Iron-Deficient Rats

Young (21 days) and adult (48 days) Sprague-Dawley rats were fed a semi-synthetic diet low in iron prepared from milk powder (22). The rats had free access to food and distilled water. Control animals received the same diet supplemented with ferrous ammonium sulphate but were restricted to the amount of diet that was consumed by the iron-deficient group in order to keep their weights similar to iron-deficient groups. All animals were kept in 12h light and 12h dark cycle. The duration of feeding the iron-deficient diet was determined by the behavioural response to apomorphine administration (2 mg/kg i.p.) measured at weekly intervals, as were haemoglobin and serum iron concentrations (7, 11).

Neurotransmitter Binding Site Assay

When the animals showed signs of iron-deficiency (Hb < 10 g/dl and serum iron < 1.4 µg/ml) their behavioural response to apomorphine (2 mg/kg) was examined for 30 minutes after the injection of the agonist. At the end of this period they were killed, brains were removed and dissected into specific regions for assay of neurotransmitter binding sites.

Specific ^3H-spiroperidol binding was measured in vitro in membranes prepared from the caudate nucleus according to the procedure described by Creese et al (9). Specific binding was defined as the difference between the total counts in the absence of unlabelled haloperidol and the counts obtained in the presence of 10 µM haloperidol. Specific α- and β-adrenergic binding sites were estimated in the membrane fractions from the cortex using the radioligands ^3H-WB4101 and ^3H-DHA according to the methods of Greenberg et al. (15a) and Bylund and Snyder (6) respectively. Specific cholinergic muscarinic binding site in the hippocampus and caudate nucleus were determined by the procedure described by Yamamura et al. (32) using ^3H-QNB for specific and excess oxotremorine for non-specific binding.

RESULTS

Dopaminergic Mediated Circadian Rhythms
During Iron-Deficiency

Glover and Jacob (14) reported that nutritional iron-deficiency in rats results in the reduction of 24h spontaneous motor activity and reversal of circadian rhythm. That is, while control rats were more active in the dark period, iron-deficient animals showed a significantly higher level of motor activity in the light period. We have confirmed these results (40) and extended them to the studies of circadian rhythms of apomorphine (2.5 mg/ kg) evoked stereotyped behaviour and d-amphetamine (15 mg/kg) induced hypothermia (33-36), in rats kept in 12h light - 12h dark cycles. In control rats the behavioural and body temperature responses due to apomorphine and d-amphetamine respectively show circadian rhythm (33-36,40). The greatest effects are seen in the dark period and they are significantly different (p < 0.01) from the smaller changes recorded in the light period (Fig. 1). Iron-deficient rats also show biphasic stereotyped behaviour and hypothermia in reaction to apomorphine and d-amphetamine; however, in contrast to control rats the greatest and smallest effects are observed in light and dark period respectively and their overall responses to these drugs are significantly (p < 0.01) diminished (40). These studies led us to examine the effect of duration of the iron-free diet on the response to d-amphetamine. Initially, at day 0 on the iron-deficient diet, d-amphetamine produced hypothermia (Fig. 2), similar to that observed in the control rats. With increasing time on the iron-free diet, however, there was a gradual diminution and phase reversal of d-amphetamine-induced hypothermia. Thus iron-deficient rats exhibited a significantly greater (p < 0.01) inhibition of d-amphetamine-induced hypothermia in the dark period as compared to the light period.

d-Amphetamine fails to induce hypothermia in rats lesioned in the region of the olfactory turbercule, but induces hypothermia in rats with striatal lesions (33,36). The hypothermic effect of d-amphetamine is apparently mediated by the release of DA in the mesolimbic (nucleus accumbens) pathways (33,35,36). Drugs that increase the availability of DA or stimulate DA central receptors (e.g. apomorphine, L-Dopa and amphetamine) cause hypothermia, whereas drugs that decrease the availability of DA or block the interaction of DA with its receptors (e.g. pimozide, haloperidol and chlorpromazine) not only fail to produce hypothermia, but also block the hypothermic effect of d-amphetamine. The finding that d-amphetamine-induced hypothermia in iron-deficient rats was almost completely blocked by simple iron-deficiency, an effect similar to the action of neuroleptics (e.g. haloperidol) strongly suggested a diminution of DA receptor function in the iron-deficient rats (37,40).

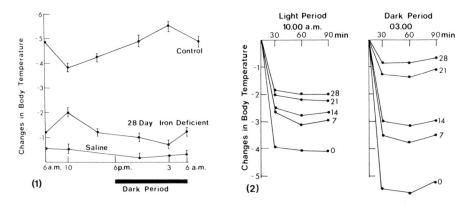

FIG. 1. Circadian rhythm of d-amphetamine (15 mg/kg) induced hypothermia in control and iron-deficient rats kept at an ambient temperature of 4°C (40).

FIG. 2. The hypothermic effect of d-amphetamine (15 mg/kg) in rats on iron-deficient diet for 0 to 28 days. Rats were kept at an ambient temperature of 4°C and colonic temperature was recorded for 90 min. after receiving d-amphetamine at the times indicated in the light and dark period (40).

Specific Binding of ^{3}H-Spiroperidol in
Brains of Iron-Deficient Rats

The effects of iron-deficiency, in young (21-day-old) and adult (48-day-old) rats, on their body weight, haemoglobin and serum iron concentrations, behavioural response to apomorphine and ^{3}H-spiroperidol binding site are shown in Table 1. It is obvious that the younger animals are more susceptible to the induction of iron-deficiency as compared to adults by virtue of the duration on iron-deficient diet, the reduction in haemoglobin and serum iron concentrations. In both groups there were significant reductions of the behavioural response to apomorphine (2 mg/kg, I.P.) and specific ^{3}H-spiroperidol binding in membrane fractions from caudate nucleus.

The dissociation constant (K_D) and the densities of ^{3}H-spiroperidol binding sites (B_{max}) were determined by measuring the specific binding of ^{3}H-spiroperidol at various concentrations ranging from 0.125 to 10 nM. The analysis of the data by the method of Scatchard revealed only a single component for specific ^{3}H-spiroperidol binding in control and iron-deficient young (21-day-old) rats. The dissociation constants (K_D) of specific binding for both groups were similar; however, the maximum number of binding sites calculated was significantly (57%) lower in the iron-deficient groups of rats (Table 2).

TABLE 1.   The characteristics of young and adult control and
iron-deficient rats

	Young (21 days)		Adult (48 days)	
	Control	ID†	Control	ID†
Duration of diet (weeks)	4	4	7	7
Body weight (g)	150±6	134±7	343±11	326±9
Haemoglobin (g/dl)	14.1±1.2	5.9±0.6**	16±0.3	10.4±0.7*
Serum iron (µg/ml)	3.3±0.3	0.76±0.07*	2.8±0.2	0.87±0.16*
Apomorphine (2mg/kg) movement/40 min	1614±72	798±159*	1398±189	214±91**
³H-spiroperidol binding (pmoles/g tissue)	25.1±4	12.7±1.6**	19.5±1.2	10.6±1.3*

Membrane fractions prepared from caudate nucleus were incubated
with 1nM ³H-spiroperidol in the presence or absence of 10µM haloperidol for determination of specific and non-specific spiroperidol binding. * (p < 0.001); ** (P < 0.01). † Iron-deficient.

H-Spiroperidol Binding Sites and Time on Iron-Deficient Diet

The diminution of specific ³H-spiroperidol binding sites as
measured in the caudate nucleus, is reversible if rats (21-day-
old) made iron-deficient (4 weeks) are fed iron supplemented
(control) diet for 2 weeks (Table 2). Not only does the ³H-spiroperidol binding return to control values but so also do the
behavioural response to apomorphine and the concentration of
haemoglobin and serum iron. A single intraperitoneal injection
of iron-dextran (5mg/kg) to iron-deficient groups of rats was not
able to restore spiroperidol binding sites in caudate nucleus or
the behavioural response to apomorphine 3 days after the injection. These results would suggest that either the dose of iron-
dextran was not sufficiently high or the time needed for iron to
act is longer than 3 days. The latter suggestion is the most
likely explanation since, as will be discussed later, iron-
deficiency decreases brain protein synthesis. Its reversal by
iron repletion is a time-dependent process with a half-life of
6-8 days (16,31).
We have examined ³H-spiroperidol binding sites in the caudate
nucleus of rats maintained on iron-deficient diet for various

TABLE 2.   Scatchard analysis of specific ^{3}H-spiroperidol binding in the caudate nucleus

Treatment	K_D (nM)	B_{max} (pmole/g tissue)	Apomorphine-induced behaviour
Control	0.72±0.2	45±9	1614±72
Iron-deficient	0.68±0.1	19±2*	789±159*
Iron-repleted	0.81±0.1	38±6	1462±300

In iron-repleted experiments rats (21-day-old) had received low iron diet for 4 weeks: they then received iron supplemented (control) diet for 2 weeks. The behavioural response is expressed as total movements during the first 40 min after apomorphine (2mg/kg i.p.) (3). *Significantly different from control and iron-repleted groups (P < 0.01).

periods. It is apparent that the reduction in the ^{3}H-spiroperidol binding sites is dependent on the time during which the rats are fed iron-deficient diet (Table 3), and this is correlated with the reduction in serum iron and behavioural response to apomorphine (2.0mg/kg).

Effect of Iron-Deficiency on Adrenergic and Cholinergic Binding Sites

The specific binding of ^{3}H-WB4101, ^{3}H-DHA and ^{3}H-QNB, which bind to α_1- and β-adrenergic and to cholinergic muscarinic binding sites, respectively, were measured in various membrane preparations from brains of iron-deficient and control rats as described in the Methods section. The membranes were incubated with various concentrations (0.2-2μM) of each ligand in the presence or absence of unlabelled noradrenaline or oxotremorine (100 μM final concentration). Specific binding was calculated from the difference in binding between incubations conducted in the presence or absence of unlabelled neurotransmitter. Scatchard analysis of the data for each radioligand indicated the existence of a single binding site component in control and iron-deficient groups. It is apparent that iron-deficiency has no effect on the K_D or B_{max} of α_1- and β-adrenergic and cholinergic muscarinic binding sites (Table 4) Although not presented, similar results were obtained for the binding of ^{3}H-QNB in the caudate nucleus.

Effect of Haemolytic Anaemia on ^{3}H-Spiroperidol Binding Sites

It was deemed essential to establish whether the reduction of ^{3}H-spiroperidol binding sites in the membrane fractions of

TABLE 3. ^{3}H-spiroperidol binding sites in caudate nucleus of rats kept on iron-deficient diet for various times

Time (week)	0	1		2		4	
	Control	Control	ID*	Control	ID*	Control	ID*
Haemoglobin (g/dl)	9.9±0.4	12.3±0.3	8.4±0.3	13.1±0.3	7.0±0.4	13.4±0.7	5.7±0.5
		$P < 0.01$		$P < 0.001$		$P < 0.001$	
Serum iron (µg/ml)	2.2±0.2	3.8±0.3	1.6±0.2	3.8±0.3	1.0±0.05	3.6±0.1	1.0±0.1
		$P < 0.001$		$P < 0.001$		$P < 0.001$	
Apomorphine response**	926±60	1136±139	823±107	1580±140	1017±60	1378±94	625±98
		NS		$P < 0.05$		$P < 0.01$	
^{3}H-spiroperidol binding (pmol/g)†	19.3±1.5	20.9±0.4	19.1±0.8	23.8±0.9	18.1<1.6	24.1±1.1	17.1±1.0
		NS		$P < 0.05$		$P < 0.01$	

* Iron-deficient group
** Response to apomorphine (2mg/kg I.P.) was measured as motor activity in individual rats and is expressed as movements/40 min. after receiving the drug.
† Spiroperidol binding was estimated according to the procedure described in Table 1.

TABLE 4. Effects of iron deficiency on brain α-and β-adrenergic and cholinergic muscarinic binding sites

Ligands (Brain region)	Control		Iron-Deficient	
	K_D	B_{max}	K_D	B_{max}
^{3}H-WB4101 (cortex)	0.89±0.07	6.8± 0.6	0.99±0.04	7.9± 0.2
^{3}H-DHA (cortex)	0.34±0.02	8.9± 0.5	0.37±0.02	9.0± 0.3
^{3}H-QNB (hippocampus)	0.24±0.04	82.1±14	0.21±0.05	74.8±20
^{3}H-QNB (caudate)		114±7.7		112±7.2

K_D and B_{max} were calculated from the Scatchard plot and are expressed as nM and pmoles/g tissue, respectively. ^{3}H-QNB binding in the caudate nucleus was measured at 1nM and is expressed as pmoles/g tissue.

caudate nucleus from iron-deficient rats is due to anaemia or iron-deficiency per se. Rats receiving the control diet were treated chronically with phenylhydrazine(daily subcutaneous injections of 50 mg/kg for one week) followed by 3 weeks of daily injection of 30 mg/kg. Haemoglobin concentration and the behavioural response to apomorphine were examined at weekly intervals and compared to control rats. At the end of the 4th week, rats were killed and serum iron and ^{3}H-spiroperidol binding in the caudate nucleus were measured. Although phenylhydrazine treatment markedly reduced the haemoglobin concentration (45%) as compared with control animals, the serum iron level, the behavioural response to apomorphine and the ^{3}H-spiroperidol binding in the caudate nucleus were not affected (Table 5).

DISCUSSION

Rats made nutritionally iron-deficient exhibit decreased spontaneous and drug (amphetamine,apomorphine and 5-methoxy-N,N-dimethyltryptamine) induced motor activity (14,37,39,40). They also have reduced brain iron content (10,37). Restoration of normal or drug-induced behaviours and brain iron content can be achieved by placing the iron-deficient rats on iron supplemented diet for 8 days or more (3,40). Since in most studies motor activity was examined,Leibel et al. (20) suggested that the diminished drug-induced behavioural response in iron-deficient rats is related to a peripheral effect of the iron-deficiency due to anaemia. Although this might be true for locomotor activity (12), it cannot explain centrally-mediated inhibition of d-amphetamine-

TABLE 5. Effects of chronic phenylhydrazine treatment

	Control	Phenylhydrazine*
Weight	233±19 (5)	266±31 (5)
Haemoglobin (g/100ml)	12.7±1.2(5)	7.1±0.5**(5)
Serum iron (μg/ml)	3.1±0.9(5)	4.7±0.7 (5)
Movements during 40 min after apomorphine (2mg/kg)	1065±150(4)	1028±183 (4)
Specific ³H-spiroperidol binding (pmoles/g tissue)	20.7±3 (5)	22.6±3 (5)

* Rats were injected subcutaneously with phenylhydrazine (50mg/kg) for one week followed by 3 weeks of daily injection (30mg/kg).
** P < 0.01.

induced hypothermia in iron-deficient rats pretreated with DA antagonists haloperidol or chlorpromazine (33-36).

The biochemical and behavioural studies of Youdim et al. (37, 39,40,41) had indicated that the alterations of DA-mediated behaviours in iron-deficient rats might be due to postsynaptic dopamine receptor changes. The cerebral DA binding sites have been classified into two groups, one type being linked to adenylate cyclase (D_1 receptor) and the other not dependent on the activation of cyclic nucleotides (D_2 receptor) (17,29). Apomorphine is thought to act on both types of dopamine receptors (17). Although it was shown that the behavioural response to apomorphine is greatly decreased in iron-deficient rats, the basal activity of caudate nucleus DA-sensitive adenylate cyclase and its response to increasing concentration of DA was unchanged. In the present and previous (3) studies the specific ³H-spiroperidol binding is markedly decreased in iron-deficient rats. The reduction in the binding caused by iron-deficiency is due to a decrease in the number of binding sites without any change in the affinity of ³H-spiroperidol for its binding site (3). The effect of iron-deficiency seems to be specific for the D_2 binding site, as neither α- and β-adrenergic binding sites nor cholinergic muscarinic binding sites were affected. The reduction in the D_2 binding sites parallels the behavioural response to apomorphine. Moreover, when iron-deficient rats are fed the diet supplemented with iron for two weeks not only the behavioural response to apomorphine but also the number of ³H-spiroperidol binding sites are restored almost to control values. Therefore the reduction of the behavioural responses of iron-deficient rats to drugs, such as apomorphine and amphetamine, is due to a central effect at the level of diminution of the dopaminergic receptor number.

There is further evidence to support this conclusion. As in the livers from rats chronically treated with neuroleptics

(haloperidol and fluphenazine), prolactin binding sites in the
livers of iron-deficient rats are greatly induced (1,2,4). The
upregulation of prolactin binding sites in both cases have been
shown to be the result of increased serum prolactin because
chronic treatment of rats with physiological doses of prolactin
produces similar effects in the liver and lung (1,4). Although
^{3}H-spiroperidol binding sites in the pituitary and nucleus accumbens of iron-deficient animals have not been estimated, the
increased liver prolactin binding sites (2) and the inhibition of
amphetamine-induced hypothermia (40) in these animals have been
attributed to the diminished dopamine D_2 binding sites and function in the above brain regions, respectively (3).

   The mechanism by which iron-deficiency diminishes the DA D_2
binding sites is unclear. In vitro studies using iron-chelators
and iron salts have indicated that iron is not simply part of the
receptor to which ^{3}H-spiroperidol binds. Neither chelating
agents nor iron-salts, except at very high concentrations ($>10^{-5}$M)
affect the binding of ^{3}H-spiroperidol to membrane fractions from
caudate nucleus of control and iron-deficient rats (unpublished
data). The possibility that iron-deficiency may cause some conformational changes in the DA D_2 receptor seems unlikely because
of unchanged ^{3}H-spiroperidol binding K_D. However, it has been
suggested that iron may be important for the synthesis of the
receptor (3). There is overwhelming evidence that iron-deficiency
interferes with protein synthesis and that iron is important for
the incorporation of ^{14}C-amino acids into proteins of brain (8,16,
28,31). These results are rather important in light of the finding
that haemolytic anaemia in rats (produced by chronic phenylhydrazine treatment) is without effect on brain protein synthesis (31).
Furthermore, these animals also show normal behavioural responses
to apomorphine and amphetamine and do not have diminished ^{3}H-
spiroperidol binding sites in the caudate nucleus.

SUMMARY: BIOCHEMICAL AND BEHAVIOURAL SIMILARITIES OF IRON-DEFICIENT AND NEUROLEPTIC-TREATED RATS

   It has been demonstrated that nutritional iron-deficiency induced in rats results in the reduction of DA D_2 receptor binding
sites, leading to down-regulation of dopaminergic activity similar
to that observed in neuroleptic-treated animals. The following
observations are common to both conditions:
   (a) Decreased behavioural response to pre- and post-synaptic-
       ally DA and serotonin acting drugs, amphetamine, apomor-
       phine and 5-methoxy-N,N-dimethyltryptamine.
   (b) Inhibition of amphetamine or apomorphine induced hypother-
       mia in rats kept at an ambient temperature of 4°C.
   (c) Increased sleeping time to phenobarbitone which cannot be
       attributed to the rate of drug metabolism (5,38).
   (d) Upregulation of prolactin binding sites in the liver as a
       result of increased serum prolactin.
Additionally, nutritional iron-deficiency lowers brain iron and

interferes with protein synthesis in this organ, which could explain the reduction of DA D_2 receptor number and function. Given the fact that the highest brain concentrations of iron are found in dopaminergic structures (see 42 for review), and the essential role of intact dopaminergic systems to attentional and learning processes (15b,30), the resultant behavioural changes due to the reduction of dopaminergic activity in iron-deficient animals may go some way to explain the adverse effects on cognition, behavioural patterns, learning and attention, event-related potentials (ERPs) and EEG changes reported in iron-deficient children (19-28,30).

REFERENCES

1. Amit, T., Ben-Harari, R.R.,and Youdim, M.B.H. (1982): Brit. J.Pharmac., 74:955-956P.
2. Ashkenazi, R., Ben-Shachar, D., and Youdim, M.B.H. (1982): Brit.J.Pharmac., 74:762-763P.
3. Ashkenazi, R., Ben-Shachar, D., and Youdim, M.B.H. (1982): Pharmac.Biochem.Behav., in press.
4. Barkey, R.J., Shani, J., Lahav, M., Amit, T., and Youdim, M.B.H. (1981): Mol.Cell.Endocrin. 21:129-138.
5. Becking, G.C., (1972): Biochem.Pharmacol., 21:1585-1594.
6. Bylund, D.B., and Snyder, S.H. (1976): Mol.Pharmacol., 5: 568-580.
7. Caraway, W.T. (1963):Clin.Chem., 9:188-196.
8. Chase, M.S., Gubler, C.J., Cartwright, G.E., and Wintrobe, M.M. (1952): J.Biol.Chem., 199:757-765.
9. Creese, I.L., Stewart, K., and Snyder, S.H. (1979): Eur.J. Pharmac., 60:55-66.
10. Dallman, P.R., Simes, M.A., and Manies, E.C. (1975): Br.J. Haemat., 31:209-215.
11. Drabkin, D.L.,and Austin, J.H. (1935): J.Biol.Chem., 112: 51-65.
12. Edgerton, V.R., Bryant, S.L., and Gillespie, C.A. (1972): J.Nutr., 102:381-393.
13. Garby, L. (1973): In:Clinics in Haematology, edited by S.T. Callender. W.B.Saunders, London, pp. 245-257.
14. Glover, J., and Jacobs, A.C. (1972): Brit.Med.J., 2:627-628.
15a. Greenberg, D.A., U'Prichard, D.C. and Snyder, S.H. (1976): Life Sci., 19:69-76.
15b. Iversen, S.D. (1977): In:Handbook of Psychopharmacology, Vol. 8. Drugs, Neurotransmitters and Behavior, edited by L.L. Iversen, S.D. Iversen and S.H. Snyder. Plenum Press, New York, pp. 333-384.
16. Jacobs, A., and Wordwood, M., editors (1974): Iron in Biochemistry and Medicine. Academic Press, London.
17. Kebabian, J.W., and Calne, D.B. (1979): Nature, 277:93-96.
18. Kessner, J., and Kalk,L.(1973): Strategy for Evaluating Health Services. Institute of Medicine, National Academy of Sciences, Washington,D.C.

19. Leibel, R.L., Greenfield, D., and Pollitt, E. (1978): In: Nutrition: Pre and Postnatal Development, edited by M. Winick. Plenum Press, New York, pp.383-405.
20. Leibel, R.L., Greenfield, D. and Pollitt, E. (1979): Brit. J. Haemat., 41:145-150.
21. Lazoff, B., Billenham, G., Viteri, F.E., and Urrutia, J.I. (1982): In: Iron Deficiency: Brain Biochemistry and Behavior, edited by E. Pollitt and R.L. Leibel. Raven Press, New York, pp. 183-194.
22. McCall, M.G., Newman, G.E., O'Brien, J.R.P., Valberg, L.S., and Witts, L.J. (1962): Brit.J.Nutr., 16:29-304.
23. Oski, F.A. (1979): Am.J.Dis.Chid., 133:315-322.
24. Oski, F.A., and Honig,A. (1978): J.Pediat., 92:21-23.
25. Pollitt, E., and Leibel, R.L. (1976): J.Pediat., 88:372-381.
26. Pollitt, E., and Leibel, R.L., editors (1982): Iron-Deficiency: Brain Biochemistry and Behavior. Raven Press, New York.
27. Pollitt, E., Viteri, F., Saco-Pollitt, C., and Leibel, R.L. (1982): In: Iron-Deficiency Brain Biochemistry and Behavior, edited by E. Pollitt and R.L. Leibel. Raven Press, New York, pp.195-208.
28. Porter, R., and Fitzsimons,D.W., editors (1977): Iron Metabolism. Elsevier,Amsterdam, pp.222.
29. Spano, P.F., Memo,M., Stefanini, E., Fresia, P., and Trabuochi, M., (1980): In:Neurotransmitters and Peptide Hormones, edited by G. Pepeu, M.J. Kuhar and S.J. Enna, Raven Press, New York, pp 243-257.
30. Tucker, D.M., and Sandstead, H.H. (1982): In: Iron-Deficiency Brain Biochemistry and Behavior, edited by E. Pollitt and R.L. Leibel. Raven Press, New York, pp. 161-183.
31. Weisenberg, E., Halbreich, A., and Mager, J. (1980): Biochem.J., 188:633-641.
32. Yamamura, H.I., Kuhar, M.J., Greenberg, D., Snyder, S.H. (1974): Brain Res., 66:541-546.
33. Yehuda, S. (1979): Commun.Psychopharmac., 3:115-120.
34. Yehuda, S., and Wurtman, R.J. (1972): Life Sci., 11:851-859.
35. Yehuda, S., and Wurtman, R.J. (1972): Nature, 240:477-478.
36. Yehuda, S., and Wurtman, R.J. (1975): Eur.J.Pharmac., 30: 154-158.
37. Youdim, M.B.H., and Green,A.R. (1977): In: Iron Metabolism, edited by R. Porter and D.W. Fitzsimons, Elsevier, Amsterdam, pp 201-237.
38. Youdim, M.B.H., Green, A.R., and Aronson, J. (1977): In: Anaemia in General Practice. Abbott Laboratories Ltd. (publishers) U.K.pp 37-42.
39. Youdim, M.B.H., Green, A.R., Bloomfield, M.R., Mitchell, B.D. Heal, D.J., and Grahame-Smith, D.G. (1979): Neuropharmacology, 19:259-267.
40. Youdim, M.B.H., Yehuda,S., Ben Uriah, Y. (1981): Eur.J. Pharmac., 74:295-301.

41. Youdim, M.B.H., Yehuda, S., Ben-Shachar, D., and Ashkenazi, R. (1982): In: Iron Deficiency: Brain Biochenistry and Behaviour, edited by E. Pollitt and R.L. Leibel. Raven Press, New York, pp 39-57.

42. Youdim, M.B.H., Ashkenazi, R, Ben-Shachar, D., and Yehuda, S. (1982): In: Parkinson's Disease: Advances in Neurology, edited by G. Hassler. Raven Press, New York (in press).

CNS Receptors—From Molecular
Pharmacology to Behavior, edited by
P. Mandel and F. V. DeFeudis.
Raven Press, New York © 1983.

Muscarinic Receptor Subclasses: Evidence from Binding Studies

N. J. M. Birdsall, E. C. Hulme, J. Stockton, A. S. V. Burgen, C. P. Berrie, R. Hammer, E. H. F. Wong, and M. J. Zigmond

*Division of Molecular Pharmacology, National Institute for Medical Research,
London NW7 1AA, England*

Muscarinic receptors are present in a wide variety of tissues, their activation leading to physiological responses as diverse as secretion, contraction of smooth muscle, vasodilation, and the regulation of the force and rate of heart muscle contraction. Furthermore muscarinic acetylcholine receptors are the predominant acetylcholine receptors in the central nervous system being involved in central motor mechanisms, memory, vestibular function as well as in processes which regulate mood and awareness. There is an equally large number of different biochemical and electrophysiological responses that have been implicated as being directly or closely linked to activation of this receptor. These include regulation of adenylate and guanylate cyclase, increased turnover of phosphatidylinositol and its phosphorylated derivatives, changes in membrane potential and conductance to several ions (K^+, Na^+, Ca^{++}, Cl^- ions) as well as the mobilisation of internal calcium. The number of responses and putative mechanisms poses the question of whether there is only one receptor protein linked directly to a single effector system, any diversity in whole tissue response resulting from post activation mechanisms which are presumably cell- or tissue-specific in nature. The other possibilities are that there is one receptor protein linked directly to different effectors or that there are different receptor binding proteins. The first hypothesis implies that the binding properties of the receptor, measured directly in an appropriate binding assay or estimated pharmacologically in whole tissue, should not vary from tissue to tissue. The other two possibilities predict that agonists and antagonists which sense the differences in binding protein structure or receptor-effector coupling could be found. Such drugs would exhibit a selective mode of action on a receptor subclass.

Selective Antagonists

Our original binding studies indicated that muscarinic antagonists bound to an apparently uniform population of binding sites on membrane preparations from the rat cerebral cortex (12). The measured affinities agreed quantitatively with those estimated by antagonism of contraction of ileal smooth muscle. These findings suggested that the antagonist binding properties of muscarinic receptors in the brain and ileum were similar. However, we have found that a novel antagonist, pirenzepine, binds to cortical muscarinic receptors with a considerably higher potency than that found in smooth muscle (9). Differences in pirenzepine binding properties of the receptors are found in other tissues (Table I) whereas there is only a small variation in the affinity of the 'classical' muscarinic antagonist N-methylscopolamine (NMS) (9).

TABLE I. The binding of pirenzepine to muscarinic receptors
in different tissues

	IC_{50} *M	Hill coefficient
Cerebral cortex	$5x10^{-8}$	0.7
Hippocampus	$3x10^{-8}$	0.8
Medulla-pons	$4x10^{-7}$	1.0
Submandibular	$1x10^{-7}$	0.8
Parotid	$3x10^{-7}$	1.0
Atria	$7x10^{-7}$	1.0
Stomach wall	$1x10^{-6}$	1.0
Fundic mucosa	$2x10^{-7}$	0.8

* Values are determined by competition experiments as described in reference 9, and are corrected for the occupancy of the radioligand.

A further difference between pirenzepine and classical muscarinic antagonists is that it does not exhibit simple mass action binding curves in all tissues. Evidence for this is the fact that the Hill coefficient (nH) is less than 1 in, for example, the cerebral cortex and sublingual gland (Table I). Using non-linear least squares curve fitting procedures it has been possible to explain this data by the existence of high affinity ($4-5 \times 10^{7}$ M^{-1}) and low affinity ($1-4 \times 10^{6}$ M^{-1}) pirenzepine binding sites whose proportions vary from tissue to tissue. These high affinity sites can be demonstrated directly using ^{3}H-pirenzepine which has been shown to bind with an

affinity of 5×10^7 M^{-1} to 60-70% of the total binding sites
for classical muscarinic antagonists in the cerebral cortex
(Stockton et al., unpublished results). Similarly, the tissue
selectivity found for pirenzepine in competition experiments is
found in direct binding experiments with ^{3}H-pirenzepine (Table
II). A much higher occupancy of ^{3}H-pirenzepine is found in
tissues, such as cerebral cortex, hippocampus and the sub-
mandibular gland, where the IC_{50} for pirenzepine binding (Table
I) is low (< 10^7 M) and the Hill coefficient is less than 1,

TABLE 2. Receptor occupancy of 10^{-9} M ^{3}H-pirenzepine in
different tissues[†]

	Occupancy %
Cerebral cortex	4.5
Hippocampus	5.2
Medulla-pons	1.2
Atria	<0.5*
Submandibular	2.5

[†] The total number of muscarinic receptor sites was determined
with 10^{-8} M ^{3}H-NMS.

* No specific ^{3}H-pirenzepine binding could be detected.

than in the medulla-pons and atria where low affinity pirenzepine
sites predominate, and the Hill coefficients are close to 1
(Table I). The binding profile found in vitro is in accord with
the known pharmacological selectivity of pirenzepine found in
vivo and in vitro. For example, pirenzepine inhibits gastric
secretion at lower doses than those needed to affect smooth
muscle contraction or heart rate (13,15). Although the IC_{50}
value in the fundus mucosa is relatively low, the Hill coefficient is less than 1 suggesting the presence of high affinity
pirenzepine sites which may be responsible for the high
sensitivity of the gastric mucosa to the action of pirenzepine in
antagonising vagally-induced secretion.
    We have also found that a number of muscarinic antagonists
such as atropine or NMS have lower affinities for muscarinic
receptors in the rat myocardium when compared to values found in
the cerebral cortex. The greatest difference (∿ 10-fold) is
shown by 4-diphenylacetyl-N-methylpiperidine methiodide (Di-4),
a drug which was shown by Barlow et al. (1) to have the greatest
selectivity in antagonising muscarinic responses in the heart
and smooth muscle. An example of a drug with the converse
selectivity to Di-4 is gallamine which is known to block the

inotropic and chronotropic actions of muscarinic agonists in the
heart (but not other muscarinic responses) at doses comparable
to those producing neuromuscular blockade (14,16). Binding
studies show that the interaction of gallamine with conventional
agonists and antagonists is not competitive (in agreement with
the whole tissue pharmacological studies (8)). Gallamine binds
to a novel binding site, distinct from the site to which acetylcholine and atropine bind, and allosterically decreases the
binding of agonists and antagonists to the conventional site (3).
In agreement with the reported pharmacological studies, the
effects of gallamine on the binding of muscarinic ligands are
much greater in the heart than in other tissues. We have now
found a number of drugs besides gallamine which bind to the
allosteric site, as well as drugs which bind to both the
conventional and the allosteric site (Zigmond et al., unpublished
results).

Selective Agonists

We have demonstrated the existence of subclasses of binding
sites (SH, H, L) which may be discriminated by potent agonists
(2,6,10) and have shown that the proportions of these sites may
vary between different tissues (6). However it has not been
certain whether these sites represent different receptors,
different states of receptor-effector coupling of one system or
a combination of both phenomena. We have now found that an
agonist, McN-A-343, which was reported some time ago to have a
selective pharmacological action on ganglionic muscarinic
receptors (17), differs from other muscarinic agonists in the
way it binds to muscarinic receptors. In the rat cerebral
cortex, it behaves as a competitive agonist, discriminating
between SH, H and L sites but in the myocardium, it binds non-
competitively with conventional antagonists (in contrast to
conventional muscarinic agonists) and behaves in some respects
like gallamine, although it is not certain that both drugs bind
to the same allosteric site (4).

Modulation of the binding properties of muscarinic receptors
Further evidence for muscarinic receptor heterogeneity may be
obtained from the variations between tissues in the ability of
ligands, which interact with the receptor or an associated
protein, to modify the binding properties of the receptors. For
example, in the myocardium and to a lesser extent in some brain
regions, magnesium ions will induce a conversion of L to H and
H to SH sites which is partially or completely antagonised by
GTP or GTP analogues (11). This type of modulation of agonist
binding, seen for a number of other receptor systems, is in
accord with the hypothesis that Mg^{2+} and GTP change the interaction between the receptor and a guanine nucleotide binding
protein, and in fact the linkage between muscarinic receptor
activation and inhibition of adenylate cyclase can be

demonstrated in broken cell preparations.

However in other tissues such as bovine heart conduction tissue and the hypothalamus, no effect of GTP could be observed (7), suggesting that these receptors are linked to a different effector mechanism.

Chemical modification of muscarinic receptors provides a method of distinguishing between receptor subtypes (5,18). The reaction of membranes with p-chloromercuribenzoate (PCMB) at 10^{-4}-10^{-3} M concentrations modified sulphydryl group(s) on muscarinic receptors to produce large changes in the agonist and antagonist binding properties. The heterogeneity in binding of potent agonists is eliminated and the intrinsic differences in agonist and antagonist binding observed in different tissues are largely removed. The heterogeneity in agonist binding can be restored by dithioerythritol treatment of the PCMB-treated receptors from the cerebral cortex, but not from the myocardium or medulla-pons. In contrast, the effects of PCMB on antagonist binding are reversed in all the tissues examined.

Discussion

The subclassification of a receptor system must depend primarily on the evidence of the selective pharmacological actions of certain drugs. Binding studies can complement these studies by providing a quantitative confirmation of the pharmacological findings. Even if no selective drugs exist, binding studies may provide evidence of receptor heterogeneity, by demonstrating a selective modulation of the binding properties of a receptor subpopulation by, for example, chemical modification or ligands which are involved in directly-linked effector mechanisms. Caution must be exerted, however, in any subclassification based predominantly on the results of binding studies. In such cases it is not known whether the subpopulations of binding sites each represent a discrete functional receptor system or whether they represent different conformational states of the same receptor system.

There is evidence both from pharmacological and binding studies that pirenzepine is a selective antagonist which has a low affinity for muscarinic receptors in the heart and smooth muscle and has a considerably higher affinity for some muscarinic receptors in sympathetic ganglia, the central nervous system and certain secretory glands. On the other hand there are antagonists, for example Di-4, which have a different pattern of selectivity from that of pirenzepine, exhibiting a higher affinity for muscarinic receptors in smooth muscle and the cerebral cortex than in the heart. Gallamine exhibits a converse selectivity to Di-4 and is most potent on myocardial muscarinic receptors. However it is not a competitive antagonist and binds to a different binding site from that to which conventional agonists and antagonists bind. It is possible, at least in the myocardium, that the selective muscarinic agonist McN-A-343 interacts with this site. The selective actions of McN-A-343 may therefore depend on its binding to the allosteric receptor site in one tissue and to the conventional site on muscarinic receptors in another tissue. Backing-up the evidence of the selective actions of certain drugs are the findings that sulphydryl reagents have differing effects on muscarinic receptors in different tissues. This may be due to the receptor subclasses having a different chemical structure or to their being linked to different effectors.

The available evidence therefore clearly points to the existence of subclasses of muscarinic receptors. At the present time, the differing patterns of selectivity exhibited by the selective antagonists makes a precise definition of the sub-classes difficult. Nevertheless there is the prospect of the development of further novel and selective drugs.

References

1. Barlow, R.B., Berry, K.J., Glenton, P.A.M., Nicolau, N.M., and Soh, K.S. (1976): Brit.J. Pharmacol., 58:613-620.

2. Birdsall, N.J.M., Burgen, A.S.V., and Hulme, E.C. (1978): Molec. Pharmacol., 14:723-736.

3. Birdsall, N.J.M., Burgen, A.S.V., Hulme, E.C., and Stockton, J. (1981): Brit. J. Pharmacol., 74:798P.

4. Birdsall, N.J.M., Burgen, A.S.V., Hulme, E.C., Stockton, J., and Zigmond, M.J. (1983): Brit. J. Pharmacol., (in press).

5. Birdsall, N.J.M., Burgen, A.S.V., Hulme, E.C., and Wong, E.H.F. (1980): Brit. J. Pharmacol., 68:142P.

6. Birdsall, N.J.M., Hulme, E.C., and Burgen, A.S.V. (1980): Proc. Roy. Soc. Lond., 207B:1-13.

7. Burgen, A.S.V., Birdsall, N.J.M., and Hulme, E.C. (1981): In: Cell Membrane in Function and Dysfunction of Vascular Tissue, edited by E. Godfraind and P. Meyer, pp. 15-26. Elsevier/North Holland Biomedical Press, Amsterdam.

8. Clark, A.L., and Michelson, F. (1976): Brit. J. Pharmacol., 58:323-331.

9. Hammer, R., Berrie, C.P., Birdsall, N.J.M., Burgen, A.S.V., and Hulme, E.C. (1980): Nature, 283:90-91.

10. Hulme, E.C., Birdsall, N.J.M., and Burgen, A.S.V. (1975): INSERM, 50:49-70.

11. Hulme, E.C., Birdsall, N.J.M., Berrie, C.P., and Burgen, A.S.V. (1980): In: Neurotransmitters and their Receptors, edited by U.Z. Littauer, Y. Dudai, I. Silman, V.I. Teichberg and Z. Vogel, pp. 241-250. John Wiley & Sons Ltd., Chichester.

12. Hulme, E.C., Birdsall, N.J.M., Burgen, A.S.V., and Mehta, P. (1978): Molec. Pharmacol., 14:737-750.

13. Jaup, B.H. (1968): Scand. J. Gastroenterol., 16:Suppl.68.

14. Laity, J.H.L., and Garg, B.K. (1962): J. Pharm. Pharmacol., 14:371-373.

15. Matsuo, Y., and Seki, A. (1979): Arzneimittelforschung, 29: 1028-1035.

16. Riker, W.F., and Wescoe, W.C. (1951): Ann. N.Y. Acad. Sci., 54:373-394.

17. Roszkowski, A.P. (1961): J. Pharmac. exp. Ther., 132:156-170.

18. Wong, E.H.F. (1981): PhD Thesis, C.N.A.A.

CNS Receptors—From Molecular
Pharmacology to Behavior, edited by
P. Mandel and F. V. Defeudis.
Raven Press, New York © 1983.

[3H]Pirenzepine Specifically Labels a High Affinity Muscarinic Receptor in the Rat Cerebral Cortex

Henry I. Yamamura, Mark Watson, and William R. Roeske

*Departments of Pharmacology, Biochemistry, Psychiatry, and Internal Medicine, and
The Arizona Research Laboratories, University of Arizona Health Sciences Center,
Tucson, Arizona 85724*

Recent studies of the muscarinic receptor have provided ample evidence for apparent heterogeneity of agonist binding sites (2,5–8,11,12). Under appropriate conditions (guanine nucleotides and ions), a heterogeneous population of high affinity agonist binding sites in the rat heart can be interconverted to a homogeneous population of low affinity sites with a Hill coefficient of one (6,11,12). These data support the hypothesis that the differences among the various agonist binding sites of the muscarinic receptor are due to environmental membrane constraints and not to the existence of a molecularly heterogeneous population of receptors (3,7,11,12).

A most unexpected finding is the apparent heterogeneity of antagonist binding sites of the muscarinic receptor. Previous pharmacological studies have shown significant differences between antagonist potencies in the ileum and atria (1) and in the ileum and the ganglia (4), thus implying the presence of different classes of muscarinic receptors in these tissues. Recently such differences have also been noted between these tissues using biochemical techniques of radioligand binding studies (9,10).

Pirenzepine, a nonclassical muscarinic antagonist, was among the first drugs used to show antagonist heterogeneity. Pirenzepine/[3H]-antagonist competition curves were characterized with Hill coefficients of less than one in several peripheral and central tissues (9,10). The potency of pirenzepine for inhibiting antagonist binding to muscarinic receptors in different tissues varied by a factor of about 30, with heart and smooth muscle receptors being of lowest affinity and cerebral cortical, and hippocampal receptors showing the highest affinity (9,10). These binding data have been explained by the existence of three subclasses (A, B, & C) of muscarinic receptors. It has been

proposed that A sites possess the highest affinity (~20 nM), B
sites are of intermediate affinity (~200 nM) and that C sites
have the lowest affinity (~1000 nM) for pirenzepine (9,10).
  We have recently examined the specific binding of [³H]pirenze-
pine of high specific activity to muscarinic receptors in the rat
cerebral cortex (13). Briefly, the methodology is as follows:
aliquots of a 5% cerebral cortical homogenate were incubated with
varying concentrations of [³H]pirenzepine (75 Ci/mmole, New
England Nuclear, Boston, MA) in 50 mM Na/K PO₄ buffer, pH 7.4 at
0-4°C for 120 min, at which time equilibrium was achieved. Termination of the incubation was achieved by centrifuging the incubation medium at 27,000 x g for 20 min to separate bound from
free [³H]pirenzepine. Non-specific binding was determined using
atropine at 1 μM concentration. Specific and non-specific [³H]-
pirenzepine binding in a typical experiment using rat cerebral
cortex is shown in Fig. 1.

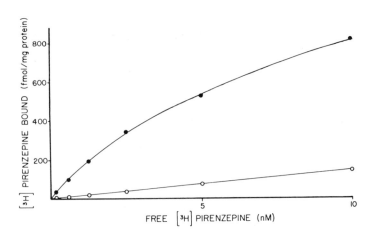

FIG. 1. A representative experiment of specific (●) and non-
specific (o) binding of [³H]pirenzepine to rat cerebral cortical
homogenates. (Reprinted by permission.)

Non-specific binding is shown to increase linearly with increasing concentrations of [³H]pirenzepine, while specific binding of
[³H]pirenzepine shows a downward concavity. Non-linear least
squares regression analysis yielded an average dissociation constant (K_d) value of 6.2 nM and a receptor density (B_{max}) of 1.1
pmole/mg protein. The average Hill coefficient of five separate
experiments was 0.98, which is consistant with simple mass action

behavior. Interestingly, when specific binding of [³H]pirenze-
pine was performed using rat cerebellar and heart homogenates,
only minimal amounts of specific binding of [³H]pirenzepine was
obtained under these conditions. Specific [³H]pirenzepine binding in these tissues at a concentration of 60 nM was only about
5% of the value obtained in the cerebral cortex.

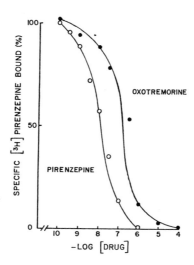

FIG. 2. Inhibition of [³H]pirenzepine binding by pirenzepine (o)
and oxotremorine (•) in rat cerebral cortical homogenates.

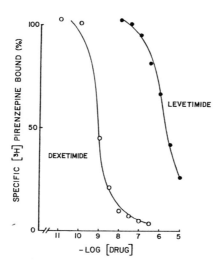

FIG. 3. Stereospecific inhibition of [³H]pirenzepine by dexetimide (o) and levetimide (•) in rat cerebral cortical homogenates.

We also determined the pharmacological and stereospecificity
of [³H]pirenzepine binding in the rat cerebral cortex. Fig. 2
shows the inhibition of [³H]pirenzepine by oxotremorine and
pirenzepine, while Fig. 3 illustrates the stereoselectivity of
[³H]pirenzepine binding. These data are summarized in Table 1
(modified from reference 13).

TABLE 1. The effects of muscarinic cholinergic drugs on the inhibition of [³H]pirenzepine in the rat cerebral cortex

Drug	IC_{50} (nM)	Hill Slope
Pirenzepine	11.8	0.93
Atropine	1.5	1.1
Dexetimide	1.2	1.2
Levetimide	1955	0.8
Oxotremorine	237	0.6
Carbachol	33,000	0.7

It can be seen from Table 1 that both pirenzepine and atropine
were effective inhibitors of [³H]pirenzepine binding with IC_{50}
values of 11.8 and 1.5 nM, respectively. Dexetimide, a potent
muscarinic antagonist, was also very effective in inhibiting
[³H]pirenzepine binding, being about 1500 times more effective
than its enantiomer, levetimide, thus illustrating the stereospecificity of the binding site. Muscarinic agonists, on the other
hand, were less effective in inhibiting [³H]pirenzepine binding
with IC_{50} values of 237 nM for oxotremorine and 33 μM for carba-
chol. In general, the Hill coefficients were one for the muscarinic antagonists and less than one for the muscarinic agonists.

The results of these studies with radiolabelled pirenzepine of
high specific activity clearly demonstrate the presence of a
unique high affinity binding site for this drug in the rat cerebral cortex. Preliminary examination of rat cerebellar and heart
homogenates show much less specific [³H]pirenzepine binding.
This implies that either there is a lower density of high affinity binding sites in these tissues, or that these tissues have a
lower affinity muscarinic binding site. The demonstration of
both pharmacological specificity and stereospecificity strongly
point to the fact that we are indeed specifically labelling the
pharmacologically relevant muscarinic cholinergic receptor in
this brain region. Further studies however, are presently being
done to determine whether distinct populations of antagonist
binding sites exist.

ACKNOWLEDGMENT

Portions of this study were supported in part by USPHS grants
MH-30626, MH-27257, and Program Project Grant HL-20984, a
Research Scientist Development Award Type II (MH-00095) from the

National Institute of Mental Health to H.I. Yamamura, and a Research Career Development Award (HL-00776) from the National Heart, Lung, and Blood Institute to W.R. Roeske. We sincerely appreciate the secretarial assistance of Alice Barrett.

REFERENCES

1. Barlow, R.B., Berry, K.J., Glenton, P.A.M., Nikolaou, N.M., and Soh, K.S. (1976): A comparison of affinity constants for muscarinic-sensitive acetylcholine receptors in guinea-pig atrial pacemaker cells at 29°C and in ileum at 29°C and 37°C. Br. J. Pharmac., 58:613-620.

2. Birdsall, N.J.M., Burgen, A.S.V., and Hulme, E.C. (1978): The binding of agonists to brain muscarinic receptors. Mol. Pharmacol., 14:723-736.

3. Birdsall, N.J.M., Hulme, E.C., and Burgen, A.S.V. (1980): The character of muscarinic receptors in different regions of the rat brain. Proc. R. Soc. Lond., 207:1-12.

4. Brown, D.A., Forward, A., and Marsh, A. (1980): Antagonist discrimination between ganglionic and ileal muscarinic receptors. Br. J. Pharmac., 71:362-364.

5. Ehlert, F.J., Roeske, W.R., and Yamamura, H.I. (1982): Regulation of the muscarinic receptors by guanine nucleotides, ions, and dopaminergic agonists. In: Pharmacological and Biochemical Aspects of Neurotransmitter Receptors, edited by H. Yoshida and H.I. Yamamura (in press) J. Wiley & Son, New York.

6. Ehlert, F.J., Roeske, W.R., and Yamamura, H.I. (1982): Muscarinic Cholinergic Receptor Heterogeneity. Trends in Neuroscience, (in press).

7. Ehlert, F.J., Roeske, W.R., and Yamamura, H.I. (1982): The nature of muscarinic receptor binding. In: Handbook of Psychopharmacology, edited by L. Iversen, S. Iversen, and S.H. Snyder, (in press) Plenum Press, New York.

8. Fields, J.Z., Roeske, W.R., Morkin, E., and Yamamura, H.I. (1978): Cardiac muscarinic cholinergic receptors. J. Biol. Chem., 253:3251-3258.

9. Hammer, R. (1982): Subclasses of muscarinic receptors and pirenzepine further experimental evidence. Scad. J. of Gastroenterology, 17 Supp. 72 59-65.

10. Hammer, R., Berrie, C.P., Birdsall, N.J.M., Burgen, A.S.V., and Hulme, E.C. (1980): Pirenzepine distinguishes between different subclasses of muscarinic receptors. Nature, 283:90-92.

11. Roeske, W.R., Ehlert, F.J., Barritt, D.S., Yamanaka, K., Rosenberger, L.R., Yamamda, S., Yamamura, S., and Yamamura, H.I. (1982): Recent advances in muscarinic receptor heterogeneity and regulation. In: Molecular Pharmacology of Neurotransmitter Receptor Systems edited by T. Segawa, H.I. Yamamura, and K. Kuriyama. Raven Press, New York (in press).

12. Roeske, W.R. and Yamamura, H.I. (1980): Muscarinic choliner-

gic receptor regulation. In: Psychopharmacology and Biochemistry of Neurotransmitter Receptors edted by H.I. Yamamura, E. Usdin, and R.W. Olsen, Elsevier/North-Holland Biomedical Press, New York, pp. 101-114.

13. Watson, M., Roeske, W.R., and Yamamura, H.I. (1982): [³H]Pirenzepine selectively identifies a high affinity population of muscarinic cholinergic receptors in the rat cerebral cortex, Submitted.

CNS Receptors—From Molecular
Pharmacology to Behavior, edited by
P. Mandel and F. V. Defeudis.
Raven Press, New York © 1983.

Discrimination of Heterogeneous Serotonin₁ Receptors by Indolealkylamines

D. L. Nelson, B. Weck, and W. Taylor

Department of Pharmacology and Toxicology, Collge of Pharmacy, University of Arizona, Tucson, Arizona 85721

Use of the ligand-binding technique to study receptors for serotonin (5-hydroxytryptamine, 5-HT) in the central nervous system (CNS) has resulted in the classification of the sites measured by this technique into subgroups based on their pharmacological selectivity. Thus, two principal groups of sites have been distinguished, the serotonin₁ (S_1 or 5-HT₁) sites and the serotonin₂ (S_2 or 5-HT₂) sites (16,20). The 5-HT₁ sites are defined by the high-affinity binding of ³H-5-HT (K_d = 1-4nM) to brain membranes (3,11,16) while the 5-HT₂ sites are defined by the binding of ³H-spiperone in rat frontal cortex (16,20) or by the binding of ³H-ketanserin (8). While 5-HT interacts with both of these sites, it is approximately 150-1000 times less potent at the 5-HT₂ sites (8,10,18,20). In addition to the 5-HT₁ and 5-HT₂ sites another site defined by the binding of ³H-5-HT (K_d = 14-20 nM) has been described which has been suggested to exist on glial membranes (2).

Both the 5-HT₁ and 5-HT₂ sites have properties which are consistent with those that would be expected for functional receptors. For example, the pharmacology of both sites is appropriate for 5-HT receptors with the 5-HT₁ sites generally having higher affinity for agonists and the 5-HT₂ sites having higher affinity for antagonists (1,6,20). Correlations have been shown between the ability of antagonists to inhibit binding to 5-HT₂ sites and their ability to inhibit both tryptamine-induced convulsions and hydroxytryptophan-induced head twitches in rats and mice (7,18), and it also appears that many peripheral actions of 5-HT, especially in the vasculature, are due to actions at 5-HT₂ receptors (24). In addition, the numbers of 5-HT₁ and 5-HT₂ sites can be regulated by procedures which alter central serotonergic function or activity. Administration of antidepressants, for example, results in a decrease in the numbers of $5-HT_2$ sites in the brain (17), and procedures which either increase or decrease the availability of 5-HT at central 5-HT receptors decrease or increase respectively the numbers of $5-HT_1$ sites (9,11,12,19,22). Correlations have also been proposed between the different binding sites and the 5-HT receptors measured electrophysiologically. Thus, Peroutka et al. (18) have suggested that the $5-HT_1$ site may represent the central 5-HT receptors which cause inhibition of neuronal firing and that the $5-HT_2$ sites may represent receptors responsible for the excitatory effects of 5-HT.

While it has been possible to establish correlations between $5-HT_2$ sites defined by ligand binding and physiologically functional receptors, e.g., by evaluating the central actions of tryptamine (7) and hydroxytryptophan (18) and the peripheral actions of 5-HT in the vasculature (24), such direct correlations of $5-HT_1$ sites with function have not been made. Thus, the evidence suggesting that the $5-HT_1$ binding sites may represent functional serotonergic receptors remains somewhat minimal and includes primarily the following: 1) the pharmacology of the sites seems appropriate, i.e., both 5-HT agonists and antagonists inhibit the high-affinity binding of ^3H-5-HT; 2) the numbers of $5-HT_1$ sites can be increased or decreased following appropriate alterations in central serotonergic activity; and 3) based on a limited number of compounds, the pharmacology of the $5-HT_1$ sites resembles that of the inhibitory 5-HT receptors measured electrophysiologically. Therefore, it would be desirable to be able to directly compare the potency of compounds as agonists or antagonists at 5-HT receptors which mediate physiological responses with their potencies at the $5-HT_1$ binding sites. However, there are several factors which make such comparisons difficult. First, the $5-HT_1$ sites are not homogeneous. While saturation studies with ^3H-5-HT reveal a single population of high-affinity sites apparently having identical affinity for 5-HT, the use of other drugs has revealed that the $5-HT_1$ sites are actually heterogeneous. For example, the logit-log plots for the inhibition of ^3H-5-HT by many drugs have slopes less than unity (11). The neuroleptic spiperone, in fact, produces biphasic inhibition curves of ^3H-5-HT binding in rat brain which has resulted in the classification of two types of $5-HT_1$ sites, $5-HT_1$-A (K_i spiperone = 2-13 nM) and $5-HT_1$-B (K_i spiperone = 35,000 nM)(13,15). More recent investigations suggest that classifying $5-HT_1$ sites into only two groups based on their affinities for certain neuroleptics may actually be an oversimplification. Examination of other species and other classes of drugs has revealed that the $5-HT_1$ sites may be composed of at least three different subgroups (14). Thus, it becomes apparent that if one wishes to compare the pharmacology of a functional 5-HT receptor with that of the $5-HT_1$ sites, it will first be necessary to develop the means of examining drug potencies at the individual subgroups of $5-HT_1$ sites.

A second difficulty in trying to compare the pharmacology
of 5-HT₁ sites with functional 5-HT receptors is the lack of
specific 5-HT₁ antagonists. In general 5-HT agonists are much
more potent at 5-HT₁ than 5-HT₂ sites. Thus, all indoleamines
which have been examined are 30 to several thousand fold more
potent at the 5-HT₁ compared to the 5-HT₂ sites (1,10,20). In
addition, the piperazine-type 5-HT agonists MK 212 and trifluor-
ophenylpiperazine are also more potent at the 5-HT₁ sites (1).
The exception to date seems to be quipazine which has been reported to be equipotent at both sites (1). The situation,
however, is reversed for the antagonists, i.e., all 5-HT antagonists that have been examined are at least as potent at 5-HT₂
sites as at 5-HT₁ sites and in most cases are actually much more
potent at the 5-HT₂ sites (1,6,20).
     Therefore, it seems that the characterization of 5-HT₁
sites and their eventual comparison with functional 5-HT receptors will depend upon the development of compounds, both agonists and antagonists, that are relatively selective for individual subpopulations of 5-HT₁ sites. Our approach to the problem of developing such compounds has been to concentrate on the
indoleamines. There are several reasons for this. First, as
mentioned above, the indoleamines as a class appear to have much
greater affinity for the 5-HT₁ than the 5-HT₂ sites. Thus, they
provide a basic structure that discriminates between these two
classes of sites. Second, they not only appear to differentiate
between 5-HT₁ and 5-HT₂ sites, but certain indoleamines also
discriminate between different types of 5-HT₁ sites. For example, we have demonstrated that both psilocybin and 5-methyoxy-
N,N-dimethyltryptamine differentiate at least two different populations of 5-HT₁ sites (14). In addition, it appears that
appropriate structural modifications can be carried out which
result in indoleamines that can act as 5-HT antagonists, e.g.,
Woolley and Shaw described the synthesis of a number of indoleamines which acted as 5-HT antagonists in peripheral tissues
(26). Thus, indoleamines seem promising as a class of compounds
for the development of 5-HT₁ subtype specific agonists and
antagonists.
     One of our primary concerns in examining these compounds
has been to systematically determine how structural modifications affect the affinities of these agents for the 5-HT₁ sites.
The present discussion illustrates an example of how simple
structural changes (in this case the addition of substituents to
the primary amino group of tryptamine) can alter the ability of
indoleamines to recognize 5-HT₁ sites.

MATERIALS AND METHODS

The measurement of ³H-5-HT binding was carried out essentially as described previously (15). In the present study whole
rat cortex dorsal to the rhinal sulcus was used. The tissue was
homogenized in 40 volumes of cold 50 mM Tris-HCl buffer (pH 7.4)

using a Brinkman Polytron (setting 5 for 15 sec). The homogenate was then centrifuged at 48,000 x g for 10 min and the pellet
was resuspended. This process was repeated three additional
times with a 10-min incubation (37°C) of the suspension between
the second and third resuspensions. The final pellet was resuspended in 50 volumes of the buffer for use in the binding
assay. Each assay tube (final volume = 2 ml) contained the
following: 500 μl of membrane suspension, 10 μM pargyline, 4 mM
$CaCl_2$, 50 mM Tris, ^{3}H-5-HT (1.8 nM), and added drugs for a final
pH of 7.4. The incubation (7 min at 37°C) was terminated by
vacuum filtration through Whatman GF/B filters followed by
three, 5-ml washes with cold buffer. The filters were dried and
radioactivity in the filters was measured by liquid scintillation spectrometry. Specific ^{3}H-5-HT binding was defined as the
difference between binding in the absence and presence of either
1 μM unlabeled 5-HT or 1 μM metergoline and represented 60-80%
of total bound radioactivity.

Metergoline was a gift from Farmitalia Carlo Erba. N,N-
Diisopropyltryptamine, 1-[2-(3-indolyl)-ethyl]-piperidine, and
4-[-2(3-indolyl)-ethyl]-morpholine were synthesized in our laboratory. All other tryptamines were obtained from Sigma Chemical Company.

RESULTS AND DISCUSSION

For the present discussion a series of tryptamines was examined to determine the effects of changing the substituents at
the alpha-amino group on the ability of these compounds to recognize 5-HT$_1$ sites. The structures, names, and abbreviations
used for these are shown in Table 1.

Tryptamine (which lacks the 5-hydroxyl group of serotonin)
was found to have an IC$_{50}$ value for inhibiting ^{3}H-5-HT binding
that was about 35-60 fold greater than that of unlabeled 5-HT.
Addition of methyl or ethyl groups to the amino group resulted
in little change in the IC$_{50}$ values (Table 1). Increasing the
bulk of the added alkyl groups to form DIPT, however, resulted
in a large (5-7 fold) increase in the IC$_{50}$ value. Changing the
alkyl groups to form the ring systems in PDT and MLT resulted in
little change in the IC$_{50}$ values compared to DIPT.

While the IC$_{50}$ values can provide some information about
the overall potencies of these compounds, they do not give a
complete picture of the interaction of the tryptamine analogues
with the 5-HT$_1$ sites. The reason for this is that the inhibition curves produced by these compounds are not simple monophasic curves, as can be seen in Fig. 1. Panel A of Fig. 1 contrasts the curves produced by tryptamine and DMT with the monophasic curve produced by the 5-HT antagonist metergoline which
gives a logit-log plot having a slope of unity. As can be seen
from this figure, the tryptamine curve tended to form a plateau
at higher concentrations with about 25% of the sites showing
resistance to inhibition by tryptamine. Addition of two methyl

TABLE 1.   Potency of tryptamine analogues for inhibiting the
binding of ^{3}H-5-HT

$$\text{CH}_2\text{-CH}_2\text{-R}$$

R	COMPOUND	IC_{50} (nM)[a]
$-NH_2$	Tryptamine (TRYP)	176 ± 27
$-N(CH_3)_2$	N,N-Dimethyltryptamine (DMT)	137 ± 30
$-N(C_2H_5)_2$	N,N-Diethyltryptamine (DET)	176 ± 42
$-N\begin{smallmatrix}CH(CH_3)_2\\CH(CH_3)_2\end{smallmatrix}$	N,N-Diisopropyltryptamine (DIPT)	961 ± 272
$-N\bigcirc$	1-[2-(3-indolyl)-ethyl]-piperidine (PDT)	1000 ± 78
$-N\bigcirc O$	4-[2-(3-indolyl)-ethyl]-morpholine (MLT)	1421 ± 262

[a]IC_{50} values are given as the mean $\pm$ S.E.M. and were each
derived from 4-5 separate experiments.

groups to tryptamine to form DMT resulted in a significant
change in the shape of the inhibition curve. Thus, the DMT
curve more closely resembled a monophasic curve, and was able to
completely inhibit all specific ^{3}H-5-HT binding. Lengthening
the alkyl substituents to form DET resulted in only small
changes in the shape of the curve (Fig. 1-B). Increasing the
bulk of these substituents to form DIPT, however, produced a
large change in the curve (Fig. 1-B). This shift in potency
appeared to be primarily confined to concentrations between
10^{-7} and 3×10^{-5} M. Changing the alkyl substitutions to produce
piperidyl or morpholinyl heterocycles (PDT and MLT) resulted in
compounds that produced inhibition curves that were very similar
to DIPT (Fig. 1-C). The inhibition curves produced by DIPT, PDT
and MLT were all distinctly biphasic.

The curves produced by tryptamine and its analogues were
subjected to nonlinear regression analysis (15) to determine
whether they were consistent with recognition of a single or
multiple sites. Each curve shown in Fig. 1 was analyzed for
its ability to fit both one-site and two-site models as pre-

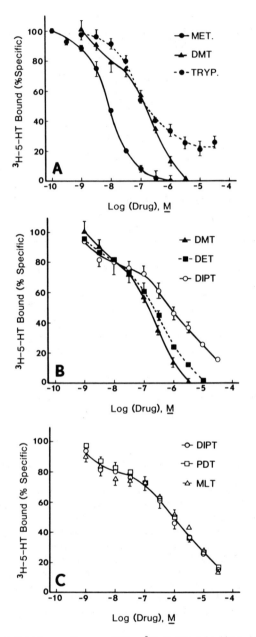

FIGURE 1. Inhibition of specific ³H-5-HT binding by analogues
of tryptamine. ³H-5-HT binding is expressed as the percent of
specific binding occurring in the absence of inhibitors, and
each point represents the mean ± S.E.M. from 4-5 separate experiments. The drug abbreviations correspond to those used in
Table 1 with the addition of the antagonist metergoline (MET).

viously described (15). All of the curves except for DMT fit a
two-site model significantly (p<.01) better than a one-site
model. The parameter estimates from the appropriate models are
shown in Table 2. K_1 and K_2 represent the K_d values of the
tryptamines for high- and low-affinity sites respectively estimated by the two-site model. B_1 and B_2 represent the proportions of specific binding occurring at these sites.

The data from the present study indicate that relatively
small changes in structure can produce significant changes in
the ability of tryptamines to recognize the 5-HT₁ sites and that
it is possible to produce tryptamines which show good discrimination between different populations of these sites. It also
provides us with some information regarding the structural requirements for recognition of these sites. Thus, while about
25% of the ³H-5-HT binding sites are quite resistant to inhibition by tryptamine, alkylation to form DMT or DET results in
compounds which readily inhibit all specific ³H-5-HT binding.
While addition of methyl or ethyl groups seemed to facilitate
recognition by one population of 5-HT₁ sites, as compared to
tryptamine, increasing the size of the substituents to form
DIPT, PDT or MLT seemed to decrease affinity for one of the
populations. This was shown by the fact that there was a shift
to right in the curve for concentrations greater than 3 x 10⁻⁸M
while there was no change at lower concentrations.

The findings here are in agreement with previous studies
which have demonstrated that the high-affinity binding of ³H-5-
HT is to a heterogeneous population of sites (13,14,15). In
fact, the curves for several of the tryptamine analogues suggested a very complex interaction with the 5-HT₁ sites.
Although the inhibition curves for DIPT, PDT, and MLT fit a two-
site model significantly better than a one-site model, it was
noted that the computer-generated curves for the two-site model
did not really fit the observed data points as well as would be
expected if the curves actually represented a two-site model.
Therefore, the inhibition curves generated by these three compounds were also analyzed according to a three-site model. Even
though the curves do not really contain enough data points for a
good three-site analysis, it was found that DIPT and PDT did fit
a three-site model significantly better than a two-site model.
This suggestion that the 5-HT₁ sites might represent more than
two separate populations is also in agreement with previous
studies comparing different species and various drugs (14).

TABLE 2. Parameters for the inhibition of ^{3}H-5-HT binding by tryptamine analogues

DRUG	K_1 (nM)[a]	K_2 (nM)	B_1 (%)	B_2 (%)
TRYP	33.4	>10,000	73	27
DMT	84.5	–	93	–
DET	2.6	268	28	71
DIPT	31.3	4356	37	61
PDT	89.2	7321	48	44
MLT	48.9	4606	28	57

[a] See text for definitions of K_1, K_2, B_1 and B_2.

The finding that certain tryptamines, i.e., DIPT, PDT and MLT, produce biphasic curves for the inhibition of ^{3}H-5-HT binding suggests that they or similar analogues might be useful as radioactively labeled ligands for 5-HT$_1$ sites. Since they exhibit such a large difference in affinities between the different populations of 5-HT$_1$ sites, it should be possible to label the high-affinity population of sites without labeling the sites with lowest affinity. Such ligands would have an advantage over ^{3}H-5-HT in that the labeled sites should be less heterogeneous than those measured using ^{3}H-5-HT, which would be of benefit in studies trying to correlate the pharmacology of the binding sites with functional receptors.

While the compounds examined for the present study all interact with 5-HT$_1$ sites, a number of questions remain regarding their activity in physiological systems. Tryptamine certainly has physiological activity, although there have been numerous studies suggesting that it may act at receptors other than 5-HT receptors (4,5,27), and DET and DMT have long been regarded as hallucinogens (21) and are active at certain peripheral receptors such as those found in the rat fundus (23). Recently, DIPT has also been shown to be psychoactive in man (21). We have been looking for physiological measures of serotonergic activity to determine whether the properties of the 5-HT$_1$ sites can be correlated to any functional 5-HT receptors, and recently we have begun to examine the rat fundus as one possible system. This tissue is very sensitive to 5-HT and can be stimulated by a wide variety of 5-HT analogues (23). However, the receptors which mediate the response to 5-HT do not appear to be 5-HT$_2$ receptors, i.e., the response to 5-HT is not blocked by the specific 5-HT$_2$ antagonist ketanserin (25). Preliminary results in our laboratory have shown that both DIPT and PDT stimulate the rat fundus, although they are 10-100 times less potent than 5-HT. Further studies are under way to determine whether MLT has an effect on this system, as well as to determine the potencies of various 5-HT antagonists for comparison with 5-HT$_1$ sites.

One of the major goals of the synthesis and testing of indoleamines and related compounds is the development of agents having high affinity for 5-HT$_1$ sites, but which recognize only specific populations of these sites. At present ^{3}H-5-HT is the only labeled ligand available that is specific for 5-HT$_1$ sites, and its usefulness seems somewhat limited by the fact that it appears to label a very heterogeneous group of sites. The present work, however, suggests that it should indeed be possible to develop indoleamines that will be useful as radioactively labeled ligands which bind to specific subtypes of the 5-HT$_1$ sites.

Supported by NIH grant NS 16605 and a PMA grant.

REFERENCES

1. Blackshear, M. A., Steranka, L. R., and Sanders-Bush, E.
    (1981): Eur. J. Pharmacol., 76: 325-334.
2. Fillion, G., Beaudoin, D., Rousselle, J. C., Deniau, J. M.,
    Fillion, M. P., Dray, F. and Jacob, J. (1979):
    J. Neurochem., 33, 567-570.
3. Fillion, G., Fillion, M. P., Spirakis, C., Bahers, J. M.,
    and Jacob, J. (1976): Life Sci. 18: 65-74.
4. Jones, R. S. G. (1982): Neuropharmacology, 21: 209-214.
5. Kellar, K. J. and Cascio, C. S. (1982): Eur. J. Pharmacol.,
    78: 475-478.
6. Leysen, J. E., Awouters, F., Kennis, L., Laduron, P. M.,
    Vandenberk, J., and Janssen, P. A. J. (1981): Life Sci.,
    28: 1015-1022.
7. Leysen, J. E., Niemegeers, C. J. E., Tollanaere, J. P., and
    Laduron, P. M. (1978): Nature, 272, 168-171.
8. Leysen, J. E., Niemegeers, C. J. E., Van Nueten, J. M., and
    Laduron, P. M. (1982): Mol. Pharmacol., 21: 301-314.
9. Maggi, A., U'Prichard, D. C., Enna, S. J. (1980): Eur. J.
    Pharmacol. 61: 91-98; 1980.
10. Middlemiss, D. N., Carroll, J. A., Fisher, R. W., and
    Mounsey, I. J. (1980): Eur. J. Pharmacol. 66: 253-254.
11. Nelson, D. L., Herbet, A., Bourgoin, S., Glowinski, J., and
    Hamon, M. (1978): Mol. Pharmacol. 14: 983-995.
12. Nelson, D. L., Herbet, A., Pichat, L., Glowinski, J. and
    Hamon, M. (1979): Naunyn-Schmiedenberg's Arch. Pharmacol.
    310: 25-33.
13. Nelson, D. L., Pedigo, N. W., and Yamamura, H. I. (1981):
    J. Physiol. (Paris), 77: 369-372.
14. Nelson, D. L., Schnellmann, R., and Smit, M. (1982): In:
    Molecular Pharmacology of Neurotransmitter Systems,
    edited by T. Segawa, H. I. Yamamura, and K. Kuriyama,
    (in press).   Raven Press, New York.
15. Pedigo, N. W., Yamamura, H. I., and Nelson, D. L. (1981):
    J. Neurochem., 36: 220-226.
16. Peroutka, S. J. and Snyder, S. H. (1979): Mol. Pharmacol.
    16: 687-699.
17. Peroutka, S. J. and Snyder, S. H. (1980): Science, 210:
    88-90.
18. Peroutka, S. J., Lebovitz, R. M., and Snyder, S. H. (1981):
    Science, 212: 827-829.
19. Savage, D. D., Frazer, A. and Mendels, J. (1979): Eur. J.
    Pharmacol., 58, 87-88.
20. Seeman, P., Westman, K., Coscina, D., and Warsh, J. J.
    (1980): Eur. J. Pharmacol., 66: 179-191.
21. Shulgin, A. T. and Carter, M. F. (1980): Commun. Psycho-
    pharmacol., 4: 363-369.
22. Steigrad, P., Tobler, I., Waser, P. G., and Borbely, A.,
    (1978) Naunyn-Schmiedenberg's Arch. Pharmacol., 305,
    143-148.

23. Vane, J. R. (1959): Brit. J. Pharmacol., 14: 87-98.
24. Van Nueten, J. M., Janssen, P. A. J., Van Beek, J.,
    Xhonneux, R., Verbeuren, T.-J., and Vanhoutte, P. M.
    (1981): J. Pharmacol. Exp. Ther., 218: 217-230.
25. Van Nueten, J. M., Xhonneux, R., Vanhoutte, P. M., and
    Janssen, P. A. J. (1981): Arch. Int. Pharmacodyn.,
    250: 328-329.
26. Woolley, D. W. (1962): The Biochemical Bases of Psychoses,
    pp. 93-102. John Wiley and Sons, Inc., New York.
27. Woolley, D. W. and Shaw, E. (1957): J. Pharmacol. Exp.
    Ther., 121: 13-17.

CNS Receptors—From Molecular
Pharmacology to Behavior, edited by
P. Mandel and F. V. DeFeudis.
Raven Press, New York © 1983.

Reciprocal Modulations of Central 5-HT Receptors by GTP and Cations

M. Hamon, C. Goetz, and H. Gozlan

Groupe NB, INSERM U-114, Collège de France, F-75005 Paris, France

Binding studies with radioactive ligands related to serotonin (5-HT) have led to the discovery of two specific binding sites $5-HT_1$ and $5-HT_2$ in brain (9,21). The $5-HT_1$ site is labelled by ^3H-5-HT and exhibits higher affinity for agonists than for antagonists. In contrast, the $5-HT_2$ site labelled by ^3H-spiperone, ^3H-mianserin, ^3H-ketanserin and ^3H-metergoline binds preferentially the antagonists. Although both classes of sites undergo adaptive changes expected for true receptors following treatments affecting chronically central serotoninergic synapses (9,17), only the $5-HT_2$ site would correspond to a 5-HT receptor in brain (13). Indeed, the relative efficacy of various 5-HT agonists and antagonists to displace ^3H-spiperone from its specific binding site is perfectly correlated with their potency in evoking and preventing respectively 5-HT-dependent behaviours (13,21). In contrast, such relationships have not been found with drugs acting on the $5-HT_1$ site; in spite of previous interpretations (20, 21), the detailed comparison of the respective characteristics of the $5-HT_1$ site and 5-HT-sensitive adenylate cyclase demonstrated that these two biochemical markers are not associated in brain membranes (8,9,12,16, 18).

The apparent lack of functional correlate of $5-HT_1$ site led Laduron and Ilien (13) to postulate that this site is more likely a recognition site for indolic compounds instead of a true receptor. However, a rapid survey of the pharmacological properties of the $5-HT_1$ site reveals that numerous indoles (17) and even 5-hydroxyindoles (1) are unable to displace ^3H-5-HT specifically bound to brain membranes. Furthermore, these indoles are precisely those compounds which are inactive in biological tests classically used for identifying 5-HT agonists and antagonists. In contrast, non-indolic compounds (8-OH-N,N-DPAT, TFMPP...see table 3) capable of evoking 5-HT-dependent biological responses inhibit

the specific binding of ^{3}H-5-HT onto 5-HT$_1$ sites (8,9).
Accordingly, the 5-HT$_1$ site should not be considered
only as a recognition site for indoles. Instead, numerous observations strongly suggest that it does correspond to a functional 5-HT receptor in the CNS (8,9);
in particular, guanine nucleotides and cations affect
the specific binding of ^{3}H-5-HT onto brain membranes
similarly to that of various ligands onto well identified receptors (3-5,19,23,25). As will be described,
such in vitro modulations of 5-HT$_1$ sites can even be
used to assess the agonist or antagonist properties of
new compounds.

EFFECTS OF GUANINE NUCLEOTIDES ON 5-HT$_1$ SITES

It is now well established that GTP and GppNHp inhibit the specific binding of ^{3}H-5-HT onto rat brain membranes (15,20). The maximal effect corresponding to
60% inhibition is reached with 0.1-0.5mM of each nucleotide. Scatchard analyses reveal that GTP and GppNHp
decrease both the apparent affinity for ^{3}H-5-HT and
the number (Bmax) of 5-HT$_1$ sites in brain membranes (15).
Since GTP effects on agonist binding are generally
ascribed to allosteric interactions between a GTP-bin-
ding protein and a receptor coupled to adenylate cyclase (22), Peroutka et al (20) concluded that the 5-HT$_1$
site likely corresponds to the 5-HT receptor associated
with this enzyme in brain. However, Nelson et al (18)
noted that only µM concentrations of GTP are required
for the optimal coupling of 5-HT receptors with adenylate cyclase whereas almost mM concentrations of the
nucleotide are necessary for reducing ^{3}H-5-HT binding.
However, the comparison of effective GTP concentrations
would be meaningful only if GTP undergoes similar metabolic processes under the different experimental conditions selected for measuring ^{3}H-5-HT binding and adenylate cyclase activity. Obviously, this is not the case
since Ca^{2+} added to the assay mixture for binding studies (1,18) stimulates the activity of nucleotidases (11)
whereas the chelation of the cation by EGTA in the adenylate cyclase assay largely protects GTP from catabolism (18). The crucial role played by Ca^{2+} regarding
the effective concentrations of GTP is simply demonstrated by the fact that only µM concentrations of the
nucleotide are required for reducing ^{3}H-5-HT binding in
the absence of the cation (fig.1). However, catabolism
even occurs under this condition since the addition of
0.1mM ATP or GMP, two competitive inhibitors of the nucleotidases (11), promotes the GTP-induced reduction of
^{3}H-5-HT binding (fig.1). Consequently, when GTP degradation is completely blocked, the same range of concentrations is necessary for the activation of 5-HT-sensi-

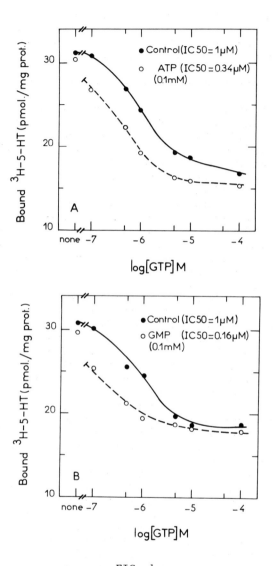

FIG. 1
Promoting effect of ATP (A) and GMP (B) on the GTP-induced
inhibition of ^{3}H-5-HT binding onto rat hippocampal membranes
The specific binding was measured with 0.8 nM of ^{3}H-5-HT and
various concentrations of GTP in the absence (●) or the presence
of ATP (0.1 mM, o, A) or GMP (0.1 mM, o ,B). Each point is the
mean of triplicate determinations.

tive adenylate cyclase and the reduction of ^{3}H-5-HT
binding (15). Nevertheless, this similarity is not enough to conclude that the 5-HT$_1$ site belongs to the receptor coupled to adenylate cyclase in brain (see below).

EFFECTS OF CATIONS ON 5-HT$_1$ SITES

As illustrated in table 1, several di- and trivalent
cations increase the specific binding of ^{3}H-5-HT onto
5-HT$_1$ sites. Trivalent cations are the most effective
since half maximal stimulation is observed with 15-20
µM of La^{3+} or Mn^{3+}. Among divalent cations, Co^{2+}, Ba^{2+}
and Mn^{2+} are only 2-3 times less efficient than trivalent cations whereas Ca^{2+} and particularly Mg^{2+} are
markedly less potent. All divalent cations are not able
to increase ^{3}H-5-HT binding since, in contrast to those
listed in table 1, Fe^{2+} and Zn^{2+} reduce the ligand binding (-31% and -88% at 1mM, respectively). Similarly,
monovalent cations decrease the specific binding of ^{3}H-
5-HT onto brain membranes (-44% and -51% with 100mM Na$^+$
and K$^+$, respectively).

The cations listed in table 1 are also those which
interact with the Ca^{2+} channel in membranes (7). Accordingly, their effects on ^{3}H-5-HT binding might result
from the possible association of the 5-HT$_1$ site with a
Ca^{2+}ionophore. Indeed, alterations in Ca^{2+} fluxes due
to 5-HT receptor stimulation have been already described in invertebrates (2). Whether this occurs also in
the rat brain deserves further investigation.

Numerous reports mention the ability of Ca^{2+} to uncouple
receptors and adenylate cyclase (see 15). Therefore, its
promoting action on ^{3}H-5-HT binding might well correspond to a symmetrical modulation when compared to the
inhibitory effect of GTP, which in contrast favours the
association of receptors with adenylate cyclase (22).
Experiments with kainic acid-induced lesions of intrinsic neurones in the rat striatum have shown, however,
that the GTP effect on ^{3}H-5-HT binding can be altered
without any change in the stimulatory action of Ca^{2+}.
These differential effects of kainic acid treatment
have been interpreted in a model with Ca^{2+} and GTP
acting on regulatory sites unrelated to a putative 5-HT
receptor-adenylate cyclase complex (15).

Scatchard analyses revealed that di- and trivalent
cations induce changes in 5-HT$_1$ sites which are exactly
the reverse to those evoked by GTP: an increase in both
their apparent affinity for ^{3}H-5-HT and their number in
brain membranes. The enhanced affinity results at least
partly from a reduction in the rate of dissociation of
^{3}H-5-HT from its binding site ($k_{-1}=0.11\pm0.01$min^{-1} at
25°C without Ca^{2+}; $k_{-1}=0.087\pm0.005$min^{-1} with 5mM Ca^{2+} at
25°C).

TABLE 1. Characteristics of cation-induced increases in ^{3}H-5-HT binding onto rat hippocampal membranes

Cation	EC50 (μM)	Maximal increase (%)	
La^{3+}	17.2	+90	
Mn^{3+}	19.7	+260	($\pm$86)
Co^{2+}	40.0	+162	
Ba^{2+}	52.2	+62	
Mn^{2+}	69.1 $\pm$ 10.9	+165	($\pm$21)
Ca^{2+}	157.3 $\pm$ 18.0	+77	($\pm$4)
Mg^{2+}	420.0	+63	($\pm$9)

For each cation, EC50 corresponds to the concentration producing half maximal increase in ^{3}H-5-HT binding. The maximal effect is expressed as a percentage over ^{3}H-5-HT binding observed in the absence of any cation. Each value is the mean of 2-5 separate determinations. SEM is given for the mean results from at least 4 independent determinations.

DIVALENT CATION-GUANINE NUCLEOTIDE INTERACTIONS ON ^{3}H-5-HT BINDING

Since GTP converts the $5-HT_1$ site into another binding site with lower affinity for ^{3}H-5-HT whereas divalent cations such as Ca^{2+} and Mn^{2+} exert the reverse action, experiments were carried out to investigate whether the same regulatory subsite is involved in both types of modulations.

A first series of experiments consisted of examining the GTP-induced inhibition of ^{3}H-5-HT binding in the absence or the presence of divalent cations. As illustrated in fig.2, Ca^{2+} strongly reduces the efficacy of GTP to inhibit ^{3}H-5-HT binding onto hippocampal membranes. Similar shifts in the IC_{50} value of GTP were observed with Mg^{2+}, Mn^{2+} and Ba^{2+} (unpublished observations). The curves obtained (fig.2) strongly suggest that a competitive interaction exists between GTP and Ca^{2+} (or other divalent cations). This first observation led us to study the fate of GTP under these experimental conditions. We found that ^{3}H-GTP binds to a specific site ($K_D=0.4\mu$M) in brain membranes (11); Ca^{2+} reduces this binding by stimulating the catabolism of the label-

led nucleotide by low Km $(5\mu M)$ membrane-bound nucleotidases (11). Furthermore, the formation of complexes
between Ca^{2+} and ^3H-GTP also likely accounts for the
lower binding of the nucleotide in the presence of the
cation (11). As a result, the concentration of ^3H-GTP
available for specific binding sites is much less in
the presence than in the absence of Ca^{2+}. Ignoring this
fact led to Scatchard plots indicative of an apparent
competitive inhibition of ^3H-GTP binding by Ca^{2+}. However, all divalent cations do not affect ^3H-GTP binding
as Ca^{2+} does since, for instance, Mn^{2+} reduces the number of ^3H-GTP binding sites in hippocampal membranes
without changing their apparent K_D. Such differential
effects suggest that more than one cation site is involved in the modulation of GTP-induced inhibition of
^3H-5-HT binding. Subsequent experiments confirmed that
GTP and cations affect $5-HT_1$ sites by acting on different subsites:
- as shown in table 1, Mn^{3+} is more potent than Mn^{2+}

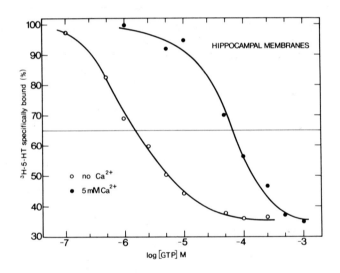

FIG.2
Effect of Ca^{2+} on the inhibition of ^3H-5-HT binding
onto hippocampal membranes due to GTP

Binding assays were carried out with 1.0nM of ^3H-5-HT and various
concentrations of GTP in the absence (o) or the presence (●) of
5mM $CaCl_2$. ^3H-5-HT specifically bound is expressed in percent of
that found when no GTP was added. Each point is the mean of
quadruplicate determinations.

TABLE 2. Effects of N-ethylmaleimide pretreatment
on the sensitivity of ^{3}H-5-HT specific binding to GTP and Mn^{2+}

	^{3}H-5-HT specifically bound (fmol./mg prot)			
Addition	Control	(%)	NEM	(%)
none	159 ± 5		81 ± 4	
GTP (0.1mM)	66 ± 3	(-58)	60 ± 5	(-26)
Mn^{2+} (1mM)	456 ± 10	(+187)	76 ± 4	(-6)

Hippocampal membranes were preincubated for 10 min at 37°C in the
absence ("control") or the presence of 1mM N-ethylmaleimide
("NEM"). The specific binding of ^{3}H-5-HT was then measured with
5nM of ^{3}H-5-HT and either 0.1mM GTP or 1mM $MnCl_2$. Each value is
the mean $\pm$ SEM of 3 experiments. The percent change due to GTP or
Mn^{2+} is indicated in parentheses.

for promoting the specific binding of ^{3}H-5-HT onto hippocampal membranes. However, in the range of concentrations acting on $5-HT_1$ sites, Mn^{2+} markedly reduces
^{3}H-GTP binding whereas Mn^{3+} remains almost inactive.
Accordingly, the effect of Mn^{3+} cannot be ascribed to a
competitive interaction at the GTP site.
- even in the case of Mn^{2+}, its interaction with the
GTP binding site is likely not responsible for its stimulating effect on ^{3}H-5-HT binding: using N-ethylmaleimide pretreated membranes (in which the number but not
the apparent affinity of $5-HT_1$ sites is markedly reduced), we observed that Mn^{2+} was no longer active whereas GTP still evoked a significant (but less pronounced)
decrease of ^{3}H-5-HT binding onto the remaining $5-HT_1$
sites (table 2). These data confirmed that GTP and Mn^{2+}
(and other divalent cations) affect the specific binding of ^{3}H-5-HT by acting on different modulatory sites.
Furthermore, they demonstrated that SH groups play a
crucial role in the Mn^{2+}-induced shift in the $5-HT1$ site
affinity. Those involved in the GTP-induced conversion
of $5-HT_1$ sites into lower affinity sites appear less
sensitive to blockade by N-ethylmaleimide (table 2).

GTP AND Mn^{2+}-INDUCED MODULATIONS OF 5-HT$_1$ SITES AS A PROBE FOR SELECTING NEW AGONISTS AND ANTAGONISTS

Mn^{2+} was chosen in these investigations because its effects on 5-HT$_1$ sites are more pronounced than those of other divalent cations, notably Ca^{2+} (table 1).

Experiments consisted of measuring the efficacy of known agonists and antagonists to displace ^3H-5-HT from its specific 5-HT$_1$ sites in hippocampal membranes in the presence or the absence of Mn^{2+} (optimal concentration: 1mM) or GTP (optimal concentration: 0.1mM). As illustrated in table 3, GTP increases by 2-7 fold the concentration of a given agonist producing half inhibition (IC50) of ^3H-5-HT binding. In contrast, Mn^{2+} decreases IC50 values by 3-10 fold. As a result, the ratio of the IC50 value measured in the presence of GTP to that measured in the presence of Mn^{2+} (IC50$_{GTP}$/IC50$_{Mn}2+$) is $\geq$ 10 with a given agonist.

Although Mn^{2+} slightly reduces the efficacy of most antagonists to displace ^3H-5-HT from its specific sites, the ratio IC50$_{GTP}$/IC50$_{Mn}2+$ remains close to unity with these compounds (table 3). This is notably the case with quipazine, often considered however as a direct 5-HT agonist acting on postsynaptic receptors in the CNS (see 10). Data in table 3, together with reports concerning the quipazine effects both on the superior cervical ganglion and the spinal cord (14) and on the presynaptic control of ^3H-5-HT release from brain cortex slices (24), confirm that this drug is in fact a 5-HT antagonist. The clearcut agonist properties of quipazine *in vivo* likely result from its presynaptic actions, all contributing to increase 5-HT in the synaptic cleft (10). Since the affinity of the 5-HT$_1$ site is about 350 times higher for 5-HT than for quipazine (table 3), stimulation of 5-HT receptors due to higher amounts of 5-HT released from presynaptic terminals probably prevails over any possible blockade by quipazine. The disappearance of the agonist effects of quipazine following the selective degeneration of serotoninergic terminals (by 5,7-dihydroxytryptamine treatment, for instance) further confirms that such effects depend only on the presynaptic actions of the drug (see 9,10).

Another interesting feature presented in table 3 concerns the possible relationships between the GTP (or Mn^{2+})-induced changes in 5-HT$_1$ sites and the hypothetical coupling of these sites with adenylate cyclase. Indeed, the GTP-induced shift in IC50 values occurs with all agonists independently of their efficacy regarding 5-HT-sensitive adenylate cyclase. In particular, it has to be noted that the GTP effect is more pronounced with RU24969 than with 5-HT although the former compound is

TABLE 3. Effects of GTP and Mn^{2+} on the apparent affinity of ^{3}H-5-HT binding sites for various agonists and antagonists

Compound		IC50 (nM)			
		—	GTP	Mn^{2+}	R
Agonists					
8-OH-N,N-DPAT	(+)	74.8	369.2	7.9	46.7
RU 24969	(0)	20.2	130.2	5.4	24.1
Bufotenine	(+)	10.9	75.9	3.2	23.7
5-HT	(+)	6.0	22.3	1.5	14.9
TFMPP	(0)	190.0	406.0	40.0	10.2
5-MDMT	(+)	21.8	71.9	8.1	8.9
Antagonists					
Metergoline	(-)	7.8	12.4	17.4	0.7
Pizotifen	(-)	334.0	366.0	516.0	0.7
Methiothepin	(-)	165.0	243.0	162.0	1.5
Methysergide	(-)	52.0	102.6	61.7	1.7
Other drugs					
Quipazine	(0)	2120	1832	2094	0.9
d-LSD	(+,-)	8.2	59.5	2.2	27.0

IC50 values are the concentrations of drugs reducing by half the specific binding of ^{3}H-5-HT onto rat hippocampal membranes. Binding assays were carried out with 2-3nM of ^{3}H-5-HT in the absence or the presence of 0.1mM GTP or 1mM $MnCl_2$. R is obtained by dividing the IC50 value in the presence of GTP by that determined in the presence of $MnCl_2$. Each value is the mean of at least 3 separate determinations.
The effect of a given drug on the activity of 5-HT-sensitive adenylate cyclase is indicated by : (+):stimulation ; (-) : inhibition ; (0)= no effect.
8-OH-N,N-DPAT = 8-hydroxy-N,N-dipropyl-2-aminotetralin ; RU 24969 = 5-methoxy-3-(1,2,3,6-tetrahydro-4-pyridinyl)1H indole; TFMPP = trifluoromethylphenylpiperazine ; 5-MDMT= 5-methoxy-N,N-dimethyltryptamine.

totally inactive on 5-HT-sensitive adenylate cyclase (6). As already discussed (8,9,15), GTP-induced reduction in the apparent affinity of binding sites for agonists may therefore occur in the absence of any association with adenylate cyclase.

CONCLUSIONS

Like numerous other receptor types, the 5-HT$_1$ site
is modulated in opposite directions by guanine nucleotides and divalent cations. GTP (and its poorly metabo-
lizable analogue GppNHp) decreases,whereas cations like
Ca^{2+}, Mn^{2+}, Ba^{2+} enhance the apparent affinity of
this site for ^{3}H-5-HT and other agonists. In contrast,
divalent cations slightly reduce the apparent affinity
of the 5-HT$_1$ site for antagonists and GTP does not significantly alter the antagonist-5-HT$_1$ site interaction.
Neither the modulation by GTP nor that due to divalent
cations seems to depend on the possible association of
the 5-HT$_1$ site with adenylate cyclase. Apparently, distinct subsites are involved in the respective effects
of GTP and cations. These observations confirm that the
high affinity binding site for ^{3}H-5-HT behaves as numerous receptor types in the CNS (3-5,19,23,25).
One important application of the GTP- and cation-induced modulations of the 5-HT$_1$ site is the development
of a simple binding test for selecting new agonists and
antagonists. This test is based on the observation that
the IC50$_{GTP}$/IC50$_{Mn^{2+}}$ ratio is $\geq$ 10 with agonists whereas it does not differ from unity with antagonists. So
far, it has been successfully used for identifying a
new potent 5-HT agonist: 8-OH-N,N-DPAT (table 3). Subsequent studies revealed that this tetralin derivative
stimulates 5-HT-sensitive adenylate cyclase activity
and inhibits the K$^+$-induced release of ^{3}H-5-HT from
rat cortex slices (unpublished observations). Accordingly, 8-OH-N,N-DPAT exerts agonist properties both on
post- and presynaptic 5-HT receptors.
Not only the 5-HT$_1$ site but also the 5-HT$_2$ site selectively labelled by tritiated antagonists is modulated by guanine nucleotides and di-and trivalent cations.
Thus, GTP significantly reduces the affinity of the
5-HT$_2$ site for agonists without affecting that for antagonists (8,9,12). In contrast, Mn^{2+}and Mn^{3+}increase
the apparent affinity of ^{3}H-spiperone binding sites for
agonists (8,9). However, the modulations of 5-HT$_2$ sites
are generally less pronounced than those of 5-HT$_1$ sites
(8,9); this may explain why some authors (20) deny their
existence.

ACKNOWLEDGEMENTS

This research has been supported by grants from
INSERM, DRET and Rhône-Poulenc S.A.

REFERENCES

1. Bennett, J.P.Jr, and Snyder, S.H. (1976): <u>Mol.Pharmacol.</u>,
   12:373-389.

2. Berridge, M.J., and Heslop, J.P. (1981): Brit.J.Pharmacol., 73:729-738.
3. Chang, R.S.L., and Snyder, S.H. (1980): J.Neurochem., 34: 916-922.
4. Childers, S.R., and Snyder, S.H. (1980): J.Neurochem., 34: 583-593.
5. Creese, I., Prosser, T., and Snyder, S.H. (1978):Life Sci., 23:495-500.
6. Euvrard, C., and Boissier, J.R. (1980): Eur.J.Pharmacol.,63: 65-72.
7. Gould, R.J., Murphy, K.M.M., and Snyder, S.H. (1982): Proc. Natl.Acad.Sci.USA, 79:3656-3660.
8. Hamon, M. (1982):In:Methods in Neurobiology, edited by P.J. Marangos, I. Campbell and R.M. Cohen, Academic Press, New-York (in press).
9. Hamon, M., Bourgoin, S., El Mestikawy, S., and Goetz, C. (1982): In:Handbook of Neurochemistry, edited by A. Lajtha, Plenum Publ. Corp., New York (in press).
10. Hamon, M., Bourgoin, S., Enjalbert, A., Bockaert, J., Héry, F., Ternaux, J.P., and Glowinski, J. (1976): Naunyn-Schmiedeberg's Arch.Pharmacol., 294: 99-108.
11. Hamon, M., Mallat, M., El Mestikawy, S., and Pasquier, A. (1982): J.Neurochem., 38:162-172.
12. Hamon, M., Nelson, D.L., Herbet, A., and Glowinski, J. (1980): In: Receptors for Neurotransmitters and Peptide Hormones, edited by G. Pepeu, M.J. Kuhar, and S.J. Enna, pp.223-233. Raven Press, New York.
13. Laduron, P.M., and Ilien, B. (1982): Biochem.Pharmacol., 31: 2145-2151.
14. Lansdown, M.J.R., Nash, H.L., Preston, P.R., Wallis, D.I., and Williams, R.G. (1980): Brit.J.Pharmacol., 68:525-532.
15. Mallat, M., and Hamon, M. (1982): J.Neurochem, 38: 151-161.
16. Nelson, D.L., Herbet, A., Adrien, J., Bockaert, J., and Hamon, M. (1980): Biochem.Pharmacol., 29:2455-2463.
17. Nelson, D.L., Herbet, A., Bourgoin, S., Glowinski J., and Hamon, M. (1978): Mol.Pharmacol., 14:983-995.
18. Nelson, D.L., Herbet, A., Enjalbert, A., Bockaert, J., and Hamon, M. (1980): Biochem.Pharmacol., 29:2445-2453.
19. Pasternak, G.W., Snowman, A.M., and Snyder, S.H. (1975) : Mol.Pharmacol., 11: 735-744.
20. Peroutka, S.J., Lebovitz, R.M.,and Snyder,S.H.(1979): Mol.Pharmacol., 16:700-708.
21. Peroutka, S.J., Lebovitz, R.M., and Snyder, S.H. (1981): Science, 212:827-829.
22. Rodbell, M. (1980):Nature (Lond.), 284: 17-22.
23. Rouot, B.M., U'Prichard, D.C., and Snyder, S.H. (1980): J.Neurochem., 34: 374-384.
24. Schlicker, E., and Göthert, M. (1981):Naunyn-Schmiedeberg's Arch.Pharmacol., 317:204-208.
25. Wei, J.W. and Sulakhe, P.V. (1980): Eur.J.Pharmacol., 62: 345-347.

CNS Receptors—From Molecular
Pharmacology to Behavior, edited by
P. Mandel and F. V. DeFeudis.
Raven Press, New York © 1983.

Modulation of an Adenylate Cyclase-Linked Serotonin (5-HT$_1$) Receptor System in a Neuroblastoma x Brain Explant Hybrid Cell Line (NCB-20) by Opiates, Prostaglandins, and α$_2$-Adrenergic Agonists

Elizabeth Berry-Kravis and Glyn Dawson

Departments of Biochemistry and Pediatrics, Joseph P. Kennedy, Jr. Mental Retardation Research Center, University of Chicago; and Wyler Children's Hospital, Chicago, Illinois 60637

[^{3}H]Serotonin ([^{3}H]5-hydroxytryptamine, [^{3}H]5HT) (3,9,10), and [^{3}H]-lysergic acid diethylamide (LSD) (1,2) have been shown to bind with nanomolar affinity to a site in the central nervous system which has been classified as 5HT$_1$ (19). Serotonin agonists (5-methoxytryptamine, bufotenine, and other tryptamine derivatives) are more potent displacers of [^{3}H]5HT binding to 5HT$_1$ sites than are serotonin antagonists (cyprohepta-dine, mianserin, spiperone, and other neuroleptics).

Binding of agonists to 5HT$_1$ sites is regulated by guanine nucleotides (18) and a high degree of correlation is observed between drug inhibition of serotonin-sensitive adenylate cyclase systems previously described in brain (8) and inhibition of [^{3}H] serotonin binding to 5HT$_1$ receptors (20) suggesting linkage of 5HT$_1$ receptors to adenylate cyclase. Synaptic inhibition is believed to be mediated through such 5HT$_1$ receptors, whereas excitation is probably mediated through non-adenylate cyclase-linked 5HT$_2$ receptors (20).

A preliminary report on a mouse neuroblastoma x Chinese hamster brain hybrid cell line, NCB-20, has suggested the presence of a serotonin-sensitive adenylate cyclase as well as serotonin binding sites (16). Studies in this laboratory (4) confirm the existence of these binding sites and suggest that the higher affinity site has the characteristics of a 5HT$_1$ receptor. The existence of other neurotransmitter binding sites and adenylate cyclase-linked systems in the clonal hybrid cell line suggested that it could be used to study CNS neurotransmitter interactions at the molecular level.

EXPERIMENTAL PROCEDURES

Cell Culture Conditions

Mouse neuroblastoma cell line N4TG1 was obtained from Dr. A. Gilman (University of Virginia, Charlottesville, Virginia), mouse neuroblastoma x rat glioma hybrid cell line NG108-15 was from Dr. W.A. Klee (National Institutes of Health, Bethesda, Maryland); and mouse neuroblastoma x 18-day Chinese hamster embryo brain explant hybrid cell line NCB-20 was from Dr. J. Minna (Veterans Administration Hospital, Washington, DC). Cells were cultured on 100 mm Falcon plastic dishes (for binding assays) and in Costar 35 mm plastic tissue culture wells (for cyclic AMP determinations), in modified Eagle's medium supplemented with 10% Newborn (Bobby) calf serum as described previously (17).

Crude Cell Membrane Preparations

Cells were harvested mechanically and crude membrane fractions obtained as described previously (4). Pellets were stored at -80°C, until use in binding assays, with no loss of activity over periods as long as six months.

Ligand Binding Assays

Crude membrane pellets were resuspended in 50 mM Tris HCl buffer, pH 7.4, containing 0.1 mM ascorbate and 10μ M pargyline hydrochloride, to give a protein content ranging from 1 to 3 mg/ml as determined by the method of Lowry et al. (15). Aliquots (200 μl) of this membrane preparation were then added to triplicate test tubes containing 20 μl of 5-[³H]hydroxytryptamine and 20 μl of test drugs or buffer. After incubation for 15 minutes at 37°C, 1.0 ml aliquots of ice-cold 50 mM Tris-HCl, pH 7.4, were added to each test tube and the contents were rapidly filtered under vacuum through Whatman GF/C glass microfibre filters, washed, and the bound radioactivity was determined by liquid scintillation counting as described previously (4). Non-specific binding was measured in the presence of a large excess (1 mM) of unlabelled 5-hydroxytryptamine and subtracted from total bound radioactivity to give specific binding.

Measurement of Cyclic AMP Levels

5-Hydroxytryptamine and other neurotransmitters/drugs were used in solutions prepared fresh and added to monolayer cultures growing in Costar 35 mm tissue culture wells. 3-Isobutyl-1-methylxanthine (IBMX) was added to all plates at the same time as 5HT to prevent breakdown of cyclic AMP by phosphodiesterase. After 30-minute incubations, culture medium was removed and 0.2 ml of 6% trichloroacetic acid was added to each well (4). Cyclic AMP levels were determined by radioimmunoassay via competition with an [¹²⁵I] cyclic AMP derivative for binding to anti-cyclic AMP anti-

sera in 50 mM acetate buffer, pH 4.75, according to the method
of Harper (11).

RESULTS AND DISCUSSION

Binding of [^{3}H]5-Hydroxytryptamine to Neurotumor Cell Lines

NCB-20 cells were found to bind [^{3}H]5HT rapidly, with saturation occurring by 10 minutes at 37° (4). Binding isotherms
were subjected to Scatchard analysis and a non-linear Scatchard
plot was obtained, with high and low affinity components of K_D =
180 nM and 3000 nM, respectively (FIG. 1). There were about
ten times as many apparent low affinity binding sites (B_{max} =
9.8 pmol/ mg protein) as there were apparent high affinity binding sites (B_{max} = 1000 fmol/mg protein). Binding isotherms could
be saturated by binding [^{3}H]5HT to NCB-20 cell membranes in the
presence of 1 μM spiperone (FIG. 1). Scatchard analysis of these
binding curves gave a linear Scatchard plot with K_D = 200 nM
and B_{max} = 1200 fmol/mg protein corresponding to the high affinity
binding site observed on the non-linear Scatchard plot. This
suggested that the low affinity [^{3}H]5HT binding site was possibly
a high affinity neuroleptic binding site. [^{3}H]spiperone was
found to bind with high affinity to NCB-20 cell membranes, K_D =
10-30 nM (Berry-Kravis, manuscript in preparation).
   In contrast, N4TG1 cells did not bind [^{3}H]5HT except at extremely high [^{3}H]5HT concentrations and this was most likely
attributable to filter binding (FIG. 1). In all subsequent
studies, the concentration of [^{3}H]5HT was kept below 1 μM to
eliminate the possibility of the filter binding artifact. NG108-
15 cells were found to bind [^{3}H]5HT with very low affinity such
that binding could not be measured without filter binding interference. This binding was found to be saturable, by a centrifugation method for separation of bound and unbound ligand, with
a K_D of approximately 4 μM (Berry-Kravis, unpublished results).
This is consistent with the data of MacDermot et al. (16) which
gave evidence for a serotonin receptor on NG108-15, presumably
of low affinity, that mediated cell depolarization and acetylcholine release.

Inhibition of [^{3}H]5HT Binding

[^{3}H]5HT binding to NCB-20 cell membranes took place at sufficiently low concentrations to label only the higher affinity
binding site, as indicated by Hill plots of the competition of
5HT against [^{3}H]5HT binding with an average slope of 1.14
(Berry-Kravis, unpublished results). A K_i value of 280 nM was
obtained for 5HT competition in good agreement with K_D value
of 180 nM obtained from Scatchard analyses of [^{3}H]5HT binding.
A drug potency series was constructed from studies on the inhibition of high affinity [^{3}H]5HT binding (Table 1). Serotonin
agonists, tryptamine derivatives (5,6-dihydroxytryptamine,
5-methoxytryptamine and 5HT), as well as the LSD derivative methy-

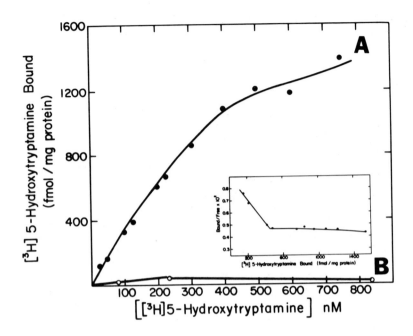

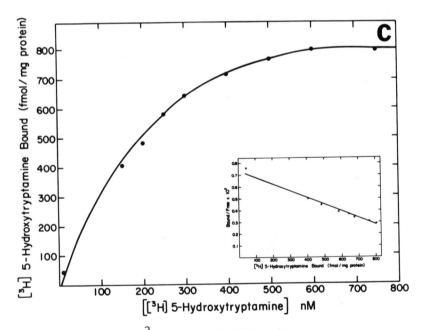

FIG. 1A. Binding of [³H]5HT to NCB-20 cells
     B. Binding of [³H]5HT to N4TG1 cells
     C. Binding of [³H]5HT to NCB-20 cells in presence of
         1 µM spiperone.

sergide, were ten times more potent as inhibitors than traditional 5HT antagonists such as cyproheptadine, mianserin, clozapine, and spiperone. These results are comparable to those previously reported for brain (19) (Table 1). All classical serotonin antagonists were significantly more potent than the pure $5HT_2$ antagonist ketanserin (13). Dopamine agonists and antagonists, norepinephrine, opiates and opioid peptides, all had very little potency in displacing the high-affinity [^{3}H]5HT binding, despite the presence of high affinity binding sites for all these ligands on NCB-20 cells.

TABLE 1. Comparison of Pharmacological Properties of $5HT_1$ Receptor in NCB-20 Cells and Rat Frontal Cortex

Competitor	NCB-20 Apparent K_i (nM)	Brain Apparent K_i (nM)
5HT Agonists		
5,6-Dihydroxy-tryptamine	54 + 8	300 + 4
5-Hydroxytryptamine	280 + 37	4 + 1
Methysergide	430 + 52	88 + 10
5-methoxytryptamine	620 + 69	11 + 3
5HT Antagonists		
Cyproheptadine	2210 + 140	1500 + 150
Clozapine	5040 + 210	1000 + 150
Mianserin	6900 + 100	860 + 110
Spiperone	34500 + 20000	730 + 70
Ketanserin	not detectable	—
Other Neuroactive agents		
Dopamine	86000 + 12000	20000 + 2700
Norepinephrine	104000 + 35000	
Chlorpromazine	260000 + 120000	

	IC_{50} (nM) (100 μM)		K_i (nM)	
	−Gpp (NH) p	+Gpp (NH) p	−GTP	+GTP (1mM)
5HT	410 + 60	*1040 + 120	2.1 + 0.1	*4.5 + 0.2
Cyproheptadine	3250 + 200	3550 + 350	—	—
Clozapine	7400 + 310	6950 + 350	1100 + 200	1200 + 200
Spiperone	—	—	650 + 100	690 + 200

*p<0.01

Regulation of [^{3}H]5HT Binding by Guanine Nucleotides, Cations and Ascorbate

Guanine nucleotides were found to decrease agonist, but not antagonist binding, in the same manner as reported for 5HT receptors in rat brain homogenates (18) (Table 1). Sodium ions were found to increase binding as much as 20 percent over a wide range of concentrations (100 µM to 100 mM). Potassium ions, however, did not significantly change binding levels. The divalent cations tested had varying effects. Calcium appeared to increase and magnesium to decrease binding to a small extent, while manganese increased binding by almost 40 percent (4).

GTP reversed sodium, calcium and manganese stimulated increases in binding, while Gpp(NH)p reversed sodium and calcium effects, but when combined with manganese resulted in dramatic binding increases of about 160 percent over controls and 100 percent over samples incubated with manganese. [^{3}H]5HT binding was found to be ascorbate-dependent (4), with ascorbate concentrations of 1 mM or higher giving large reductions in binding. This inhibition of binding was much more dramatic for NCB-20 than the inhibition of binding to brain preparations by ascorbate.

5HT-Stimulated Increases in Intracellular Cyclic AMP

5HT, in the presence of IBMX, produces a 4 to 5-fold stimulation of intracellular cyclic AMP levels in NCB-20 cells (FIG 2). EC_{50} values from 250 to 600 nM for 5HT have been found with an average of 360 ± 150. This is consistent with K_a values of 400–800 nM reported by MacDermot et al. (16) for 5HT activation of adenylate cyclase in NCB-20.

MacDermot et al. (16) observed that the 5HT stimulation of adenylate cyclase in NCB-20 membranes was potentiated by guanine nucleotides, which contrasts with our observation that guanine nucleotides inhibited 5HT binding at the $5HT_1$ site (as previously reported for brain (18)). This difference could be explained by the existence of a guanine nucleotide binding site on the receptor itself as well as on the GTP binding protein (as previously proposed for the glucagon receptor (21)) or a common GTP binding protein regulating both receptor and adenylate cyclase activity (as in the case of the β-adrenergic receptor (14)). Sodium ions may exert their stimulatory effect on 5HT binding by interacting with a specific site on the receptor and in doing so negate the effects of GTP and Gpp(NH)p. In contrast, manganese ions (but not other divalent cations such as calcium and magnesium) block the GTP effect but stimulate binding in the presence of Gpp(NH)p. This is consistent with a specific role for Mn^{2+} in stimulating GTP hydrolysis (6). Inhibitory neurotransmitters or neuromodulators such as enkephalin are believed to inhibit adenylate cyclase by first activating GTP hydrolysis (12), whereas 5HT binding to a $5HT_1$ site might be expected to inhibit GTP hydrolysis.

Reversal of 5HT-Stimulated Cyclic AMP Synthesis by Enkephalin

The expression of both δ (enkephalin) and σ (phencyclidine, ethylketocyclazocine) receptors on NCB-20 cells (17) suggested a system for observing mutual antagonism between enkephalin action (which inhibits adenylate cyclase activity) and serotonin stimulation of adenylate cyclase. Short-term treatment with [$_D$Ala^2$_D$Leu^5] enkephalin results in slight lowering of basal cyclic AMP levels and a lowering of 5HT-stimulated cyclic AMP levels by 50% (FIG. 2A), but after 6 hr of continuous exposure to enkephalin, the 5HT-

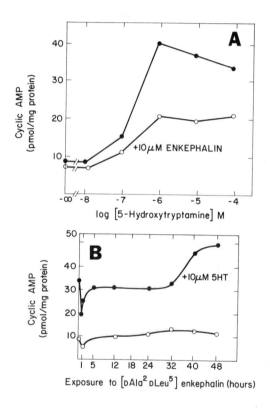

FIG. 2A. Effect of 5HT on the level of intracellular cyclic
AMP, following 30 min culture in the presence (O) or
absence (●) of 10 μM[$_D$Ala^2$_D$Leu^5]enkephalin.
B. Effect of 30 min 10 μM 5HT exposure (●) on the level
of intracellular cyclic AMP, following continuous
exposure to 10 μM [$_D$Ala^2$_D$Leu^5]enkephalin for up to
48 hr; (O), no 5HT added (enkephalin effect on basal
levels).

stimulated cyclic AMP level was restored to normal. Prolonged

[$_D$Ala^2$_D$Leu^5] enkephalin treatment (32–48 hr) resulted in a supersensitivity to 5HT (FIG. 2B). This is reminiscent of the observed
supersensitivity of guinea pig ileum to 5HT (presumably mediated
via 5HT$_2$ receptors) following chronic <u>in</u> <u>vivo</u> morphine treatment
(25).
    The long-term effect of [$_D$Ala^2$_D$Leu^5] enkephalin was seen more
graphically when 5HT dose response curves were constructed after
different periods of opioid exposure. It can be seen from
FIG. 3A that increasing exposure time to [$_D$Ala^2$_D$Leu^5] enkephalin

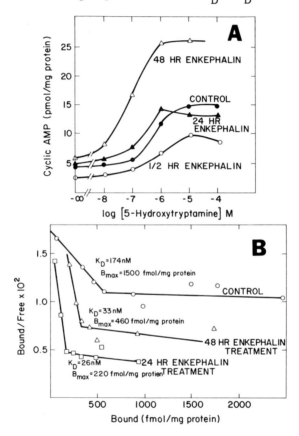

FIG. 3A.   Cyclic AMP level in NCB-20 cells following treat-
           ment with 5HT for 30 min following continuous ex-
           posure to [$_D$Ala^2$_D$Leu^5]enkephalin.
      B.   Scatchard analysis of [^{3}H]5HT binding to NCB-20
           membranes following exposure to [$_D$Ala^2$_D$Leu^5]enkephalin.

resulted in decreasing EC$_{50}$ values for 5HT stimulation of cyclic
AMP synthesis and that after 48-hr treatment, the three-fold
maximal stimulation of cyclic AMP synthesis observed in controls
was increased to a five-fold stimulation.

Several factors could be involved in this supersensitivity phenomenon, but one clear-cut observation has been that prolonged opiate treatment increases the affinity of the 5HT₁ receptor for [³H]5HT from a K_D of 175 nM at 0 hr, to 25 nM at 24 hr and 30 nM at 48 hr (FIG. 3B). Surprisingly, the treatment reduced the actual number of binding sites seven-fold over the first 24 hr but then caused a doubling of the high affinity sites over the next 48 hr. Other important components of the coupling to adenylate cyclase have not yet been investigated.

Effect of Prolonged Opiate Treatment on the Cyclic AMP Response to Other Drugs and Neurotransmitters

It has been repeatedly observed since 1974 (23) that opiates reverse the PGE₁ stimulation of adenylate cyclase in NG108-15 hybrid neurotumor cells. We have confirmed this in NCB-20 cells (FIG. 4) and show the reversal of this effect over a 24-48 hr period, with no apparent evidence of supersensitivity to PGE₁.

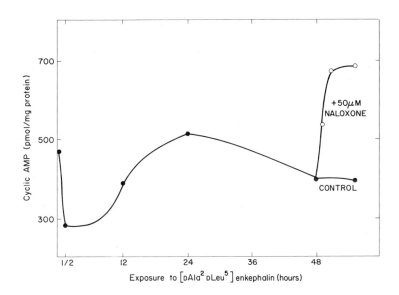

FIG. 4.   Cyclic AMP level in NCB-20 cells treated with 10 μM PGE₁ for 30 min: after continuous exposure to [ᴅAla²ᴅLeu⁵]enkephalin for 55 hr (●), and after 50 μM naloxone treatment in the 48th hr of [ᴅAla²ᴅLeu⁵]enkephalin exposure (O).

One explanation of this difference in the effect of long-term enkephalin treatment on PGE$_1$ and 5HT-mediated increases in cyclic AMP level is that the two drugs stimulate adenylate cyclase through different mechanisms in these cells. Evidence for this comes from an observation that the stimulation by PGE$_1$ and 5HT was synergistic. Thus, even though PGE$_1$ alone increased the cyclic AMP level of the cell over 100-fold, 10^{-5}M 5HT further increased the stimulation to 150-fold (FIG. 5).

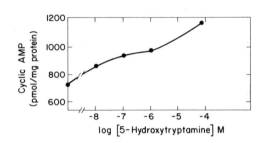

FIG. 5.   Effect of 5HT on the level of intracellular cyclic AMP following 30 min culture in the presence of 10μ M PGE$_1$.

The supersensitivity to 5HT after 48 hr of opiate treatment may be compared to the burst of cyclic AMP synthesis seen when the antagonist naloxone is added to opiate "tolerant" NCB-20 cells which have undergone 48 hr exposure to opiates (FIG. 4). This has been shown previously in NG108-15 cells by Sharma et al. (24) and has been claimed to be biochemical equivalent of the onset of withdrawal symptoms in opiate-addicted individuals given naloxone. It may reflect some alteration in membrane structure similar to that which results in the supersensitivity to 5HT.

Some type of alteration in membrane structure may also occur after long-term exposure to other ligands which inhibit adenylate cyclase through different receptors. Clonidine which has been shown to inhibit adenylate cyclase through an α_2-adrenergic receptor present on NG108-15 cells (22) also reduces both basal and 5HT-stimulated cyclic AMP levels in NCB-20 cells. Long-term exposure to clonidine does not appear to result in a tolerance phenomenon as with opiates. Basal levels do not return to normal over an incubation period of as long as 60 hr (FIG. 6). 5HT-stimulated levels do return to normal following 24-48 hr clonidine exposure although supersensitivity does not occur in a 60-hr time period.

In conclusion, the NCB-20 clonal cell line, formed by fusing a mouse neuroblastoma cell line N18TG2 with an explant of Chinese hamster embryonic brain neurons, expresses a number of adenylate cyclase-linked CNS neurotransmitter receptor systems not found in the parental neuroblastoma cell line. The study of antagonism and synergism between these different systems should permit greater understanding of CNS receptor mechanisms.

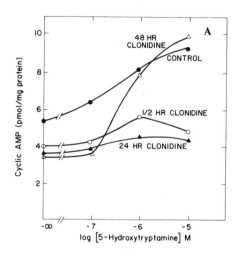 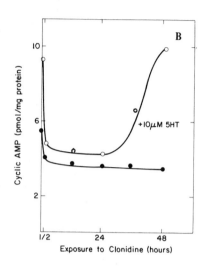

FIG. 6A. Cyclic AMP level in NCB-20 cells following treatment
with 5HT for 30 min following continuous exposure to
1 µM clonidine for 0 hr (●), 1/2 hr (O), 24 hr (▲),
and 48 hr (△).

   B. Effect of 30 min 10 µM 5HT exposure (O) on the level
of intracellular cyclic AMP following continuous exposure to 1 µM clonidine for up to 48 hr; (●), no 5HT
added (effect of clonidine on basal levels).

ACKNOWLEDGEMENTS

   We would like to thank Daniel Cermak for excellent technical
assistance in tissue culture and Dr. R.W. McLawhon for helpful
discussions. Supported by USPHS grants HD-06426, HD-09402,
HD-04583, and DA-02575. E. Berry Kravis is a recipient of
Medical Scientist Training Grant GM-07281 and G. Dawson is a
Joseph P. Kennedy, Jr. Scholar.

REFERENCES

1. Bennett, J.L. and Aghajanian, G.K. (1974): Life Sci. 15,
    1935-1944.
2. Bennett, J.P., Jr. and Snyder, S.H. (1975): Brain Res. 94,
    523-544.
3. Bennett, J.P., Jr. and Snyder, S.H. (1976): Mol. Pharmacol.
    12, 373-389.
4. Berry-Kravis, E. and Dawson, G. (1982): J. Neurochem.,
    in press.
5. Cheng, Y. and Prusoff, W. (1973): Biochem. Pharmacol. 22,
    3099-3108.

6.   Childers, S. and Snyder, S. (1980): <u>J. Neurochem.</u> 34, 583-593.
7.   Dawson, G., Matalon, R., and Dorfman, A. (1972): <u>J. Biol.</u>
     <u>Chem.</u> 247, 5944-5951.
8.   Enjalbert, A., Bourgoin, S., Hamon, M., Adrien, J., and
     Bockert, J. (1978): <u>Mol. Pharmacol.</u> 14, 2-10.
9.   Fillion, G., Fillion, M.-P., Spirakis, C., Bahers, J.-M., and
     Jacob, J. (1976): <u>Life Sci.</u> 18, 65-70.
10. Fillion, G.B., Rousselle, J.-C., Fillion, M.-P., Beaudoin, D.M.,
     Goiny, M.R., Deniau, J.M., and Jacob, J.J. (1978):
     <u>Mol. Pharmacol.</u> 14, 50-59.
11. Harper, J. and Brooker, G. (1975): <u>Cyclic Nucl. Res.</u> 1, 207-
     218.
12. Koski, G. and Klee, W. (1981: <u>Proc. Natl. Acad. U.S.A.</u> 78,
     4185-4189.
13. Leyson, J.E., Niemegers, C.J.E., Van Nueten, T.M.,
     Laduron, P.M. (1982): <u>Mol. Pharmacol.</u> 21, 301-314.
14. Limbird, L., Gill, D.M., and Lefkowitz, R. (1980): <u>Proc.</u>
     <u>Natl. Acad. Sci. U.S.A.</u> 77, 775-779.
15. Lowry, O.H., Rosebrough, N.J., Farr, A.L., and Randall, R.J.
     (1951): <u>J. Biol. Chem.</u> 193, 265-275.
16. MacDermot, J., Higashida, H., Wilson, S., Matsuzawa, H.,
     Minna, J., and Nirenberg, M. (1979): <u>Proc. Natl. Acad.</u>
     <u>Sci. U.S.A.</u> 76, 1135-1139.
17. McLawhon, R., West, R., Miller, R., and Dawson, G. (1981):
     <u>Proc. Natl. Acad. Sci. U.S.A.</u> 78, 4309-4313.
18. Peroutka, S.J., Lebovitz, R.M., and Snyder, S.H. (1979):
     <u>Mol. Pharmacol.</u> 16, 700-708.
19. Peroutka, S.J. and Snyder, S.H. (1979): <u>Mol. Pharmacol.</u>
     16, 687-699.
20. Peroutka, S.J., Lebovitz, R.M., and Snyder, S.H. (1981):
     <u>Science</u> 212, 827-829.
21. Pramod, L., Welton, A., and Rodbell, M. (1977): <u>J. Biol.</u>
     <u>Chem.</u> 252, 5942-5946.
22. Sabol, S. and Nirenberg, M. (1979): <u>J. Biol. Chem.</u> 254,
     1913-1920.
23. Sharma, S., Nirenberg, M., Klee, W. (1975): <u>Proc. Natl.</u>
     <u>Acad. Sci. U.S.A.</u> 72, 590-594.
24. Sharma, S., Klee, W.A., and Nirenberg, M. (1975): <u>Proc.</u>
     <u>Natl. Acad. Sci. U.S.A.</u> 72, 3092-3096.
25. Shultz, R. and Goldstein, A. (1973): <u>Nature</u> 244, 168-169.

CNS Receptors—From Molecular
Pharmacology to Behavior, edited by
P. Mandel and F. V. DeFeudis.
Raven Press, New York © 1983.

Role and Localization of Serotonin$_2$ (S$_2$)-Receptor-Binding Sites: Effects of Neuronal Lesions

*J. E. Leysen, *P. Van Gompel, *M. Verwimp,
and †C. J. E. Niemegeers

Department of *Biochemical Pharmacology and †Pharmacology, Janssen Pharmaceutica,
B-2340 Beerse, Belgium

In 1977, the neuroleptic ^{3}H-spiperone was found to label specific binding sites in frontal cortical tissue. These sites showed the features of serotonergic receptor sites: 1) serotonin appeared to be the only neurotransmitter which revealed binding affinity at micromolar order, which is likely to be the physiological concentration of serotonin in synaptic clefts, 2) potent serotonin antagonists showed binding affinities of nanomolar order, and 3) a highly significant correlation was found between the binding affinities of drugs and their potencies to antagonize serotonin-mediated behavioural excitation (11,12). The sites were later designated as 5 hydroxytryptamine$_2$ (5 HT$_2$) or serotonin$_2$ (S$_2$)-receptor sites because they were found to be distinct from sites labelled by ^{3}H-5 HT, which were called 5 HT$_1$ or S$_1$-receptor sites (14). The investigation of the S$_2$-receptor binding sites was hampered by the lack of specific ligands to label the sites: ^{3}H-spiperone labels with high affinity both S$_2$- and dopamine receptor sites (12,8), ^{3}H-LSD (14) and ^{3}H-metergoline (3) label S$_1$-, S$_2$- and dopamine receptor sites, and ^{3}H-mianserin (15) labels S$_2$- and histamine$_1$ receptor sites. Recently, a new class of serotonin antagonists was introduced, with ketanserin as the prototype (7,16). ^{3}H-Ketanserin approved to be a particularly suitable and selective ligand to study the S$_2$-receptor binding in vitro (13) and in vivo (5). Using ^{3}H-ketanserin as the ligand, the role of the S$_2$-receptor binding sites in serotonin-mediated behavioural excitation was further substantiated and clear evidence was provided that S$_2$-receptor sites also mediate serotonin-induced vasoconstriction (6,13).

In this paper, the specificity of ^{3}H-ketanserin to label S$_2$-receptor sites in various brain areas is illustrated and the regional distribution of the sites in the central nervous system of four animal species is investigated. The cellular localization of the S_2-receptor sites in rat forebrain areas is explored by examining the effects of various types of neuronal lesions.

MATERIALS AND METHODS

Drug binding and regional distribution studies were carried out using female Wistar rats (150 g), female Pirbright guinea pigs (300 g), male New Zealand rabbits (3 kg) and mongrel dogs. Tissue dissection and preparation was as previously described (13).

Neuronal lesions were performed on male Wistar rats (150 g) by stereotaxic injection of neurotoxins. Animals were anaesthetized with 2.5 mg/kg i.p. alfentanil or with 30 mg/kg i.p. etomidate. A David Köpf stereotaxic apparatus was used and coordinates were according to König and Klippel (4); they are indicated in the legends to the tables and refer to the stereotaxic zero point.

In vitro binding assays using ^{3}H-ketanserin were carried out as previously described (13) using per assay 2 ml of a washed membrane preparation from the mitochondrial plus microsomal fraction (M+L+P), suspended in Tris HCl buffer 50 mM, pH 7.7 (5 mg original wet weight of tissue per ml, protein content 56.5 + 3.3 mg/g tissue, mean + S.D., n = 15). Specific ^{3}H-ketanserin binding was given by the difference between the total binding and the binding in the presence of 1000-fold excess methysergide over the ^{3}H-ketanserin concentration. The rapid filtration procedure using a 40-well multividor (Janssen Scientific Instruments, Beerse, Belgium) and GF/B glass fibre filters was applied.

Binding assays using ^{3}H-haloperidol, ^{3}H-WB4101 or ^{3}H-pyrilamine were as previously described (7). Uptake of neurotransmitters was estimated using ^{3}H-neurotransmitters at a concentration of 10 nM and a freshly prepared mitochondrial fraction of brain tissue suspended in Krebs Henseleit solution (5 mg original wet weight of tissue per ml, protein content 58.5 + 2.2 mg/g tissue, n = 15). Incubations were run for 5 min at 25° C and stopped by the rapid filtration procedure in the same way as in binding studies. To define specific uptake the following blanks were measured and subtracted from total uptake of radioactivity: uptake in the presence of 10^{-6} M chlorimipramine for ^{3}H-5 HT uptake, in the presence of 10^{-6} M desimipramine for ^{3}H-norepinephrine (NE) uptake, in the presence of 10^{-5} M cocaine for ^{3}H-dopamine (DA) uptake and uptake at 0° C for ^{3}H-glutamic acid (GLU) uptake.

Enzymatic activities, protein and catecholamines were measured as previously described (9). Drugs were kindly supplied by the companies of origin. Radioactive materials were: ^{3}H-ketanserin (spec. act. 22.3 Ci/mmole), ^{3}H-WB4101 (spec. act. 27 Ci/mmole), ^{3}H-pyrilamine (spec. act. 27.3 Ci/mmole), ^{3}H-5 hydroxytryptamine (spec. act. 11.1 Ci/mmole), ^{3}H-norepinephrine (spec. act. 41.8 Ci/mmole), ^{3}H-dopamine (34.4 Ci/mmole) from New England Nuclear, Boston, USA; ^{3}H-haloperidol (spec. act. 22 Ci/mmole) from IRE, Fleurus, Belgium; ^{3}H-glutamic acid (spec. act.

27 Ci/mmole) from the Radiochemical Centre Amersham, U.K. The radiochemical purity of the compounds was regularly checked on thin layer chromatography and high pressure liquid chromatography and was required to be >98 % for experimental use.

RESULTS

The equilibrium binding constants (K_i-values) for various neurotransmitter antagonists and agonists for binding to S_2-, dopamine (D_2)-, α_1-adrenergic (α_1A)- and histamine$_1$ (H_1)-receptor sites are presented in Table 1. Serotonin antagonists, belonging to different chemical classes show nanomolar binding affinities for the S_2-receptor binding sites labelled with ^{3}H-ketanserin in both the pre-frontal cortex and the striatum. Amongst dopamine antagonists, spiperone binds in addition to D_2-receptor sites also with nanomolar affinity to S_2-receptor binding sites. However, more selective dopamine antagonists such as haloperidol and domperidone have only a very moderate binding affinity for the S_2-receptor sites, but they bind potently to D_2-receptor sites. The potent α_1-adrenergic antagonist, prazosin, and H_1-receptor blocker, pyrilamine, do not bind to the S_2-receptor binding sites up to micromolar concentrations, but they bind to α_1A- and H_1-receptor sites respectively with

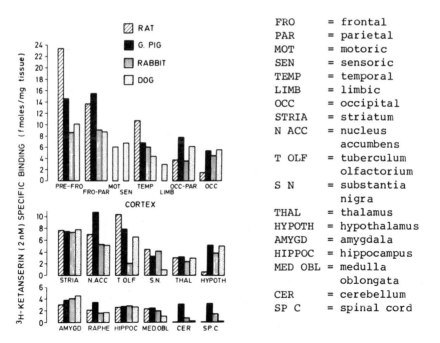

FRO	= frontal
PAR	= parietal
MOT	= motoric
SEN	= sensoric
TEMP	= temporal
LIMB	= limbic
OCC	= occipital
STRIA	= striatum
N ACC	= nucleus accumbens
T OLF	= tuberculum olfactorium
S N	= substantia nigra
THAL	= thalamus
HYPOTH	= hypothalamus
AMYGD	= amygdala
HIPPOC	= hippocampus
MED OBL	= medulla oblongata
CER	= cerebellum
SP C	= spinal cord

FIG. 1. Regional distribution of S_2-receptor binding sites in the central nervous system of 4 mammalian species.

TABLE 1. K_i-values (nM) for receptor binding sites

	S2- ³H-Ketanserin		D2- ³H-Haloperidol	α1A- ³H-WB4101	H1- ³H-Pyrilamine
	Pre-frontal cortex	Striatum	Striatum	Forebrain	Cerebellum
Serotonin antagonists					
Ketanserin	0.53	0.27	220	10	10
Cyproheptadine	0.50	0.62	31	100	2.7
Pipamperone	0.87	2.8	120	54	> 1 000
Methysergide	1.1	2.2	200	2 300	> 1 000
Dopamine antagonists					
Spiperone	0.60	0.39	0.16	10	> 1 000
Haloperidol	25	18	1.2	8.0	> 1 000
Domperidone	88	70	0.9	90	> 1 000
α1A antagonist					
Prazosin	> 1 000	> 1 000	> 1 000	0.09	> 1 000
H1 antagonist					
Pyrilamine	> 1 000	> 1 000	> 1 000	2 300	2
Serotonin agonists					
Bufotenin	120	500	9 900	–	–
Serotonin	300	2 500	11 200	–	–
5 Methoxytryptamine	740	2 000	–	–	–
Dopamine	94 000	31 000	140	16 400	–
Norepinephrine	> 100 000	> 100 000	1 600	821	–
Histamine	> 100 000	> 100 000	> 100 000	> 100 000	–

nanomolar affinity. Serotonin and its agonists reveal micromolar binding affinities for the S_2-receptor binding sites, and they are much less active at the D_2-receptor sites. Conversely dopamine, norepinephrine and histamine are virtually inactive at the S_2-receptor binding sites, and they bind with micromolar affinities to the D_2-, α_1A- and H_1-receptor sites, respectively.

The distribution of S_2-receptor binding sites, specifically labelled with ^{3}H-ketanserin, was found to be very similar in brains of rats, guinea pigs, rabbits and dogs, such as shown in Figure 1. The S_2-receptor binding sites are particularly enriched in frontal cortical areas. Substantial amounts are also detected in the mesolimbic areas, nucleus accumbens and tuberculum olfactorium, and in the dopaminergic brain area, the striatum. Other brain areas contain only a very minor amount of the sites. Although the overall density of S_2-receptor binding sites in the rat spinal cord is low, a distinct distribution could be detected: cervical part, ventral: 2.13 ± 0.09, dorsal: 1.10 ± 0.09; thoracal part, ventral: 1.71 ± 0.08, dorsal: 1.27 ± 0.07; lumbar part, ventral: 1.67 ± 0.11, dorsal: 1.08 ± 0.10, (values in fmoles/mg tissue, n = 6).

The effects of kainic acid lesions in the rat pre-frontal cortex are summarized in Table 2. Pre-frontal cortical injection of 0.5 µg kainic acid did not consistently affect the S_2-receptor binding in this area. However, administration of 3 µg and 4 µg kainic acid caused a decrease by 45 to 77 % of pre-frontal cortical S_2-receptor binding sites. Also [3]H-5 HT and ^{3}H-GLU uptake in the pre-frontal cortex were decreased but to somewhat lesser extent than the binding. GLU decarboxylase was decreased by 40 to 50 %. It was noted that kainic acid lesions in the pre-frontal cortex did not alter the activity of choline acetyltransferase in this brain area and did not affect measured receptor binding, neurotransmitter uptake or enzymatic activities in the striatum. Morphological examinations showed that after injection of the low dosage of kainic acid (0.5 µg), in the pre-frontal cortex, there was no regular loss of neurones in this area, whereas at 1, 2 and 3 weeks after injection of the high dosages (3 and 4 µg) neurones had completely disappeared in a large area around the injection site; in the immediate vicinity of the injection site revascularization and infiltration of phagocytes was apparent, and this was surrounded by an area with excessive gliosis. The influence of frontal cortical kainic acid lesions on mescaline-induced head twitches (13) was studied in bilaterally-lesioned animals. The number of head twitches, counted over a 15-min period, after i.v. injection of 20 mg/kg mescaline, was increased by 80 % in kainic acid-lesioned rats (n = 15) and by 60 % in sham-lesioned rats (n = 15) as compared to naive controls (n = 15, mean number of head twitches in controls 24 ± 12 per 15 min). Injection of the high dosages of kainic acid in the pre-frontal cortex was well tolerated by the animals (90 % survival after unilateral injection of 4 µg; 60 % survival after bilateral injection of 4 µg).

TABLE 2. Kainic acid (KA) lesions in the pre-frontal cortex

Lesion conditions	Assays in the pre-frontal cortex: control (C): fmoles/mg tissue, lesioned (L): % change				
	3H-Ketanserin specific binding at 1 nM	3H-Ketanserin specific binding at 2 nM	3H-5 HT specific uptake at 10 nM	3H-GLU specific uptake at 10 nM	GLU decarboxylase fmoles/mg tissue, min
A. Unilateral					
0.5 μg KA (n = 6) 2 weeks C		19.6 ± 0.5			
L		-(21 ± 5) %			
3 weeks C		18.1 ± 0.8			
L		-(3 ± 4) %			
3.0 μg KA (n = 3) 2 weeks C	15.8 ± 0.3	20.3 ± 0.8	103 ± 5	387 ± 13	929 ± 40
L	-(45 ± 8) %	-(46 ± 9) %	-(22 ± 11) %	-(20 ± 7) %	-(41 ± 8) %
3 weeks C	19.8 ± 0.4	24.3 ± 3.3	110 ± 7	367 ± 16	1 019 ± 50
L	-(57 ± 2) %	-(54 ± 5) %	-(26 ± 9) %	-(18 ± 7) %	-(43 ± 8) %
4.0 μg KA (n = 3) 2 weeks C	19.1 ± 1.0	25.3 ± 1.0	96 ± 1	326 ± 23	737 ± 20
L	-(65 ± 3) %	-(62 ± 2) %	-(50 ± 1) %	-(37 ± 4) %	-(52 ± 1) %
3 weeks C	17.4 ± 1.4	23.6 ± 0.6	104 ± 3	338 ± 24	1 002 ± 36
L	-(60 ± 4) %	-(60 ± 2) %	-(48 ± 4) %	-(38 ± 6) %	-(52 ± 3) %
B. Bilateral					
4.0 μg KA (n = 4) 3 weeks C	19.8 ± 1.0	27.1 ± 1.6	96.7 ± 8.7	379 ± 16	2 940 ± 220
L	-(74 ± 2) %	-(77 ± 1) %	-(44 ± 15) %	-(52 ± 1) %	-(54 ± 14) %

Kainic acid, dissolved in 0.5 μl physiological saline, adjusted to pH 6, was administered at A 10.7, L 2.0, V 5.7 above zero point. Upon sacrifice, tissues of 6-7 rats for unilateral lesions and of 3-4 rats for bilateral lesions were pooled to form 1 group, n refers to the number of groups, each group was assayed in duplicate for total activities and blanks. Controls were measured in the contralateral side of the lesion or in naive and sham-lesioned animals, various controls did not differ significantly. The following activities were not affected by any of the pre-frontal cortical lesion conditions: in the pre-frontal cortex, the choline acetyltransferase; in the striatum, 3H-ketanserin and 3H-haloperidol binding, DA, 5 HT and GLU uptake, GLU decarboxylase and choline acetyltransferase.

Injection of kainic acid (0.5 μg) in the striatum, 3 weeks prior to assays, did not consistently affect the maximal number of S_2-receptor binding sites in the striatum but caused an apparent increase in the K_D-value of ^{3}H-ketanserin specific binding (control side: B_{max} = 15.3 $\pm$ 1.2 fmoles/mg tissue, K_D = 0.9 $\pm$ 0.1 nM, lesioned side: B_{max} = 14.9 $\pm$ 3.0 fmoles/mg tissue, K_D = 2.0 $\pm$ 0.5 nM, n = 4). In the same tissue preparations, ^{3}H-haloperidol binding was reduced by 38 $\pm$ 6 % in the lesioned versus control striata. In the lesioned striata, the choline acetyltransferase was reduced by 37 %, DA uptake and 5 HT uptake were slightly increased and GLU uptake slightly decreased. In previous studies it was noted that injection in the striatum of kainic acid dosages $\geqslant$1 μg was lethal to over 75 % of the animals.

Lesioning of the serotonergic neurones originating in the raphe nuclei, by injection of 5,7 dihydroxytryptamine (8 μg, 4 weeks prior to assays) did not affect S_2-receptor binding in several brain areas, whereas 5 HT uptake was reduced by 67 to 84 %. Data are presented in Table 3. Catecholamine content, uptake and receptors in several brain areas were not affected by the raphe lesion and neither was the head twitch response of the animals to mescaline (see above).

DISCUSSION

The specific binding of ^{3}H-ketanserin, defined as that portion of the binding inhibited by 1000-fold excess methysergide, shows all the features of S_2-receptor binding sites. When ketanserin is used at nanomolar concentrations, specific binding is restricted to S_2-receptor sites and no contaminating labelling of any other neurotransmitter receptors is observed. This is demonstrated by the lack of binding affinity of selective dopamine, α_1-adrenergic, and histamine$_1$ antagonists and agonists. In contrast all potent serotonin antagonists, belonging to different chemical classes, bind to the sites with nanomolar affinities (Table 1). The selectivity of the ^{3}H-ketanserin binding allowed S_2-receptor binding sites to be clearly characterized for the first time in the dopaminergic brain area, the striatum. Features and properties of S_2-receptor binding sites in the striatum and the pre-frontal cortex were found to be similar, apart from some minor variations in the binding affinities of drugs. An important datum in favour of a neurotransmitter receptor function for the S_2-receptor binding sites is the micromolar binding affinity of serotonin itself. Hence the neurotransmitter can occupy the sites at concentrations which are likely to occur in the synaptic clefts of serotonergic neurones. This property makes it possible that the serotonin binding can be antagonized in vivo by systemically administered drugs which have nanomolar binding affinities for the sites, but which can only reach the receptor sites in very low concentrations. The allegation that the neurotransmitters themselves should have nanomolar

TABLE 3.   5,7 Dihydroxytryptamine lesions in the raphe nuclei

| | | ^{3}H-Ketanserin specific binding (n = 4) fmoles/mg tissue | | ^{3}H-5 HT (10 nM) specific uptake (n = 4) | |
		at 1 nM	at 2 nM	fmoles/mg tissue	% change versus control
Pre-frontal cortex	C	18.7 ± 0.5	25.0 ± 0.9	118 ± 6	
	L	20.9 ± 1.7	26.1 ± 1.7	29 ± 4	-(73 ± 3) %
Fronto-parietal cortex	C	11.5 ± 1.0	14.7 ± 1.4	61 ± 7	
	L	13.6 ± 0.6	16.4 ± 0.8	15 ± 2	-(77 ± 3) %
Cortex	C	8.1 ± 0.4	11.3 ± 0.8	99 ± 5	
	L	8.2 ± 0.5	11.4 ± 0.5	20 ± 2	-(77 ± 3) %
Striatum	C	8.4 ± 1.2	9.5 ± 0.4	108 ± 3	
	L	7.4 ± 0.4	9.9 ± 1.3	34 ± 4	-(67 ± 5) %
Hippocampus	C			72 ± 3	
	L			9.8 ± 1.1	-(84 ± 2) %

Rats, pretreated with desmethylimipramine (25 mg/kg i.p.,45 min beforehand) were injected with 5,7 dihydroxytryptamine (8 µg in 1 µl saline containing 0.01 % ascorbic acid):0.5 µl in the medial raphe (A 0.3, L 0, V 2.1 above zero point) and 0.5 µl in the dorsal raphe (A 0.3, L 0, V 3.9 above zero point). Animals were sacrificed after 4 weeks, tissues of 4 animals were pooled and 4 groups were formed. All brain areas were assayed for NE uptake, choline acetyltransferase, catecholamine content, and protein. The striatum was assayed for ^{3}H-haloperidol (at 2 nM) binding. The cortex and hippocampus were assayed for ^{3}H-WB4101 (at 1 and 2 nM) binding and for ^{3}H-dihydroalprenolol (at 1 and 2 nM) binding. None of the activities was found to be significantly altered in 5,7 dihydroxytryptamine-lesioned (L) compared to control (C) rats. All control values were similar in sham-lesioned and naive animals. The protein content of the tissue preparations was similar in all brain areas (see methods).

binding affinities for their receptors is a misconception, since the concentration of the neurotransmitter in the synaptic clefts is always high.

A typical distribution of S_2-receptor binding sites was found in brains of four mammalian species. Moreover, data in Table 3 demonstrate that the areas which are enriched in S_2-receptor sites: frontal cortical areas, mesolimbic areas and striatum, show marked specific uptake of 5 HT , which disappears by lesioning of the serotonergic neurones of the raphe nuclei. Hence ample serotonergic innervation of the areas enriched in S_2-receptor sites, seems to exist. Nevertheless, S_2-receptor site density and serotonergic innervation do not concur entirely, as appears by the low S_2-receptor density in the hippocampus in contrast to the marked 5 HT uptake in this area. However, the low overall S_2-receptor site densities in areas such as hippocampus, brain stem and spinal cord, which are thought to have serotonergic innervations does not necessarily detract from the possible functional importance of the S_2-receptor sites in these areas. The low number of sites may be concentrated in distinct nuclei. Existence of a regional distribution of S_2-receptor binding sites in the spinal cord could indeed be demonstrated.

At present the function of the S_2-receptor sites in the areas where they are found in great densities, such as the frontal cortex, the striatum and the mesolimbic areas is unknown. Information about the cellular localization of the sites, gained by examining the effects of various types of neuronal lesions could direct hypotheses on the functional roles of the sites. In previous studies using frontal cortical bisection, we observed a significant reduction by 28 % of S_2-receptor sites in the pre-frontal cortex area, anterior to the cut and unchanged S_2-receptor binding in the fronto-parietal cortex, posterior to the cut (10). This was taken as a possible indication for a neuronal localization of the cortical S_2-receptor binding sites. Lesions by 6-hydroxydopamine of the noradrenergic and dopaminergic neurones of the medial forebrain bundle, causing complete depletion of catecholamine content and uptake, did not cause any change in the B_{max} or K_D-values of ^3H-ketanserin binding to S_2-receptor sites in cortical or striatal brain areas. These findings virtually excluded a localization of S_2-receptor sites on dopaminergic or noradrenergic neurones of the medial forebrain bundle (10). Data from the kainic acid lesion studies, which are here reported, provide evidence that S_2-receptor binding sites are localized on neuronal cell bodies in the pre-frontal cortex. This appears from the marked reduction of S_2-receptor binding following frontal cortical injection of high dosages of kainic acid; which was morphologically shown to go along with complete disappearance of neuronal cell bodies in the injected area and excessive gliosis. A concomitant reduction of GLU uptake and GLU decarboxylase was also noted, but the choline acetyltransferase activity was unchanged in the lesioned tissue. Hence, a localization of S_2-receptor sites on glutaminergic neurones is not excluded whereas their occurrence on cholinergic neurones appears less likely. It was noted that rats tolerated well the high dosages of kainic acid (3-4 µg) which were required to cause the neuronal lesions in the frontal cortex, whereas 3 times lower dosages injected in the striatum were lethal to the greater part of animals. Small dosages of kainic acid injected in the striatum, caused destruction of neurones containing dopamine receptor sites labelled by ^{3}H-haloperidol, but did not consistently affect the S_2-receptor binding. Noteworthy is the observation that mescaline-induced head twitches were significantly enhanced in animals with bilateral pre-frontal cortex kainic acid lesions, and also in sham-lesioned animals. A possible explanation would be that the distribution of mescaline in the brain is altered by the cortical surgery. It further suggests that S_2-receptor sites localized in the frontal cortex are not involved in the head twitch phenomenon.

Extensive lesioning using 5,7-dihydroxytryptamine of serotonergic neurones originating in the raphe nuclei, causing a greater than 70 % loss of specific 5 HT uptake in various forebrain areas, appeared not to affect the S_2-receptor binding sites. Hence, S_2-receptor sites appear not to be localized on the serotonergic neurones themselves. However, so-called 'upregulation' of the sites, which is assumed to be expected in conditions of serotonergic denervation did not occur. Our findings could thus not confirm the tentative observation of Brunello et al. (1), who reported an increase in the number of S_2-receptor sites in similarly lesioned animals. In that study, ^{3}H-mianserin was used, but that requires addition of excess mepyramine, in order to detect S_2-receptor sites. The identity and quantification of the sites labelled in such conditions can be doubted. An increase in α_1-adrenergic receptors in the hippocampus, or in the cortex was not found. Hence our data are at variance with those of Consolo et al. (2), who reported an increase in ^{3}H-WB4101 specific binding in the hippocampus but not in the frontal cortex of raphe-lesioned rats.

It can be concluded that ^{3}H-ketanserin is a very suitable and selective ligand to label S_2-receptor sites. The features of the S_2-receptor binding sites are compatible with a serotonin receptor function. The S_2-receptor sites occur mostly in frontal cortical and dopaminergic brain areas, which are demonstrated to receive ample serotonergic enervation. In the frontal cortex the sites appear to be localized on neuronal cell bodies, which are destroyed by high dosages of kainic acid. These neurones could be of glutaminergic, but probably not of cholinergic nature. In forebrain areas, the sites are apparently not localized on the serotonergic neurones themselves, or on noradrenergic or dopaminergic neurones. Also, in areas which contain only low densities of S_2-receptor sites, such as the brain stem and the spinal cord, the sites are distinctly distributed and are likely to play important functional roles.

ACKNOWLEDGEMENT

Part of this work was supported by a grant from I.W.O.N.L.

REFERENCES

1. Brunello, N., Chuang, D.M., and Costa, E. (1982): Science, 215: 1112-1115.
2. Consolo, S., Ladinsky, H., Forloni, G.L., and Grombi, P. (1982): Life Sci., 30: 1113-1120.
3. Hamon, M., Mallat, M., Herbet, A., Nelson, D.L., Audinot, M., Pichat, L., and Glowinski, J. (1981): J. Neurochem., 36: 613-626.
4. König, J.F.R., and Klippel, R.A (1963): The Rat Brain: A Stereotaxic Atlas of the Forebrain and Lower Parts of the Brain Stem. Williams and Wilkins, Baltimore.
5. Laduron, P.M., Janssen, P.F.M., and Leysen, J.E. (1982): Eur. J. Pharmacol., 81: 43-48.
6. Leysen, J.E. (1981): J. Physiol. (Paris), 77: 351-362.
7. Leysen, J.E., Awouters, F., Kennis, L., Laduron, P.M., Vandenberk, J., and Janssen, P.A.J. (1981): Life Sci., 28: 1015-1022.
8. Leysen, J.E., Gommeren, W., and Laduron, P.M. (1979): Biochem. Pharmacol., 28: 447-448.
9. Leysen, J.E., Gommeren, W., and Van Gompel, P. (1981): Neurochem. Int., 3: 219-228.
10. Leysen, J.E., Geerts, R., Gommeren, W., Verwimp, M., and Van Gompel, P. (1982): Arch. Int. Pharmacodyn. Ther., 256: 301-305.
11. Leysen, J.E., and Laduron, P.M. (1977): Arch. Int. Pharmacodyn. Ther., 230: 337-339.
12. Leysen, J.E., Niemegeers, C.J.E., Tollenaere, J.P., and Laduron, P.M. (1978): Nature (Lond.), 272: 168-171.
13. Leysen, J.E., Niemegeers, C.J.E., Van Nueten, J.M., and Laduron, P.M. (1982): Mol. Pharmacol., 21: 301-314.
14. Peroutka, S.J., and Snyder, S.H. (1979): Mol. Pharmacol., 16: 687-699.
15. Peroutka, S.J., and Snyder, S.H. (1981): J. Pharmacol. Exp. Ther., 216: 142-148.
16. Van Nueten, J.M., Janssen, P.A.J., Van Beek, J., Xhonneux, R., Verbeuren, T.-J., and Vanhoutte, P.M. (1981): J. Pharmacol. Exp. Ther., 218: 217-230.

CNS Receptors—From Molecular
Pharmacology to Behavior, edited by
P. Mandel and F. V. DeFeudis.
Raven Press, New York © 1983.

The Distribution of Serotonin Binding Sites: A Comparison of ³H-Serotonin Binding in Membrane Preparations of Rat Gut and Rat Brain

*Jo Ann Heltzel and †Wolfgang H. Vogel

*Biosciences Research, 3M Center, St. Paul, Minnesota 55144; and †Department of
Pharmacology, Thomas Jefferson University, Philadelphia, Pennsylvania 19107

Many laboratories have shown high-affinity serotonin (5-HT) binding in rat brain, which is reversible, saturable, stereoselective, pharmacologically specific, temperature-dependent, and which exhibits regional receptor densities consistent with the pattern of serotonergic innervation in the CNS (1,4,7,8,12, 13,15). In the CNS the high-affinity 5-HT binding meets many of the rigid criteria set forth by Bennett (2) as binding which occurs at specific 5-HT receptor sites. Further work has correlated the activity of sites which are labelled by ³H-LSD and ³H-spiperone with the potencies of compounds which antagonize tryptamine-induced clonic seizures in rat (11) and with potencies to block 5-HT-induced contractions of rat artery in vitro (14).

However, correlations have not yet been demonstrated with CNS ³H-5-HT binding sites and relevant physiological or pharmacological 5-HT-mediated effects (14). It has been recommended that ³H-5-HT binding sites in CNS be viewed with caution, and that identification of these sites as serotonin receptor sites is somewhat premature (9). The absence of a definitive correlation of ³H-5-HT binding in CNS with relevant 5-HT-mediated effects led us to explore the nature of specific ³H-5-HT binding sites in the gut, and to compare these sites with 5-HT binding sites found in brain tissue.

Methods

Male Sprague-Dawley rats weighing 250-300 grams were decapitated. Whole brain minus cerebellum was used in all studies. Brain membranes were prepared according to the method of Bennett and Snyder (1) with modifications as previously described (7).

The proximal 60-cm section of rat gut was dissected free of attached mesentery; elements of the myenteric plexus remained intact. The gut was divided into smaller sections and flushed

several times with ice-cold 0.05 M TRIS·HCl buffer, pH 7.4. The
sections were blotted to dryness, weighed, bisected along their
longitudinal axis, and scissored into smaller pieces to ease
homogenization. Gut was homogenized in buffer using 80 mg per
ml. The homogenate was separated at 50,000 x g for 20 minutes
and resuspended in an equal volume of buffer. The resuspended
pellet was prepared by repeating this step, and could be stored
at -20°C for up to one week without loss of activity.

Serotonin binding was assayed by rapid filtration, as previously described (7) with some modification for the gut assay.
The gut homogenate was preincubated for 20 minutes in a 37°C
shaking bath to degrade endogenous 5-HT (10). The tissue concentration was reduced to 40 mg per ml using enriched buffer,
containing 10 μM pargyline and 0.1% ascorbic acid at final concentration, and reincubated for an additional 10 minutes at 37°C
to establish equilibrium conditions.

Aliquots of homogenate (0.5 ml) were incubated for two hours
at 37°C with or without 0.5 μM unlabelled 5-HT (0.1 ml) in a
final volume of 2 ml with ^{3}H-5-HT (25-30 Ci per mmole) at a concentration of 5 nM (0.1 ml). Nonspecific 5-HT binding was
measured in the presence of 0.5 μM unlabelled 5-HT; specific 5-
HT binding was measured indirectly as the difference between
5-HT bound in the presence and absence of the nonspecific binding blank. All samples were prepared in triplicate.

Following rapid filtration through glass fiber filters (GF/B)
and washing with three 5 ml portions of ice-cold buffer, the
filters were extracted by rapid shaking for 20 minutes in 10 ml
of ACS scintillation fluor (Amersham). Samples were quantitated
at 30-35% counting efficiency by liquid scintillation spectrometry.

Results

Specific 5-HT binding sites were identified in rat gut membrane homogenates using 0.5 μM unlabelled 5-HT to discriminate
nonspecific components of binding, The appropriate blank concentration was selected from the plateau of the inhibition curve
(Fig. 1) in which bound ^{3}H-5-HT was displaced by increasing concentrations of unlabelled ligand. In parallel studies in rat
brain, 2 μM unlabelled 5-HT served as the nonspecific blank.

One striking difference between 5-HT binding in brain and gut
was the time required to reach equilibrium. In gut specific 5-HT
binding was measured at 37°C at incubation periods ranging from
5-180 minutes (Fig. 2). Equilibrium was reached by 120 minutes
and remained stable throughout three hours. Additional washing
of the membrane-laden filters did not decrease specific 5-HT
binding (2.60 pmoles per gram after 3 washes versus 2.75 pmoles
per gram after 10 washes), indicating the persistence of a high-
affinity binding component. In contrast, brain membrane preparations equilibrated within five minutes and remained stable
throughout sixty minutes. In both tissues specific 5-HT binding

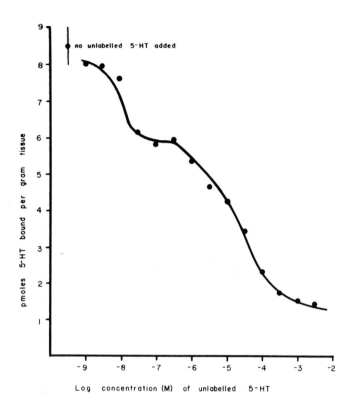

FIG. 1. Inhibition of ³H-5-HT binding by unlabelled 5-HT in rat gut. Gut membrane preparations of 20 mg tissue per sample were incubated at 37°C for two hours in the presence of 5 nM ³H-5-HT as the concentration of unlabelled 5-HT was varied between 10^{-9} and 10^{-3} M.

increased linearly as a function of tissue concentration (5 - 40 mg per sample). Similarly, specific 5-HT binding was reversible in the presence of a large excess of ligand-free buffer; as expected, reversal in the brain preparation was rapid and more prolonged in the gut preparation. In gut less than 20% of specifically-bound 5-HT remained after 2 hours at 37°C.

Saturation of specific 5-HT binding sites was observed over a concentration range of 3.5 to 35 nM ³H-5-HT in both tissues. In gut Scatchard analysis of the saturation data yielded an equilibrium dissociation constant (K_D) of 41.5 ± 1.5 nM (n=3); the apparent number of binding sites (B_{max}) was calculated to be 15.7 ± 2.0 picomoles per gram tissue. An example of the Scatchard plot is shown in Fig. 3. In the rat brain, most groups have reported K_D to fall between 1-6 nM; estimations of B_{max} are 12-20 pico-

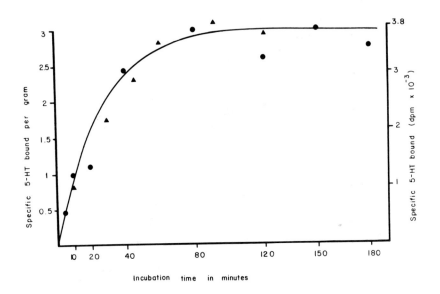

FIG. 2. Equilibrium time course of specific 5-HT binding in rat gut. Membrane preparations (20 mg tissue per sample) were incubated in the presence of 5 nM ^{3}H-5-HT at 37°C for varying time intervals. 0.5 µM unlabelled 5-HT served as the nonspecific blank; all samples were determined in triplicate. (●) and (▲) indicate the results of two experiments.

moles per gram tissue (1,4,7,8,13,15).

The pharmacologic specificity of 5-HT binding in gut was examined by competitive displacement studies with compounds known to act at presumed 5-HT receptor sites. The pharmacologic potency of each agent was determined by log-probit analysis of the displacement curve and reported as an IC_{50} value, representing the concentration which displaced 50% of specifically-bound 5-HT. IC_{50} values and the rank order of potency for each compound in both tissues is shown in Table 1.

Although the rank order of potency in gut is similar to that found in brain, gut IC_{50} values were significantly greater. Bufotenine, 2-bromo-LSD, and 5-methoxytryptamine exhibited values two to three-thousand-fold greater than those in brain, whereas methysergide, tryptamine, and N,N-diethyltryptamine were 200-800 times higher in gut. (+)-LSD and N,N-dimethyltryptamine at concentrations up to 10^{-4}M did not antagonize specific 5-HT binding in gut; however, both compounds were active in brain. For the six agents active in both tissues, a significant degree of correlation (r=0.86, p < .01) was found (Fig. 4).

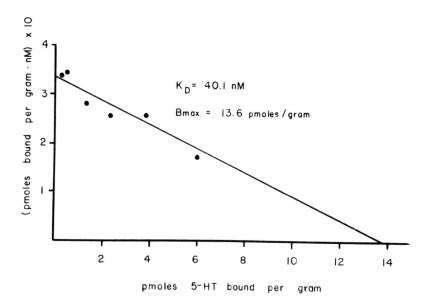

FIG. 3. Scatchard analysis of ^{3}H-5-HT binding in rat gut. Bound ^{3}H-5-HT was observed to increase as free ligand concentrations were raised between 3.5 and 35 nM. The apparent number of 5-HT binding sites (Bmax) corresponds to the x-intercept; K_D was calculated as the negative inverse of the slope of the line. The Scatchard construction suggests a single population of specific 5-HT binding sites.

Another comparison was drawn between the ability of four compounds which stimulate the contraction of rat fundus and the potency of these compounds to inhibit specific 5-HT binding in gut, shown in Table 2. Glennon et al.(6) reported apparent affinity binding constants (pA_2) calculated by Schild plot analysis based upon the concentration of an agent needed to produce 50% of a maximal contraction in the rat fundus strip. The rank ordering of IC_{50} values for the four agonists tested in the 5-HT gut binding assay was obtained as follows: bufotenine (3.9 μM) > 5-methoxytryptamine (15 μM) > tryptamine (360 μM) > N,N-diethyltryptamine (640 μM). Rank ordering using Glennon's pA_2 values showed a similar ordering, that is, bufotenine was more potent than 5-methoxytryptamine, followed by tryptamine and N,N-diethyltryptamine. Linear regression of the line of best fit determined by the least squares method yielded a regression coefficient of 0.92.

TABLE 1. Rank order of displacing agents in rat gut and brain.

	Brain IC_{50} (nM)	Rank Order	Gut IC_{50}(nM)[a]	Rank Order
Bufotenine	1.6	1	3900	1
(+)-LSD	3.9	2	$>10^5$	~8
5-Methoxytryptamine	7.9	3	15,000	2
Methysergide	74	4	59,000	3
(+)-Br-LSD	180	5	5×10^5	6
Tryptamine	1900	6	360,000	4
N,N-diethyltryptamine	3600	7	640,000	5
N,N-dimethyltryptamine	18,000	8	$>10^5$	~7

[a]IC_{50} values were measured by log-probit analysis of the inhibition curves, constructed from 4-5 values, and representing the average of 2-4 studies. In four studies (+)-LSD and N,N,-dimethyltryptamine failed to displace any measurable specific 5-HT binding in gut at concentrations up to 1×10^{-4} M.

TABLE 2. Comparison of ^{3}H-5-HT specific binding in rat gut with affinity constants obtained in contracting rat fundus.

Compound	Rank Order	Gut IC_{50} (μM)	pA2 values from ref. 6
Bufotenine	1	3.9	7.41 ± .05
5-Methoxytryptamine	2	15	6.86 ± .08
Tryptamine	3	360	6.27 ± .17
N,N-diethyltryptamine	4	640	6.00 ± .08

Affinity values (pA2) were obtained from Schild plots based upon the ability of these compounds to stimulate a contraction which was 50% of the maximum in rat fundus strips.

Discussion

Earlier work on the specific binding of ^{3}H-5-HT in rat brain established the existence of specific sites and the potency of various agents to displace bound 5-HT from these sites (1,4). We now report the characterization of specific 5-HT binding sites in rat gut. Qualitatively, there are some similarities between the specific sites in brain and gut in that one can demonstrate a finite number of specific sites, the presence of reversible binding, and a reasonable correlation between the potency of serotonin analogues with the ability of these compounds to stimulate contractions in the rat fundus.

However, a quantitative comparison of these specific 5-HT sites in brain and gut reveals a number of striking differences.

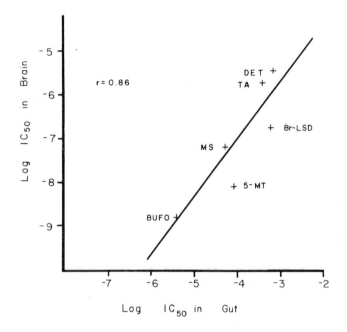

FIG. 4. Displacing potencies of various compounds on specific
[3]H-5-HT binding in rat brain and gut. IC_{50} values correspond to
the concentration of displacer which **reduces the** specific 5-HT
binding by 50%, determined by log-probit analysis. Linear regression of the line of best fit yielded a correlation coefficient of 0.86. Abbreviations are bufotenine (BUFO), 5-methoxy-
tryptamine (5-MT), methysergide (MS), tryptamine (TA), 2-bromo-
LSD (Br-LSD), and N,N-diethyltryptamine (DET).

Firstly, most laboratories have reported high-affinity ^{3}H-5-HT
binding in brain between a range of 1-6 nM (1,4,8,12,13,15),
whereas in the gut, the site showed an equilibrium dissociation
constant which was considerably higher, K_D = 40 nM. The estimate of the apparent number of sites, Bmax, was in closer agreement between the two tissues, being 12-20 picomoles per gram in
brain versus 14-18 picomoles per gram in gut.
    Using the following equation,
$$b = \frac{[Bmax]\ [Ligand]}{[K_D]\ +\ [Ligand]}$$
the kinetic values for Bmax and K_D can be estimated from the
equilibrium data, where b ≃ 2.5 picomoles bound per gram tissue
in gut. Substituting a value of K_D = 40 nM, Bmax is estimated

to be 22.5 picomoles per gram. Conversely, using the value of 15.7 picomoles per gram for Bmax obtained experimentally, K_D is approximated to be 26.4 nM. The overestimation of K_D in our gut studies is likely to be the consequence of using a rather low radioligand concentration (5 nM), which would only be expected to label 10-15% of the specific sites.

The second notable difference between 5-HT binding sites in brain and gut was the unusually prolonged time required to reach equilibrium conditions in the gut, which approached two hours. As might be expected, the reversal of specific 5-HT binding in gut also followed an extended time course. The protracted reversal of specific 5-HT binding suggests that the lengthy time course was not due to irreversible ligand binding. Furthermore, the extended time course was not the result of pre-synaptic reuptake processes since the depletion of stored 5-HT requires a longer interval. In addition, a single population of specific binding sites was identified by Scatchard analysis, indicating that the slow time course to equilibrium is occurring at a single type of binding site.

At present we can offer no insight as to the lengthy approach to equilibrium. In muscle bath preparations, serotonin can elicit a maximum contraction within a matter of seconds in spite of any diffusional barriers in the experimental model. Since the main site of serotonin production in the gut occurs in the enterochromaffin cells and since serotonin produces pronounced effects on gastrointestinal motility, it has been suggested that serotonin acts as a local hormone in gut in the control of peri-staltic activity (3). Whether the longer time course in gut would be more consistent with a hormonal rather than a neuro-transmitter role for serotonin in gut remains highly speculative.

More recently, several lines of evidence reviewed by Gershon (5) suggest that serotonin serves as the neurotransmitter in the intrinsic serotonergic innervation of the gut, commonly called the enteric nervous system. It also appears unlikely that the specific sites identified in gut are related to the intrinsic 5-HT system.

In our opinion, a more reasonable explanation for the exten-ded time course can be proposed by questioning the integrity of the preparation of the gut membrane homogenates. The con-ditions under which we sought to study specific 5-HT binding in gut may have changed the character and responsiveness of physio-logically relevant serotonin receptors. In a recent review of serotonergic binding in the CNS by Leysen (9), she suggests that membrane preparations contain many elements, some of which may be structural recognition sites which are saturable and bind related compounds with a high affinity, but bear no relation to pharmacological or physiological effects of the ligand under study.

The evaluation of the pharmacological specificity of the specific 5-HT sites in gut was studied using compounds which are known to mimic or interfere with serotonin-mediated physiological effects or behaviors. Although active in the 5-HT binding assay in brain, neither (+)-LSD nor N,N-dimethyltryptamine were able to produce measurable inhibition of specific 5-HT binding in gut. Furthermore, the remaining six compounds we tested (bufotenine, methysergide, 5-methoxytryptamine, 2-bromo-LSD, tryptamine, and N,N-diethyltryptamine) required two to three orders of magnitude greater concentrations to displace 50% of specifically-bound 5-HT in gut than in brain. Again, this discrepancy in IC_{50} values indicates that the specific 5-HT binding sites in brain and gut differ considerably.

A final comparison of gut IC_{50} values to calculated apparent affinity constants, pA_2 values, illustrated an identical rank ordering of potencies with a notable degree of correlation, r = 0.92. Again, the comparison of gut IC_{50} values to gut pA_2 suggests that the specific 5-HT binding in gut is capable of structural recognition of serotonin-related compounds, but that these sites differ from physiologically relevant receptors.

The question which must be raised by our own work in the gut, and the work of others in the CNS, is why specific 5-HT binding sites do not conform completely to the rigorous requirement for physiological and/or pharmacological relevance for the serotonin receptor. Numerous other in vitro neurotransmitter receptor sites have been identified in in vitro binding assays which fulfill all of the essential criteria. Interestingly, specific binding sites for ^{3}H-LSD and ^{3}H-spiperone in some CNS tissues appear to be physiologically relevant receptors which mediate serotonin-related effects. We respectfully suggest that the area of ^{3}H-5-HT in vitro binding requires careful reexamination of several points, such as ^{3}H-ligand stability, specific ion or cofactor requirements, and binding assay conditions. In this way, the failure to identify specific serotonin receptors in both CNS and gut tissues can be resolved.

References

1. Bennett, J.P.,Jr., and Snyder, S.H. (1976): Mol. Pharmacol., 12:373-389.
2. Bennett, J.P.,Jr. (1978): In: Neurotransmitter Receptor Binding, edited by H.I. Yamamura, S.J. Enna, and M.J. Kuhar, pp. 57-90. Raven Press, New York.
3. Erspamer, V. (1954): Pharmacol. Rev., 6:425-487.
4. Fillion, G.M.B., Rouselle, J.C., Fillion, M.P., Beaudoin, D.M., Goiny, M.R., Deniau, J.M., and Jacob, J.J. (1978): Mol. Pharmacol., 14:50-59.
5. Gershon, M.D. (1981): J. Physiol.,Paris, 77:257-265.
6. Glennon, R.A. and Gessner, P.K. (1979): J. Med. Chem., 22:428-432.
7. Heltzel, J.A., Boehme, D.H., and Vogel, W.H. (1981): Brain Res., 204:451-454.
8. Leysen, J.E., Gommeren, W., and Laduron, P. (1978): Arch. Int. Physiol. Biochim., 86:874-875.

9. Leysen, J.E. (1981): J. Physiol., Paris, 77:351-362.
10. Nelson, D.L., Herbet, A., Bourgoin, S., Glowinski, J., and Hamon, M. (1978): Mol. Pharmacol., 14:983-995.
11. Niemegeers, C.J.E. and Janssen, P.A.J. (1979): Life Sci., 24:2201-2216.
12. Peroutka, S.J. and Snyder, S.H. (1979): Mol. Pharmacol., 16:687-699.
13. Savage, D.D., Mendels, J., and Frazer, A. (1980): J. Pharmacol. Exp. Ther., 212:259-263.
14. Van Nueten, J.M., Janssen, P.A.J., DeRidder, W., and Vanhoutte, P.M. (1982): Eur. J. Pharmacol., 77:281-287.
15. Whittaker, P.M. and Seeman, P. (1978): Psychopharmacol., 59:1-5.

CNS Receptors—From Molecular
Pharmacology to Behavior, edited by
P. Mandel and F. V. DeFeudis.
Raven Press, New York © 1983.

Studies on the 'Turnover' of Central α-Adrenoceptors in the Rat Using Phenoxybenzamine

R. M. McKernan and I. C. Campbell

Department of Biochemistry, Institute of Psychiatry, London SE5 8AF England

Numerous studies have shown that α-adrenoceptors (as estimated by binding assays) can increase or decrease in density
(for review see Reisine 1981). This adaptation may occur
because of alteration in the level of transmission, e.g.
increases in [^{3}H]-WB4101 and [^{3}H]-clonidine binding after 6-OH-
dopamine lesions of the dorsal bundle (U'Pritchard et al. 1979),
or in response to drug administration, e.g. the decrease reported
in rat cortical [^{3}H]-clonidine binding after 3 weeks of antidepressant treatment (Cohen et al. 1982, Smith et al. 1981).
Although the processes involved in the up and down regulation of
other receptors is becoming clearer (Baker & Pitha 1981) the
mechanism by which α-adrenoceptors can up or down regulate is
poorly understood.

There is some variation in the time required for changes in
receptor number to become apparent. Down regulation of α-
adrenoceptors has been reported to occur in minutes, e.g. when
rat parotid cells are incubated with high concentrations of
adrenaline (Strittmatter et al. 1977), whereas α$_2$-adrenocep-
tors on the platelet are decreased in number after 4 hours of
exposure to adrenaline (Cooper et al. 1978) and α$_1$-adrenoceptors
on rat mesenteric arteries are decreased 12 hours after exposure
to adrenaline (Colucci et al. 1981). Agonist-induced desensitisation is usually readily reversible and of shorter duration
than the longer term adaptive changes seen with lesioning
studies or with drug administration.

It is of interest to investigate the rate at which these
changes occur, thus studies of α-adrenoceptor 'turnover' or

'temporal availability' may lead to further understanding of the regulation of receptor number and its alteration by drugs.

One useful approach would be to irreversibly block the receptors and measure the reappearance of binding sites. We have used phenoxybenzamine in this way, administering it in vivo and measuring the subsequent reappearance of binding sites. To assess the recovery of α_1-adrenoceptor sites the antagonist ligand [^{3}H]-prazosin has been used and to assess the recovery of α_2-adrenoceptor sites both [^{3}H]-clonidine and [^{3}H]-rauwolscine have been used since agonist and antagonist ligands may not necessarily label the same site (Bylund et al. 1981, Shattil et al. 1981).

Although binding assays yield information about the number, and affinity of receptors, they do not give any information about their function. Since α_2-adrenoceptors inhibit the release of preloaded [^{3}H]-noradrenaline from synaptosomes, we have attempted to correlate changes in this function with changes in the binding of [^{3}H]-clonidine and [^{3}H]-rauwolscine.

METHODS

Two doses of PBZ were administered 12 hours apart to male Wistar rats which were then decapitated at intervals ranging from 0.5 hours to 17 days. Cortical (or brainstem) membranes were prepared from 2-4 treated animals at each time point and from control (untreated) animals. Binding assays were carried out according to the conditions in Table 1. All assays were filtered through Gf/B filter and washed with 4 x 4ml of buffer at 4°C. B_{max} and K_d values were obtained from 6-point Scatchard plots.

TABLE 1

Ligand	Buffer	Incubation	Non-specific binding defined by
[^{3}H]-prazosin	50mM Tris 0.5mM EDTA pH7.5	20 min at 37°C	10^{-5} phentolamine
[^{3}H]-clonidine	50mM Tris 0.5mM EDTA 1mM MgCl$_2$ pH7.5	15 min at 37°C	10^{-5} adrenaline
[^{3}H]-rauwolscine	50mM Na$^+$K$^+$ PO$_4$ pH7.4	2 hr at 4°C	10^{-5} phentolamine

For superfusion studies hemi-cortices from Wistar rats were rapidly dissected and homogenised using a teflon homogeniser in 10 vols of 0.32M sucrose, this was centrifuged at 1000g for 10 mins, the supernatant was removed and then centrifuged at

12,000g for 10 min. The pellet from each hemi-cortex was very
carefully taken up in 2 ml of Krebs bicarbonate medium of the
following composition (mM): NaCl (121) KCl (1.85) $MgSO_4$ (1.15)
KH_2PO_4 (1.15) $NaHCO_3$ (25) glucose (11.1) $CaCl_2$ (1.0); pH 7.2-7.4.
The synaptosomes were incubated with 1mM ^3H-noradrenaline for
15 min, 0.5-ml aliquots of the suspension were carefully filtered
through Gf/B filters which were then transferred to superfusion
chambers and superfused with Krebs buffer as above, but containing no Ca^{2+}. The synaptosomes were stimulated with Krebs medium
containing 30mM K^+, 1.0mM $CaCl_2$ at t = 30 and t = 60. Clonidine
or clonidine + yohimbine was added to the superfusion medium
10 min before stimulation; 2-minute fractions were collected,
and the radioactivity was assayed by liquid scintillation
counting.

RESULTS

Phenoxybenzamine in vitro inhibits the binding of all three
α-adrenergic ligands with K_I values of 1.6 x 10^{-8}M, 2.8 x 10^{-6}M
and 2.1 x 10^{-6}M for [^3H]-prazosin, [^3H]-rauwolscine and [^3H]-
clonidine, respectively. (See Figure 1(a)). Thus, here phenoxybenzamine is a more potent inhibitor of $α_1$-adrenoceptors than of
$α_2$-adrenoceptors in agreement with other studies (Dubocovitch
and Langer, 1974, Borowski et al. 1977). When PBZ was administered to rats in vivo (See Figure 1(b)) and binding of these
three ligands was assessed in the cortical membranes prepared
subsequently, it was found that inhibition of binding by PBZ was
maximal after 2 administered doses of 4mg / Kg i.p. The extent
of the inhibition varied with the different ligands. The
binding of [^3H]-prazosin was inhibited by over 90% after PBZ,
but inhibition of both [^3H]-clonidine and [^3H]-rauwolscine did
not exceed 30% even with higher doses.
Since inhibition was maximal after 2 doses of PBZ of 4mg/Kg
i.p this dose regimen was used to assess the decrease and concomitant reappearance of α-adrenoceptor binding.
The half-life ($t_{\frac{1}{2}}$) for the recovery of the $α_1$-adrenoceptor
binding sites is approximately 5 and 6 days in cortex and brainstem, respectively. The 'turnover' pattern of [^3H]-clonidine and
[^3H]-rauwolscine binding sites is quite different from that of
the $α_1$ binding sites (see Figure 3). PBZ inhibits binding by
up to 30% only and the sites recover with a half-life of 12-
14 hours for [^3H]-clonidine binding and 10-12 hours for [^3H]-
rauwolscine.

(a)   <u>INHIBITION OF RADIOLIGAND BINDING BY 'IN VITRO' PBZ</u>

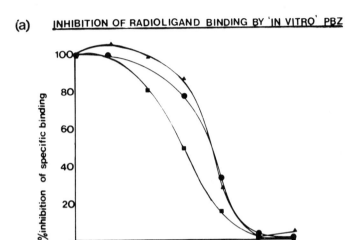

(b)   INHIBITION OF RADIOLIGAND BINDING BY 'IN VIVO' PBZ

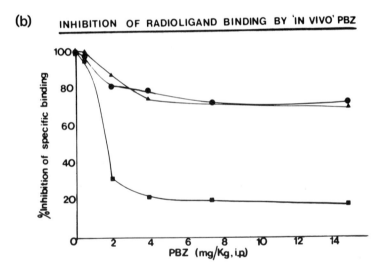

FIGURE I(a). Inhibition of specific [³H]-clonidine (▲), [³H]-rauwolscine (●) and [³H]-prazosin (■) binding by phenyoxyben-zamine (PBZ) in vitro. Figure 1(b) Inhibition of binding of the same ligands in cortices prepared from rats 3 hours after administration of phenoxybenzamine (PBZ). Each point represents the B_{max} value obtained from a six-point Scatchard plot performed on pooled cortices from 2 animals.

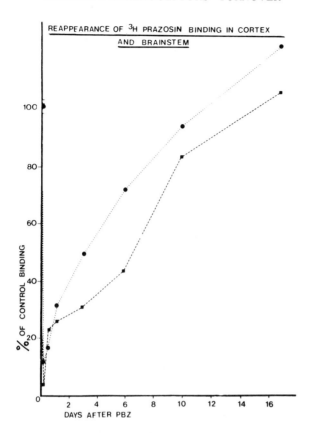

FIGURE 2.   Reappearance of [^{3}H]-prazosin binding in the
cortex (●) and brainstem (■) after PBZ (2 x 4mg/Kg i.p.) Each
point represents the B$_{max}$ from a 6-point Scatchard plot performed on pooled cortices from 3 animals. Binding is expressed
as a percentage of control values which were B$_{max}$ 7.3 pmol/g
wet wt, K$_d$ 0.414 ± 0.5nM (n = 8) in the cortex, and B$_{max}$ 5.8pmol/g
wet wt, K$_d$ 2.0 ± 0.9nM (n = 8) in the brainstem.

It seems unlikely that the smaller inhibition of [^{3}H]-
clonidine binding is due to removal of the PBZ from these sites
during the assay procedure since extensive washing of the
membranes in vitro (centrifugation and resuspension up to 6 times)
did not increase the specific binding of [^{3}H]-clonidine or [^{3}H]-
prazosin (See Figure 4).
Superfusion studies measuring the K$^+$-evoked release of preloaded [^{3}H]-noradrenaline from crude cortical synaptosomal
preparations were also performed. This was necessary to investigate whether the 30% inhibition by PBZ of the specific [^{3}H]-
clonidine binding affected the function of the α$_2$-adrenoceptor.

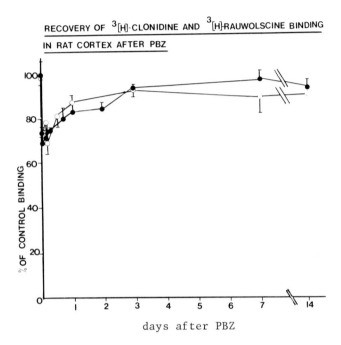

days after PBZ

FIGURE 3.   Recovery of [^{3}H]-clonidine (●) and [^{3}H]-rauwolscine (0) binding after PBZ (2 x 4mg/Kg i.p.) Each point represents the mean ± SEM of 2-4 independent experiments. In each experiment B_{max} was obtained from a 6-point Scatchard plot, and binding is expressed as a percentage of control values which were for [^{3}H]-clonidine, B_{max} 6.3 pmol/g wet wt, K_d 2.53 ± 0.18nM, (n = 25) and for [^{3}H]-rauwolscine 6.2 pmol/g wet wt, K_d 2.40 ± 0.4 (n = 19). All points from 1hr to 2 days were significantly less than control (P<0.01).

When synaptosomes were prepared from control cortices, two stimulations (S_1 and S_2) with K^+, evoked the same release of ^{3}H. This was inhibited by 35% when 1μM clonidine was present in the second stimulation (S_2), and this effect was fully attenuated by 20μM yohimbine. When synaptosomes were prepared from rats 3 hrs after the administration of PBZ the second K^+-evoked release of ^{3}H was only 65% of that released in S_1. When clonidine was added in S_2 it seemed to cause no further decrease in ^{3}H-release, nor did yohimbine attenuate the release produced by K^+ alone in S_2. When cortical synaptosomes were prepared from rats treated for 3 days with PBZ, K^+ alone still produced a smaller release of ^{3}H in S_2 compared with S_1; however, clonidine now reduced this further, and the effect was attenuated, but not significantly so, by yohimbine. (See Table 2).

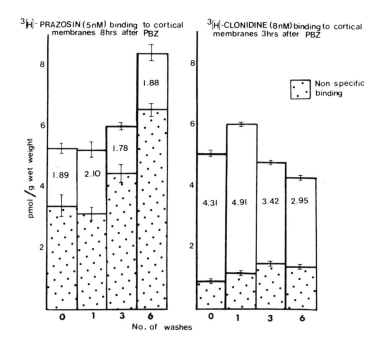

FIGURE 4. The effect of repetitive washing on the total and non-specific binding of [^{3}H]-prazosin and [^{3}H]-clonidine are shown. The numbers printed represent the specific binding (pmol/g wet wt).

TABLE 2.   Superfusion Studies

Treatment	S_1	S_2	% S_2/S_1 (n)
Control	K^+	K^+	94.5± 7 (5)
	K^+	K^++Clon	*66.7±14 (7)
	K^+	K^++Clon+Yoh	101.5± 5 (2)
3Hrs after PBZ	K^+	K^+	69.0±12 (7)
	K^+	K^++Clon	67.0±16 (13)
	K^+	K^++Clon+Yoh	63.0± 5 (6)
3 Days after PBZ	K^+	K^+	84.1±10 (7)
	K^+	K^++Clon	70.0± 8 (5)
	K^+	K^++Clon+Yoh	78.8± 7 (5)

In all cases [K^+]=30mM, [Clonidine]=1μM and [Yohimbine]=20μM

* P<0.01 compared to control.

DISCUSSION

The data presented using rat cortical membranes shows that PBZ binds to both α_1 and α_2-adrenoceptors in vitro. It has been proposed to bind in a competitive manner initially, and subsequently becomes covalently attached to the receptor (Nickerson and Gump, 1949). This may explain the fairly high K_i values obtained, considering the irreversible binding nature of PBZ. One other contributing factor may be that PBZ also interacts with a large number of other sites which would reduce its effective concentration. In fact it binds to many receptor systems; e.g. DA receptors (Lehmann and Langer 1981), cholinergic receptors (Blazso and Minker, 1980) and opiate receptors (Robson and Kosterlitz, 1979). In addition it prevents noradrenaline uptake (Cubeddu et al. 1974) and noradrenaline transport into vesicles (Carlsson et al. 1963). Despite its wide spectrum of action it is to date the only irreversible α-adrenergic antagonist readily available for studies of this kind. While the inherent problems of non-specificity are appreciated they are of greater significance in functional studies since specificity of the receptor changes measured in the 'turnover' study is a reflection of the ligand used to label the receptor and not the PBZ.

When PBZ is included in vitro it can inhibit virtually all the specific binding of each ligand. When PBZ is administered in vivo however, although it inhibits virtually all the [³H]-prazosin binding, in agreement with the in vitro studies, it inhibits only 30% of the [³H]-clonidine and [³H]-rauwolscine binding. There are several possible explanations for the inaccessibility of 70% of the [³H]-clonidine binding sites. There may be some physical barrier in vivo not present in vitro which prevents access of PBZ to the α_2-adrenoceptor sites. For example some could be intracellular or there could be steric hindrance to PBZ in reaching some sites. Alternatively,there may be pharmacologically different types of the α_2-adrenoceptor not all of which are bound by PBZ. It has been postulated that post-synaptic α_2-adrenoceptors are less susceptible to PBZ (Constantine and Lebel 1980) and that PBZ does not antagonise all the central effects of clonidine in vivo (Franklin and Herberg 1977), these reports could be of relevance to our findings. Without further experiments it is not possible to distinguish between the above alternatives.

The large difference between the rates of recovery of [³H]-prazosin and [³H]-clonidine binding sites,as demonstrated in Figures 2 and 3,could be a result of differences in the mechanism of recovery. The most likely explanation for the recovery of α_1-adrenoceptor sites seems to be the synthesis of new receptors (i.e. de novo protein synthesis). The same mechanism has been proposed for β-adrenoceptors whose recovery after an irreversible antagonist Alm-CO-CH₂Br required 8.3 days (heart) and 27 days (lung) (Baker and Pitha, 1981). For the more rapid 'turnover' of α_2-adrenoceptors other mechanisms are equally plausible. Irreversible blockade may lead to the unmasking of α-adrenoceptors that were preformed in the membrane but previously unavailable, a mechanism suggested to occur for β-adrenoceptors (Strittmatter et al. 1979) or it may be due to receptors inside the cell being inserted into the membrane, as has also been suggested for β-adrenoceptors (Kempson et al, 1978). Further experiments employing e.g. protein synthesis inhibitors will be needed to extend understanding of the mechanisms involved. The similar binding and recovery pattern of [^{3}H]-clonidine and [^{3}H]-rauwolscine suggest that in this preparation both ligands label the same site, although in many instances this is not the case (Bylund et al, 1981).

The results from the superfusion studies are surprising. Although we found a similar uptake of ^{3}H into synaptosomal fractions of control and PBZ-treated rat brains, and the release evoked by K^+ in S_1 was also similar, there was a marked reduction in ^{3}H release during S_2 in those preparations from PBZ-treated animals. We have been unable to find any previously published work on the effects of PBZ administration in vivo on the subsequent characteristics of ^{3}H-noradrenaline release from brain preparations. This may therefore be a novel observation, but it is not easy to interpret since PBZ binds to α_2-adrenoceptors and also prevents noradrenaline uptake (Cubbedu et al. 1974) particularly into adrenergic vesicles (Carlsson et al. 1963); the effect may be a composite of these changes. Regardless of the mechanism, the reduced ^{3}H efflux in S_2 makes it very difficult to assess the effect of clonidine in the PBZ-treated animals. Further experiments, perhaps using NA uptake inhibitors in the superfusate, to eliminate differences in this factor in PBZ-treated versus control preparations, will be necessary before this point is resolved. Even this may not answer the question since the uptake inhibitor DMI itself has been reported to attenuate the effect of clonidine (Pelayo et al. 1980).

If the most simple explanation of the results from PBZ-treated rats where clonidine was incorporated into the perfusate during S_2 is accepted, i.e. that a loss of presynaptic α_2 function accompanies PBZ treatment, this is of considerable interest. It implies that a 30% loss of binding sites can be associated with a near 100% loss of function. This has implications both for the physiological role of α_2 receptors and for the use of binding studies to elucidate function.

One further problem related to the use of PBZ for studying 'turnover' of receptors is that, as an irreversible antagonist, binding to many sites it may itself alter the normal pattern of receptor regulation and turnover, and results should be interpreted in the light of such knowledge. It is still however a potentially very useful technique for investigating the 'turnover' of α-adrenoceptors and its alteration by drugs.

Acknowledgements

This work was supported by the Medical Research Council of the UK. We are grateful to Dr M Lynch and Mr H Russell for advice and assistance, and to Mrs S Stanley for preparation of the manuscript.

REFERENCES

1. Baker, S. P. and Pith, J. (1982):J.Pharmac.Exp.Ther. 220(2):247-251.
2. Blazso, G. and Minker, E. (1980):Acta Pharm.Hung. 50:137
3. Borowski, E., Starke, K., Ehrl, H., and Endo T. (1977): Neuroscience. 2:285-296.
4. Bylund, D. B. (1981): Pharmacologist. 23: 534.
5. Carlsson, A., Hillarp, N. A. and Waldeck, B. (1963): Acta Physiol.Scand. 59:Suppl. 1215 1-38.
6. Cohen, R. M., Aulakh, C. S., Campbell, I. C. and Murphy, D. L. (1982): Eur.J.Pharmacol. 81:145-148.
7. Colucci, W. S., Gimbrome, M. A., and Alexander, R. W. (1981): Circ.Res. 48(1):104-111.
8. Constantine, J. W. and Lebel, W. (1980): N.S.Arch.Pharmacol. 314:101-109.
9. Cooper, B., Handin, R. I., Young, L. H. and Alexander, R. W. (1978): Nature. 274:703-706.
10. Cubbedu, L. X., Barnes, E. M., Langer, S. Z. and Weiner, N. (1974): J.Pharmac.Exp.Ther. 190:431-450.
11. Dubocovitch, M. L. and Langer, S. Z. (1974): J.Physiol. 237:505-519.
12. Franklin, K. B. J. and Herberg, L. J. (1977):Eur.J.Pharmac. 43(1):33-38.
13. Glossmann, H. and Hornung, R. (1980): N.S.Arch.Pharmacol. 314:101-109.
14. Kempson, S., Marinetti, G. V. and Shaw, A. (1978): Biochem.Biophys.Acta. 540:320-329.
15. Lehmann, J. and Langer, S. Z. (1981): Eur.J.Pharmacol. 75: 247-250.
16. Nickerson, M. and Gump, W. S. (1949): J.Pharmacol.Exp.Ther. 97: 25-47.
17. Pelayo, F., Dubocovitch, M. L. and Langer, S. Z. (1980): Eur.J.Pharmacol. 64:153-155.
18. Reisine, T. (1981): Neuroscience. 6(8):1471-1503.
19. Robson, L. E. and Kosterlitz, H. W. (1979): Proc.Roy.Soc. London Ser.B. 205:425.
20. Shattil, S. J., McDonough, M. Turnbull, J., and Insel, P. A. (1981): Mol.Pharmacol. 19: 179-183.
21. Smith, C. B., Garcia-Sevilla, J. H., and Hollingsworth, P. J. (1981): Brain Res. 210: 413-418.
22. Strittmatter, W. J., Davies, J. N. and Lefkowitz, R. J. (1977): J.Biol.Chem. 252:5478-5482.
23. Strittmatter, W. J., Hirata, F., and Axelrod, J. (1979): Science. 204:1205-1207.
24. U'Prichard, D. C., Bechtel, W. B., Rouot, B. M. and Snyder, S. H. (1979): Mol.Pharmacol. 16:47-60.

CNS Receptors—From Molecular
Pharmacology to Behavior, edited by
P. Mandel and F. V. DeFeudis.
Raven Press, New York © 1983.

Receptor Hypothesis of the Alcohol Withdrawal State

[1]Mark A. Gillman and [1]Frederick J. Lichtigfeld

Department of Experimental and Clinical Pharmacology, University of Witwatersrand Medical School, Johannesburg, South Africa; and Department of Psychiatry, Rietfontein Hospital, Transvaal, South Africa

The alcohol withdrawal state (AWS) is characterised by a well defined cluster of signs and symptoms, which are manifestations of a complex of inter-related metabolic and neurotransmitter changes, which are set in motion primarily by chronic abuse, followed by alcohol withdrawal. It is the purpose of this paper to attempt to correlate these various factors, mainly from clinical observations and where possible, also from a neuro-chemical and metabolic standpoint.

HYPOXIA

Pure oxygen (O_2) has been shown to clear approximately two thirds of the physical symptoms of the Alcohol Withdrawal State (AWS). (54).

Van Wulfften Palte (82) showed that O_2 administration could reverse acute alcoholic intoxication, in addition he was able to improve cases of delirium tremens (DT's) by the administration of 95% O_2 with 5% CO_2 (to enhance ventilation). Other workers have noted the striking resemblance between alcohol intoxication and other anoxic states (57). Dembo and Kondrashenko (22) have demonstrated that hypoxia is an important mechanism in the pathogenesis of the AWS, while Victor (80) showed that O_2 and CO_2 could ameliorate this condition. Furthermore, ethanol is known to produce a reductive state (42,55), including a keto-acidemia, linked to the conversion of NAD to NADH. Oxidized diphosphopyridine nucleotide (DPN) has also been used to treat the AWS (63). These factors emphasize the importance of tissue anoxia, with the concomitant reductive state in the production of the syndrome of AWS.

---

[1]Co-Directors, The South African Brain Research Institute.

THE OPIOIDS

Nitrous oxide (N$_2$O) at analgesic concentrations ameliorates to a large degree the mainly behavioural symptoms of AWS (54). This supports the hypothesis that the opiate receptor is directly involved in the pathogenesis of the AWS since N$_2$O has been shown both in vitro (2) and in vivo (10, 32, 61) to be an opiate agonist. Furthermore, there is cross tolerance between ethanol and N$_2$0 (49), while endorphin (27) and met-enkephalin (56) release occurs following ethanol administration. The fact that Naloxone (Nx.) can reverse and met-enkephalin can potentiate ethanol - produced analgesia and anesthesia is further evidence implicating opioids in the pathogenesis of AWS (24). There have been a number of reports showing that alcohol-induced states can be influenced by Nx. (45, 46, 73).

In our work (in preparation) using Nx. at a dose of 2 mg - 4 mg, on 18 cases of acute alcoholic intoxication, single blind, 12 cases responded positively by becoming sedated within 15 minutes of iv. administration. Interestingly, in 12 other cases where Nx. 4 mg. was given double blind, 2 subjects responded to placebo, 4 to active substance, whilst the balance (2 with Nx. and 4 with placebo) showed no response. It is possible that the placebo response was caused by an opioid - mediated mechanism (53). Furthermore, in the single blind series 4 cases not responding to Nx. administration received the lower dose.

This positive response may be related to Nx. potentiating the opioid effect of ethanol in a manner analogous to that seen with morphine (34), and N$_2$0 (32).

The bipolar response seen with morphine and N$_2$0 has led us to postulate the dual-system hypothesis of pain perception (32), and this effect may indicate that the dual-system hypothesis must be extended from pain (31) and pleasure (35) to include other states.

Although there is considerable evidence implicating opioids in the mediation of the pharmacological effects of ethanol, there is also conflicting evidence. For instance Nx. has been reported to be ineffective in reversing the effects of ethanol (36, 40, 47).

However, this lack of effect may be due to the alcohol interacting with a receptor not sensitive to Nx. (41) and/or with receptors sensitive to other neurotransmitters. It is also possible that the Nx. may have potentiated the effects of the alcohol as described above.

THE MONOAMINES

ADRENALINE AND NOR-ADRENALINE

Beta-blockers have been used successfully in decreasing the hyper-adrenergic state invariably present in the AWS., this effect being postulated to have occurred by reversing adreno-receptor supersensitivity (70). This supersensitivity is similar to that seen in rats suffering from ethanol withdrawal, however in this case the alpha-receptor was shown to be super-sensitive (28).

The possible link between the opioid system and the adrenergic system will be described later (vide infra).

DOPAMINE (DA)

DA concentrations in the brains of sober chronic alcoholics are lower than in normal controls (72), whilst intoxicated alcoholics had a large increase in DA concentrations in their brains as compared to controls. As a result of this there is an increase in the DA metabolites salsolinol and other tetrahydroisoquinolines (72), which have been shown to interact with opiate receptors (38).

In addition, a Nx.-sensitive increase in DA metabolism is found in acutely intoxicated rats indicating that an opioid mechanism participates in this increased metabolism (67). This effect was found to be particularly pronounced in the nigrostriatal system (67).

It is conceivable that in chronic alcoholism following withdrawal the DA system is exhausted with consequent DA receptor supersensitivity causing symptoms such as tremor. This exhaustion is probable since there are decreased levels of homovanillic acid in the CSF of alcoholics showing withdrawal symptoms as compared to alcoholics not showing such symptoms (75).

In acute alcoholic intoxication, the administration of Nx. may cause sedation (as we found, vide supra) by antagonism of DA effects. This could occur as a result of the antagonism by Nx. of the analeptic effect of DA (43) since the arousal effect of DA is particularly strong in opiate-mediated coma including alcoholic stupor (43).

SEROTONIN

Serotonin (5HT) has been implicated in the development of tolerance to ethanol, in that lowered levels of this neurotransmitter seem to accelerate the loss of ethanol tolerance (48).

Pycock et al (66) have shown an increase in the release of 5HT caused by the administration of opiate agents. In addition, intracisternally — administered beta-endorphin increases concen-trations of both 5HT and its metabolite 5-hydroxy Indole Acetic Acid (5HIAA) (78).

In the presence of active ethanol metabolism there is an increase of the production of the alcoholic metabolites of 5HT viz, tryphtophol and 5-hydroxytryptophol (15).

These break-down products have a sedative and hypnotic effect in mice (15). When there is an increase in the metabolism of 5HT to these alcohol metabolites, there is a concomitant shift of the metabolism of 5HT away from 5HIAA to these substances. Furthermore, the levels of the alcohol derivatives of 5HT in the CSF decline after the last drink (8), thus possibly contributing to the restlessness, agitation and insomnia seen in the AWS. In addition, there is a relative deficiency of 5HIAA in the CSF of alcoholics showing florid symptoms during withdrawal as compared to controls (75). A deficiency of 5HIAA has been correlated with depression and suicidal tendencies in non-alcoholic psychiatric conditions (3). It is suggested that the depression and suicides related to the AWS may have a similar mechanism. The changes in 5HT levels alluded to above would furthermore be aggravated by depression of opioid activity.

GAMMA-AMINOBUTYRIC ACID

Ethanol can potentiate the action of gamma-aminobutyric acid (GABA) (59), and there is evidence that GABA is involved in the mechanism of action of ethanol (60). Moreover post-mortem receptor binding studies in human alcoholic brains (76) have shown an increase in GABA-receptor numbers associated with low levels of GABA, while GABA-ergic drugs have been used to antagonise AWS in experimental animals (19) by possibly compensating for decreased GABA-ergic inhibition (80). There is evidence that the benzodiazapines act on GABA-ergic mechanisms (20). Moreover a GABA-benzodiazepine receptor interaction may also be involved in ameliorating the AWS (58), in particular since purine bases modulate this interaction (21). This is possible since there may be a purine deficiency in alcoholism related to malnourishment.

A GABA link with the opiates has also been shown, since opiates can cause the release of GABA (66).

It is possible to speculate that a decrease of endogenous and exogenous opioid substances secondary to alcohol withdrawal would cause a deficiency of GABA giving rise to hyper-reflexia, restlessness and seizures.

We further hypothesize a mechanism similar to that causing GABA supersensitivity to cause opioid receptor hypersensitivity, the effects of which will be discussed below (vide infra).

ACETYLCHOLINE (ACh)

Arousal is mediated centrally in part by cholinergic mechanisms, as a result of the release of acetylcholine (ACh) from the axons of cell bodies in the reticular formation into diffuse cortical areas (7). In addition, it has been shown that injected amphetamine causes increased levels of ACh release in the cortex (6), this effect being prevented by a neuroleptic agent (62). It is therefore adduced from this that catecholamines are involved in mediating this release of ACh, and the anatomical locus of contact between these systems appears to be in the septum (62).

ACh content in striatal structures is increased during resting tremor (14). Infusion of ACh into the globus pallidus produces resting tremor, emphasizing the importance of this structure in the production of resting tremor (68).

It has been shown that opiate administration causes a decrease in ACh release which is antagonized by Nx (23). It is therefore possible that as a result of decreased opiate content centrally at withdrawal, there would be an increase in ACh content resulting in overstimulation of the striatum and an increase in the resting tremor. It has been suggested that a rise in ACh levels in the caudate nucleus could cause DA release (51). However, we postulate DA exhaustion during AWS, resulting in a further imbalance between DA and ACh with the enhancement of the resting tremor.

This idea is further supported since an impairment in DA metabolism can result in an increase in ACh release, thereby increasing the imbalance between ACh and DA (52).

Acetyl Coenzyme A is an important precursor of ACh synthesis, and during hypoxia this substance accumulates causing further production of ACh (71). The limiting factor appears to be thiamine since there may not be enough Acetyl Coenzyme A as a result of thiamine deficiency, to produce further ACh (23). We postulate from this that the degree of resting tremor could be influenced by the thiamine status.

ACh may mediate the release of anti-diuretic hormone (ADH) (23) and it has been shown that in withdrawing alcoholics there is a raised level of ADH (26).

This raised level of ADH was positively correlated with the degree of tremor indicating that there may be an ACh effect in the production of the tremor since ACh stimulates the release of ADH (26). In addition, ADH activates the locus coeruleus (LC) noradrenergic neurones thereby aggravating further the hyper-adrenergic state (64). This work demonstrates the dynamic state of imbalance between the adrenergic and the cholinergic states in AWS. This postulate is supported by the fact that nor-adrenaline tends to decrease ACh stimulation and hence ADH release (23). This fact underlines the importance of the balance between the nor-adrenergic and cholinergic systems generally and in particular (in this case) in relation to the supra-optic nucleus of the hypothalamus with regard to the secretion of ADH (23).

Aggressive behaviour has been related experimentally to cholinergic mechanisms located in the hypothalamus (23), and in addition there is evidence that nor-adrenaline acting on the ventral tegmental area of the mid-brain can also cause violent behaviour (4); thus, an increase in cholinergic and adrenergic tone could result in the aggressive behaviour seen in AWS.

The hippocampus appears to be related to recent memory (79)

and injections of muscarinic agents here produce learning impairment (37). It is thus conceivable that recent memory loss found in AWS is mediated by this mechanism. In addition the convulsions that occur during AWS may be mediated in part by cholinergic mechanisms (23).

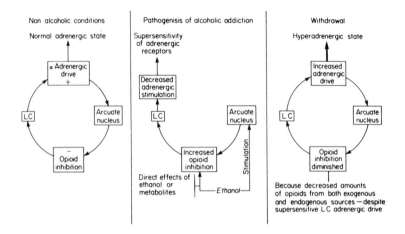

Fig. 1   The Opioid-Adrenergic Link

THE OPIOID-ADRENERGIC LINK (See Fig. 1)

The alpha adreno-receptor agonist clonidine that ameliorates the AWS (12) acts on LC neurones (1). The LC receives inhibitory opioid contacts from the arcuate nucleus of the hypothalamus (74). This reciprocal relationship could be involved in the pathogenesis of the hyperadrenergic state seen in AWS in the following manner; as a result of chronic alcoholic abuse and hence excessive opioid receptor stimulation, the adrenergic receptor is inhibited causing the adrenergic receptor to become super-sensitive, leading to the hyperadrenergic state following ethanol withdrawal. We suggest that under normal non-alcoholic conditions an increase in nor-adrenaline release causes an increase in beta-endorphin release which inhibits further nor-adrenaline secretion. It is therefore possible that this opioid - nor-adrenergic link may well be the final common pathway of all addictive withdrawal syndromes.

Thus the administration of an opiate agonist such as N_2O as shown in our work (54) inhibits the hyperadrenergic state. It is interesting to note that the administration of opium was a much employed treatment of delirium tremens in the last century (25).

A marker in alcohol withdrawal of the reductive state is the accumulation of keto acids and lactic acid. This acidosis has also been highly correlated with the intensity of hangover symptoms (84).

Seixas considered that the respiratory alkalosis that often occurred from about eight hours into the AWS might be the result of CNS sympathetic hyperactivity inducing the reactive hyper-ventilation (69). Hyperpnoea can be produced by impulses reaching the respiratory centre from the cerebral cortex as a result of emotional states, as well as from the hypothalamus (9). Thus the respiratory alkalosis that may occur during the course of the AWS may be the result of a compensatory reaction to the metabolic acidosis caused by lactic acid and keto-acids. The hyperventilation seen in these states may be, in part, of psychogenic origin as well. The hyper-adrenergic state can also compensate for the redox-state in the tissues by increasing cerebral oxygen consumption. This increase in oxygen utilisation was inhibited by Beta-Blockers, thus showing the pervasive influence of the hyperadrenergic state in the AWS syndrome (39).

The harmful consequences of the compensatory respiratory alkalosis usually associated with a low pCO_2 are:

1) Decreased cerebral blood flow aggravating cerebral anoxia by decreasing the elimination of acid metabolites (11,83)

2) Hyperventilation which increases the CSF lactate (16).

The increase of CSF lactate is directly related to severe and prolonged states of DT's (16). Under these circumstances DT's can be likened to a metabolic encephalopathy related to marked changes in the acid base balance in the CSF (18).

Thiamine deficiency is almost always present in chronic alcoholics and adds to the severity of the withdrawal symptomatology by increasing the lactate levels (65). Alcohol withdrawal seizures are associated with respiratory alkalosis (80) as well as with hypomagnesemia (80). The spectrum of metabolic disorders in AWS includes the development of ketoacidosis, with ketonuria and ketonaemia but without glucosuria (29). From the above it can be seen that the hyperadrenergic state originating centrally is further aggravated by the metabolic disorders consequent upon the reductive states.

The use of N_2O and O_2 to successfully reverse the symptoms of the AWS seems to indicate that the primary factors responsible for the pathology are tissue anoxia and an imbalance between the various neurotransmitter systems, particularly the increase in tone of both the nor-adrenergic and cholinergic systems. This increase in tone is associated with reduced activity in the opioid, serotonergic, dopaminergic and GABA-ergic systems. In the AWS there is then the unusual state of affairs where there is hyper-activity both in the cholinergic and nor-adrenergic systems occurring simultaneously as a result of release from opioid inhibition. The dopaminergic system because of its exhaustion in chronic alcoholics does not seem to react to release from opiate inhibition. The N_2O acting as an opiate agonist would tend to restore the balance by inhibiting the hyperactive systems and potentiating the hypo-active systems. These findings are based on clinical observations using N_2O and O_2 to treat AWS and as such cannot be an exhaustive review of all the myriad interactions seen in AWS.

A case in point is taurine (T) which may have a neuro-transmitter or neuromodulatory role in the CNS (50). There is excessive urinary excretion of this substance during AWS (77), which could indicate possible exhaustion of this agent in this condition.

The anti-epileptic effect of T (5) may have a role in the AWS and in fact this substance has proved beneficial in this condition (44).

Acknowledgments

This work was supported by a grant from the Anglo American Corporation. Our thanks to Mr L Kay for help with the artwork.

REFERENCES

1. Aghajanian, G. K. (1978): Nature. 276: 186-187
2. Ahmed, M. S., and Byrne, W. L. (1980): In: Endogenous and Exogenous opiate Agonists and Antagonists. Edited by E. L. Way. pp. 51-54. Pergamon. N.Y.
3. Asberg, M., Thoren, P., Traskman, L., Bertilsson, L., and Ringberger, V. (1976): Science. 191: 478-480
4. Bandler, R. J. (1971): Nature. 229: 222-223
5. Barbeau, A., and Donaldson, J. (1973): Lancet. 2: 387.
6. Bartolini, A., and Pepeu, G. (1970): Pharm. Res. Commun. 2: 23-29.
7. Bartolini, A., Weisenthal, L. M., and Domino, E. F. (1972): Neuropharmacology. 11: 113-122.
8. Beck, O., Borg, S., Holmstedt, B., Kvande, H., and Skroder, R. (1980): Acta. Pharmacol. et. toxiol. 47: 305-307.
9. Best, H. C., and Taylor, N. B. (1945): The Physiological Basis of Medical Practice. Fourth Edition. Williams and Wilkins Company. Baltimore.
10. Berkowitz, B. A., Finck, A. D., and Ngai, S. H. (1977): J. Pharmacol. Exp. Ther. 203: 539-547.
11. Berglund, M., and Risberg, J. (1981): Arch. Gen. Psychiat. 38: 351-355.
12. Bjorkqvist, S. E. (1975): Acta. Psychiat. Scand. 52: 256-263.
13. Blum, K., Hamilton, M. G., and Wallace, J. E. (1977): In: Alcohol and opiates. edited by K. Blum. pp. 203-236. Academic Press. New York.
14. Bordeleau, J. (1961): Systeme extra-pyramidal et neuro-leptiques. Psychiatriques. Montreal.
15. Bowman, W. C., and Rand, M. J. (1980): Textbook of Pharmacology. Blackwell. Oxford.
16. Brooks, B. R., and Adams, R. D. (1975): Neurology. 25: 935-

942.
17. Brooks, B. R., and Adams, R. D. (1975): Neurology. 25: 943-948.
18. Cole, M. (1969): In: Special Techniques for Neurologic Diagnosis. edited by J. F. Toole. pp. 29-48. F. A. Davis Company. Philadelphia.
19. Cooper, B. R., Viik, K., Ferris, R., and White, H. L. (1979): J. Pharmacol. Exp. Ther. 209: 396-403.
20. Costa, E., Guilotti, A., and Toffano, G. (1978): Br. J. Psychiat. 13: 248.
21. Crawley, J. N., Marangos, P. J., and Paul, S. M. (1981): Science. 211: 725-726.
22. Dembo, A. G., and Kondrashenko, V. T. (1979): Klin. Med. (Mosk). 57: 71-77.
23. DeFeudis, F.V. (1974): Central cholinergic systems and behaviour. Academic Press. London.
24. Diamond, B. J., Schwartz, B. A., Handala, H. J., Mady, V., Patel, K., and Borison, R. C. (1981): Anesthesiology: A228.
25. Dixon, E. L. (1854): Lancet. 2: 396.
26. Eisenhofer, G., Whiteside, E., Lambie, D., and Johnson, R. (1982): Lancet. 1:50.
27. Eskelson, C. D., Hameroff, S. R., and Kansell, J. S. (1980): Anesth. and Analg. 59:537-8.
28. French, S. W., and Palmer, D. S. (1973): Res. Commun. Chem. Pathol. Pharmacol. 6: 651-662.
29. Fulop, M., and Hoberman, H. D. (1975): Diabetes. 24: 785-790.
30. Gerner, R. H., Catlin, D. H., Gorelick, D. A., Hui, K. K., and Li, C. H. (1980): Arch. Gen. Psychiatry. 37: 641-647
31. Gillman, M. A., Kimmel, I., and Lichtigfeld, F. J. (1981): Neurolog. Res. 3: 317-327.
32. Gillman, M. A., Kok, L., and Lichtigfeld, F. J. (1980): Europ. J. Pharmacol. 2: 175-177.
33. Gillman, M. A., and Lichtigfeld, F. J. (1981): Brit. Med. J. 203: 64.
34. Gillman, M. A., and Lichtigfeld, F. J. (1981): J. Neurolog. Sci. 49: 41-45.
35. Gillman, M. A., and Lichtigfeld, F. J.: J. Sex Research (in Press).
36. Goldstein, A., and Judson, B. A. (1972): Science. 172: 290-292.
37. Greene, E. G., and Lomax, P. (1970): Brain Res. 18: 355-359
38. Hamilton, M. G., Hirst, M., and Blum, K. (1979): Life Sc. 25: 2205-2210.
39. Hemmingsen, R., Barry, D. I., and Hertz, M. M. (1979): In: Cerebral Blood Flow and Metabolism. edited by F. Gotoh, H. Ngai, and Y. Razaki, pp. 108-109. Acta. Neurologica Scandinavica Suppl.
40. Hemmingsen, R., and Sorensen, S. C. (1980): Acta.

Pharmacol. et toxiol. 46: 62-65.
41. Hiller, J. M., Angel, L. M., and Simon, E. J. (1981):
Science. 214: 468-469.
42. Himwich, H. W., Nahum, L. H., Rakieten, N., Fazikas, J. F.,
Du Bois, D., and Gildea, E. F. (1933): J.A.M.A. 100:
651-652.
43. Hoagland, R. J. (1965): Am. J. Med. Sci. 249: 623-635.
44. Ikeda, H. (1977): Lancet. 2: 509.
45. Jeffcoate, W. J., Cullen, M. H., Herbert, M., Hastings, A.
G. and Walder, C. P. (1979): Lancet. 2: 1157-59.
46. Jeffreys, D. B., Flanagan, R. J., and Volans, C. N. (1980):
Lancet, 1: 308-309.
47. Jorgensen, H. A., and Hole, K. (1981): Europ. J. Pharmacol.
75: 223-229.
48. Khanna, J. M., Kalant, H., Lê, A. D., Le Blanc, A. H.
(1981): Prog. Neuro-Psycholopharmacol. 5: 459-465.
49. Koblin, D. D., Deady, J. E., Dong, D. E., Eger, 11 I,
(1980): Alcohol. J. Pharm. and Exp. Ther. 213: 309-312.
50. Kruk, Z. L., and Pycock, C. J. (1979): Neurotransmitters
and Drugs. Croom and Helm. London.
51. Lalley, P. M., Rossi, G. V., and Baker, W. W. (1970): Exp.
Neurol. 27: 258-275.
52. La Rochelle, L., Bedard, P., Poirier, L. J., and Sourkes,
T. L. (1971): Neuropharmacology. 10: R73-288.
53. Levine, J. D., Gordon, N. C., and Fields, H. L. (1979):
Nature. 278: 740-741.
54. Lichtigfeld, F. J., and Gillman, M. A. (1982): S.A.M.J. 61:
349-351.
55. Lieber, C. S. (1977): In: Metabolic Aspects of Alcoholism.
edited by C. S. Lieber. page 3. MTP Press. Lancaster.
56. Medbacks, S. quoted by: Jeffcoate, W. J., Hastings, A. G.,
Cullen, M. H. and Herbert, M. (1981): Lancet. 1: 1052.
57. McFarland, R. A., and Barach, A. L. (1936). Am. J. Med. Sc.
192: 186-198.
58. Mitchell, R. (1980): Eur. J. Pharmacology. 68: 369-372.
59. Nestoros, J. N. (1980): Science. 209: 708-710.
60. Nestoros, J. N. (1980): Life Sc. 26:519-523.
61. Ngai, S. H. and Finck, A. D. (1981): Anesthesiology. 58A:
241.
62. Nistri, A., Bartolini, A., Deffenu, G., and Pepeu, G.
(1972): Neuropharmacology. 11: 668.
63. O'Hollaren, P. (1961): Western J. Surgery, Obstetrics and
Gynae. 69: 101-104.
64. Olpe, H. R. and Baltzer, V. (1981): Europ. J. Pharmacol.
73: 377-378.
65. Peters, R. A. (1967): In: Thiamine deficiency: Biochemical
Lesions and their chemical significance. edited by G. E.
W. Wolstenholme and Maeve O'Connor. pp. 1-8. J. and A.
Churchill. London.
66. Pycock, C. J., Burns, S., and Morris, R. (1981):
Neuroscience Letters. 22: 313-317.

67. Reggiani, A., Barbaccia, M. L., Spano, P. F. and Trabucchi, M. (1980): Substance and Alcohol actions misuse. 1: 151-158.
68. Ruzdik, N. and Stern, P. (1966): Med. Pharm. Exp. 14: 17.
69. Seixas, F. A. (1973): Alcoholism and the central nervous system. edited by F. A. Seixas, S. Eggleston, p. 214. Annals New York Academy, New York.
70. Sellers, E. M., Degani, N. C., Zilm, D. H. and Macleod, S. M. (1976): Lancet. 1: 94-95.
71. Schuberth, J., Sollenberg, J., Sundwall, A. and Sorbo, B. (1966): J. Neurochem. 13: 819-822.
72. Sjöquist, B., Eriksson, A., and Winblad, B. (1982): Lancet, 1: 675-676.
73. Sorensen, S. C., Mattisson, K. W. (1978): Lancet. 2: 688-689.
74. Strahlendorf, H. K., Strahlendorf, J. C., and Barnes, C. D. (1978): Brain Research. 191: 284-285.
75. Takahashi, S., Yamane, H., Kondo, H., Tani, N. and Kato, N. (1974): Folio Psychiatrica et Neurologica Japonica. 28: 347-354.
76. Tran, V. T., Snyder, S. G., Major, L. F. and Hawley, R. S. (1981): Am. Neurol. 9: 289-292.
77. Turner, F. P. and Brum, V. C. (1964): J. Surg. Res. 4. 423-431.
78. Van Loon, G. R. and De Souza, E. B. (1978): Life Sc. 23: 971-978.
79. Victor, M., Angevine, J. B., Mancall, E. L. and Fisher, M. (1961): Archs. Neurol. 5: 244-263.
80. Victor, M. (1977): In: Alcoholism and the Central Nervous System. Edited by F. A. Seixas and S. Eggleston. Ann. N.Y. Acad. Sci. pp. 235-248. N.Y. Acad. Sci.
81. Volicer, L. (1980): Brain Rs. Bull S. suppl. 2: 809-813.
82. Van Wulfften Palthe, P. M. (1926): Deutsch Ztschr f Nervenhk. 92: 79-100.
83. Wollman, H., Smith, T. C., Stephen, G. W., Colton, E. T. III, Gleaton, H. E. and Alexander, S. G. (1968): J. of Appl. Physiology. 24: 60-65.
84. Ylikahri, R. H., Pöso, A. R., Huttunen, M. O., Hillbom, M. E. (1974): Scand. J. Clin. Lab. Invest. 34: 327-336.

CNS Receptors—From Molecular
Pharmacology to Behavior, edited by
P. Mandel and F. V. DeFeudis.
Raven Press, New York © 1983.

α- and β-Adrenoceptors on Cultured Glial Cells

L. Hösli, Elisabeth Hösli, C. Zehntner, R. Lehmann, and T. W. Lutz

Department of Physiology, University of Basel, CH-4051 Basel, Switzerland

Although biochemical and autoradiographic binding studies provide good evidence that glial cells possess both α- and β-receptors (1,3,4,6), there is as yet no information on physiological
and pharmacological properties of these glial adrenoceptors.
In the present study we have tested the actions of α- and β-adrenoceptor agonists and antagonists on the membrane potential of
cultured astrocytes. Furthermore, an attempt was made to visualize binding sites for noradrenaline and α- and β-antagonists on
cultured glial cells using autoradiography.

MATERIAL AND METHODS

Explants of spinal cord, lower brain stem and cerebellum of
fetal (18-20 days in utero) and newborn rats were placed on colla-
gen-coated coverslips and grown either in Maximov double cover-
slip assemblies or in roller tubes (for details see 7,8,9). The
methods for the electrophysiological and the autoradiographic binding studies have been described in detail in previous publications (6,9).

RESULTS AND DISCUSSION

Noradrenaline (NA) and the α-agonist phenylephrine (PE) which
were added to the bathing fluid at concentrations of 10^{-7}M to
10^{-4}M caused depolarizations of most glial cells tested (Fig. 1).
These depolarizations were clearly concentration-dependent, the
threshold concentration being 10^{-7}M. They were reversibly blocked
by the α-antagonist phentolamine (10^{-5}M and 10^{-6}M). The β-antagonist atenolol, however, did not affect the depolarizations produced by NA (9). This indicates that the depolarization by these
adrenergic compounds is mediated by activation of α-receptors. In
contrast, the β-agonist isoprenaline (ISO, 10^{-6}M) produced hyperpolarizations which were antagonized by atenolol and, therefore,

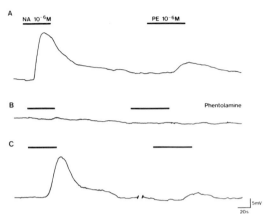

FIG. 1.   Action of the α-antagonist phentolamine on the depolarizations produced by noradrenaline (NA) and phenylephrine (PE) of a glial cell (brain stem culture, 38 days in vitro; membrane potential -69 mV).   A: Depolarizations by NA (10^{-6}M) and PE (10^{-6}M). B: After perfusion with bathing solution containing phentolamine (10^{-6}M), the depolarizations by NA and PE were blocked after 1 and 4 min respectively.   C: Recovery of the NA- and PE-depolarizations was observed 3 and 8 min after wash-out of phentolamine. Duration of perfusion with NA and PE is indicated by horizontal bars (from Hösli et al., 9).

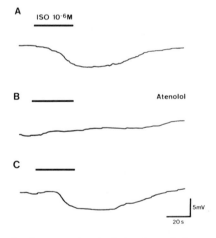

FIG. 2.   Effect of the β-antagonist atenolol on the hyperpolarization of a glial cell by isoprenaline (ISO).   A: Hyperpolarization by ISO (10^{-6}M).   B: Perfusion of the culture with atenolol (10^{-4}M) completely blocked the hyperpolarization by ISO after 2 min.   C: Recovery was observed 2 min after wash-out of atenolol. (Spinal cord culture, 28 days in vitro; membrane potential -75 mV). Duration of perfusion with ISO is indicated by horizontal bars (from Hösli et al., 9).

appeared to be due to stimulation of β-receptors (Fig. 2). During the hyperpolarization by ISO, no change in membrane resistance was observed (9). The effects of adrenergic agonists and antagonists on the glial membrane potential are similar to those observed on neurones of the central nervous system (2) and on smooth muscle preparations (5,12). Since the depolarizations by NA and PE and the hyperpolarizations by ISO were observed on the same glial cell (Fig. 3), it is suggested that α- and β-adrenoceptors coexist on the membrane of the same astrocyte.

Evidence for the existence of α- and β-adrenoceptors on glial cells was also obtained from autoradiographic studies which revealed binding sites for NA and α- and β-antagonists on cultured astrocytes (6). Fig. 4A shows binding for the β-antagonist ^{3}H-carazolol and fig. 4B illustrates glial cells labelled by the α-antagonist ^{3}H-prazosin. Glial cells also showed binding sites for the antidepressant ^{3}H-desmethylimipramine (6), a compound which is most likely associated with presynaptic noradrenergic sites (10,11).

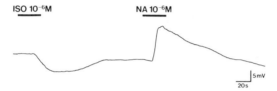

FIG. 3.   Hyperpolarization by isoprenaline (ISO, 10^{-6}M) and depolarization by noradrenaline (NA, 10^{-6}M) of the same glial cell (spinal cord culture, 19 days in vitro, membrane potential -75 mV).

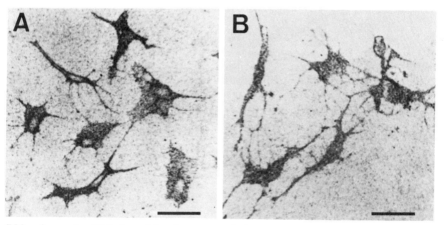

FIG. 4.   A: Glial cells in a cerebellar culture showing binding of the β-antagonist ^{3}H-carazolol (10^{-8}M, Na$^+$-free incubation medium, culture 20 days in vitro).   B: Moderately labelled glial cells after incubation with the α-antagonist ^{3}H-prazosin (10^{-8}M, Na$^+$-free incubation medium, brain stem culture 25 days in vitro). Bars 30 μm (from Hösli and Hösli, 6).

SUMMARY AND CONCLUSIONS

The action of α- and β-adrenoceptor agonists and antagonists has been studied on the membrane potential of glial cells in cultured rat central nervous system. Noradrenaline and the α-agonist phenylephrine caused a depolarization which was reversibly blocked by the α-antagonist phentolamine. In contrast, the β-agonist isoprenaline hyperpolarized the glial membrane. This hyperpolarization was not associated with measurable changes in membrane resistance and was antagonized by the β-blocker atenolol. These results suggest that the glial depolarization is mediated by activation of α-receptors, whereas the hyperpolarization is due to stimulation of β-receptors. The existence of α- and β-adrenoceptors on glial cells is further supported by autoradiographic studies showing binding of noradrenaline and α- and β-antagonists to astrocytes.

REFERENCES

1. Barovsky, K. and Brooker, G. (1980): J. Cycl. Nucleo. Res., 6: 297-307.
2. Bevan, P., Bradshaw, C.M. and Szabadi, E. (1977): Br. J. Pharmac., 59: 635-641.
3. Ebersolt, C., Perez, M. and Bockaert, J. (1981): J. Neurosci. Res., 6: 643-652.
4. Ebersolt, C., Perez, M., Vassent, G. and Bockaert, J. (1981): Brain Res., 213: 151-161.
5. Haeusler, G. and Thorens, S. (1980): J. Physiol. (Lond.), 303: 203-224.
6. Hösli, E. and Hösli, L. (1982): Neuroscience, in press.
7. Hösli, E., Möhler, H., Richards, J.G. and Hösli, L. (1980): Neuroscience, 5: 1657-1665.
8. Hösli, L., Hösli, E., Andrès, P.F. and Wolff, J.R. (1975): Golgi Centennial Symposium, Proceedings, edited by M. Santini, pp. 473-488, Raven Press, New York.
9. Hösli, L., Hösli, E., Zehntner, Ch., Lehmann, R. and Lutz, T.W. (1982): Neuroscience, in press.
10. Lee, C.M. and Snyder, S.H. (1981): Proc. Natl. Acad. Sci. USA, 78: 5250-5254.
11. Rehavi, M., Skolnick, P., Brownstein, M.J. and Paul, S.M. (1982): J. Neurochem., 38: 889-895.
12. Somlyo, A.V., Haeusler, G. and Somlyo, A.P. (1970): Science, 169: 490-491.

CNS Receptors—From Molecular
Pharmacology to Behavior, edited by
P. Mandel and F. V. DeFeudis.
Raven Press, New York © 1983.

Histamine-Induced Responses in Mammalian Brain Slices: Characterization of H_1 and H_2 Receptors

M. Garbarg, J. M. Arrang, A. M. Duchemin, T. T. Quach, C. Rose, and J. C. Schwartz

Unité 109 de Neurobiologie, Centre Paul Broca de l'INSERM, 75014 Paris, France

Histamine (HA) meets many of the essential requirements of a neurotransmitter in the mammalian brain (17). The evidence for a possible role for HA in neuronal communication in brain partly comes from the demonstration of the interaction of the amine with specific receptors. The pharmacological characterisation of biological responses to HA in various peripheral systems has led to the definition of two subclasses of receptors, termed H_1 and H_2, respectively (1).

More recently, electrophysiological and physiological approaches have allowed the identification of both classes of receptors in mammalian brain (15).

The utilisation of radioligand binding techniques to study these two classes of receptors in brain has been tried, but has met a variable success. Thus, in the case of H_2-receptors, in spite of many attempts performed with either antagonists (^{3}H-cimetidine, ^{3}H-tiotidine) or agonists (^{3}H-impromidine), this aim has not been achieved until now. In contrast, the H_1-antihistamine mepyramine was tritiated and used successfully to label HA H_1-receptors in homogenates of smooth muscle of the guinea-pig ileum (8). It has been subsequently shown in several laboratories that ^{3}H-mepyramine can be used to label H_1-receptors in particulate fractions of the brains of various animal species (2,7). Although selective lesions in the rat brain have as yet failed to allow identification of the cells bearing H_1-receptors, the ontogenetic development and the synaptosomal localisation of the labelled H_1-receptors suggest that they constitute a neuronal population of sites. This view is strengthened by the recent autoradiographic localisation of ^{3}H-mepyramine binding sites, apparently on dendrites of Purkinje cells in guinea-pig cerebellum (11). In addition to these in vitro studies, ^{3}H-mepyramine has also been used to label cerebral H_1-receptors in the living mouse (13). This simple test allows assessment not only of the apparent affinity of various compounds for H_1-receptors but also their biodisposition in the CNS. It was shown, for instance, that several tricyclic antidepressants occupy a significant fraction of H_1-receptors in brain following administration in low dosage.

On the other hand, the research aiming to uncover the physiological significance of HA in the CNS has taken advantage of the study of the HA-mediated events. In this respect, brain slices have offered many possibilities.

1. Histamine-induced glycogenolysis in mouse brain slices: Characterisation of H_1-receptors

We have recently devised a simple technique to evaluate the glycogenolytic action of various neurotransmitters on brain tissue. During incubation in the presence of ^{3}H-glucose brain slices accumulate ^{3}H-glycogen linearly with time up to 30 min,after which a plateau is maintained for at least 30 min. The addition of HA (100 μM) results in a rapid fall of the ^{3}H-glycogen content which reaches within 15 min a plateau representing 25 ± 5 % of the level in control slices (12). The ^{3}H-glycogen hydrolysis elicited by HA is clearly concentration-related (table 1).

TABLE 1. Effect of preincubation of slices from mouse cortex with histamine on histamine-induced hydrolysis of ^{3}H-glycogen and parameters of ^{3}H-mepyramine binding

Preincubation	HA-induced glycogenolysis		^{3}H-mepyramine binding	
	EC_{50} (μM)	Maximal effect (%)	Ki of HA (μM)	Maximal capacity (fmoles.mg protein^{-1})
0	4 ± 1	70 ± 5	40 ± 10	43.7 ± 2.9
HA (50 μM)	32 ± 0.6**	70 ± 4	25 ± 8	35.6 ± 2.7**

**p < 0.05
After 20 min preincubation, slices were washed three times.
For ^{3}H-glycogen hydrolysis, they were then incubated with increasing concentrations of HA.
For ^{3}H-mepyramine binding, they were homogenized in phosphate buffer before the assays (14).

The relative potencies of various agonists (dimaprit being totally ineffective) and the competitive inhibition restricted to one class of HA-receptor antagonist indicate that the HA-induced glycogenolysis is selectively mediated by typical H_1-receptors. For instance, the inactive enantiomer of chlorpheniramine is about 500-fold less potent than the active form (figure 1).

FIGURE 1. Inhibition of histamine-induced glycogenolysis by (+) and (-) chlorpheniramine in slices from mouse cerebral cortex

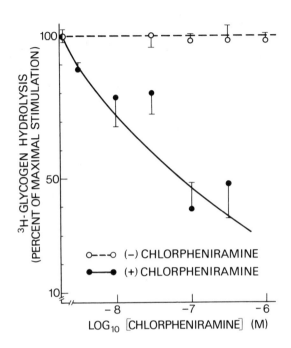

After a 30-min preincubation in the presence of ^{3}H-glucose, slices were incubated for 20 min following the addition of HA (50 μM) alone or in the presence of increasing concentrations of (+) or (-) chlorpheniramine. The response elicited by 50 μM HA in the absence of antagonist is definied as 100 % and responses in the presence of each stereoisomer are expressed relative to this value. ^{3}H-glycogen levels were 55.0 $\pm$ 5.2 and 15.9 $\pm$ 0.7 dpm.10^3.mg protein^{-1} in the absence and in the presence of HA, respectively (12). The antagonism of HA by (+) chlorpheniramine occurred with an apparent K_B value of 2 x 10^{-9} M consistent with interaction with H_1-receptors.

Furthermore, the existence of a "receptor reserve" would be consistent with the high sensitivity of this physiologic response. It appears that the HA-induced glycogenolysis involves translocation of calcium ions, as already described for a large number of actions mediated by H_1-receptors.

This model was used to investigate the desensitisation process (14). When slices were pre-exposed to HA, a shift to the right of the concentration-response curve to the amine could be subsequently observed whereas the maximal glycogenolytic response was not changed (table 1). The decrease in responsiveness to the glycogenolytic action of HA was a progressive, reversible and specific process involving only H_1-receptors.

Interestingly, the desensitisation process is accompanied by a decrease in the number of ^{3}H-mepyramine binding sites. This is not due to inhibition of ^{3}H-mepyramine binding by HA remaining in the preparation submitted to the radio-receptor assay, because the apparent affinity for the ^{3}H-antihistamine was not modified. However, the functional significance of the small decrease in the number of ^{3}H-mepyramine binding sites remains doubtful. When compared to the important shift in the concentration-response curve to HA, it might suggest that desensitisation involves changes not only at the level of H_1-receptors but also at the level of intracellular events associated with the HA-induced stimulation.

2. Histamine-stimulated cyclic AMP accumulation : characterisation of H_1 and H_2 receptors

HA receptors also mediate the formation of 3'-5' cyclic AMP in a concentration-dependent manner. Both classes of HA receptors are involved in a complex way. In cell-free preparations, a HA-sensitive adenylate cyclase has been characterized, the enzyme being coupled to typical H_2-receptors strictly identified by the inhibition constant of antagonists and relative potencies of agonists (6). In contrast, the cyclic AMP response to HA in intact brain cells is mediated by both H_1- and H_2-receptors (10). The H_1-receptors do not appear to be coupled with the adenylate cyclase but mediate an indirect stimulatory effect, perhaps through translocation of calcium ions (15). In this way, the response to a fixed concentration of HA is inhibited in a clearly biphasic manner by promethazine, a predominantly H_1-antihistamine, in increasing concentrations (figure 2).

FIGURE 2. Histamine and impromidine induced stimulation of cyclic AMP accumulation in slices from guinea-pig
hippocampus.

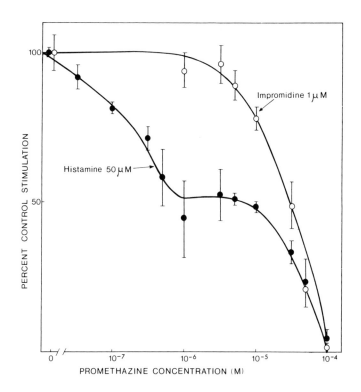

The accumulation of cyclic AMP (in pmoles.mg protein^{-1})
was 64.0 ± 2.7 in the presence of 50 μM HA and
39.7 ± 2.2 in the presence of 1 μM impromidine. Basal
levels (11.6 ± 1.3 pmoles.mg protein^{-1}) were not
altered in the presence of promethazine in concentrations up to 100 μM (3).

Among the two components of the HA response distinguished
by promethazine, the first is likely to be mediated by H_1-recep-
tors (3) whereas the second is mediated by H_2-receptors. Hence,
the Ki value of promethazine (obtained from the EC_{50} value) in
the first component is 0.022 μM and that of the second component
is 5.5 μM, a value close to the Ki value of 3.0 μM derived from

the monophasic inhibition of the response to impromidine, a specific highly selective H_2-receptor agonist(4).
    Recently a large number of structurally diverse drugs
with clinical antidepressant properties, including the so-called
"atypical" compounds,have been reported to share the ability to
act as potent inhibitors (Ki values in the range of 10 nM) of
HA-sensitive adenylate cyclase in cell free preparations from
guinea pig brain (5,9),and it has been proposed that this action
represents the molecular basis for their antidepressant activities. We have tested the possibility that the peculiar pharmacological specificity of H_2-receptors evidenced with brain homogenates depends on the kind of preparation used. For this purpose
intact slices, i.e, slices from guinea-pig hippocampus, were stimulated by impromidine (4),   thus avoiding interferences with
H_1-receptors also present in this test system.

TABLE 2. Compared potencies of various drugs as inhibitors of
         the H_2-receptor-mediated stimulation of cyclic AMP for-
         mation in slices and homogenates from guinea-pig hip-
         pocampus

Drugs	Inhibition constants (Ki, μM)	
	Slices[::]	Homogenates[#]
Antidepressants		
Clomipramine	> 10	0.05
Imipramine	> 10	0.20
Desipramine	> 10	0.30
Amitriptyline	3.5	0.04
Mianserin	10	0.06
H_1-Antihistamines		
Promethazine	3.0	0.03
Cyproheptadine	5.7	0.04
H_2-Antihistamines		
Cimetidine	0.6	0.7
Metiamide	0.8	0.9

[::]Values from (3)

[#]Values (from 5.9)

While typical H_2-antihistamines,like metiamide and cimetidine, were equally potent on cell-free and intact cell preparations,the tricyclic antidepressants were much less potent (about two orders of magnitude) as H_2-receptor antagonists on slices than on homogenates from the same tissue (16). The reasons for this difference are still not clarified but the idea that interaction with H_2-receptors represents the mode of action of antidepressants is also not substantiated by the failure of chronic treatments with mianserin to block H_2-receptors linked to cyclic AMP (Nowak, Arrang, Schwartz and Garbarg, in press).

In conclusion, brain slices have offered an in vitro model suitable for the measurement of the biological effects resulting from the interaction of HA with specific receptors and for their pharmacological characterisation. The two classes of HA receptors defined in peripheral systems are present in mammalian brain ; the H_1-receptors mediate the HA-induced glycogenolysis and are involved in the cyclic AMP response to HA whereas the H_2-receptors are directly linked to an adenylate cyclase.

REFERENCES

1. Black, J.W., Duncan, W.A.M., Durant, C.J., Ganellin, C.R., and Parsons. E.M. (1972) : Nature, 236 : 385-390
2. Chang, R.S.L., Tan Tran, V., and Snyder, S.H. (1978) : Eur. J. Pharmacol., 48 : 463-464
3. Dam Trung Tuong, M., Garbarg, M.,and Schwartz, J.C. (1980) : Nature, 287 : 548-551
4. Durant, G.J., Duncan, W.A.M., Ganellin, C.R., Parsons, M.E., Blakemore, R.C., and Rasmussen, A.C. (1978) : Nature, 276 : 403-405
5. Green, J.P. and Maayani, S. (1977) : Nature, 269 : 163-165
6. Hegstrand, L.R., Kanof, P.D., and Greengard, P. (1976) : Nature, 260 : 163-165
7. Hill, S.J., Emson, P.C., and Young, J.M. (1978) : J. Neurochem., 31 : 997-1004
8. Hill, S.J., Young, J.M., and Marrian, D.H. (1977) ; Nature, 270 : 361-363
9. Kanof, P.D. and Greengard, P. (1978) : Nature, 272 : 329-333
10. Palacios, J.M., Garbarg, M., Barbin, G. and Schwartz, J.C. (1978) : Mol. Pharmacol., 14 : 971-982
11. Palacios, J.M., Wamsley, J.K., and Kuhar, M.J. : Brain Research. (in press)
12. Quach, T.T., Duchemin, A.M., Rose, C., and Schwartz, J.C. (1980) : Mol. Pharmacol., 17 : 301-308

13. Quach, T.T., Duchemin, A.M., Rose, C., and Schwartz, J.C. (1980) : Neurosci. Letters, 17 : 49 54
14. Quach, T.T., Duchemin, A.M., Rose, C., and Schwartz, J.C. (1981) : Mol. Pharmacol., 20 : 331-338
15. Schwartz, J.C. (1979) : Life Sci., 25 : 895-912
16. Schwartz, J.C., Garbarg, M., and Quach, T.T. (1981) : Trends Pharmacol. Sci., 2 (5) : 122-125
17. Schwartz, J.C., Pollard, H., and Quach, T.T. (1980) : J. Neurochem., 35 (1) : 26-33

CNS Receptors—From Molecular
Pharmacology to Behavior, edited by
P. Mandel and F. V. DeFeudis.
Raven Press, New York © 1983.

Receptors for Lactogenic Hormones in Rabbit Hypothalamus: Properties and Regulation

Raffaele Di Carlo and Giampiero Muccioli

Institute of Pharmacology, University of Turin, 10125 Torino, Italy

It is well known that growth hormone (GH) is able to autoregulate its own secretion via the hypothalamus (14,20)with a negative feedback system (18). If GH acts directly on the hypothalamus then this target must possess specific receptors for GH. However few data are at present available on this subject.

Recently we have identified and characterized specific prolactin (PRL) binding sites in the rabbit hypothalamus (2). In the present research we report our results on the presence of GH binding sites in membranes isolated from different brain regions of the rabbit using ^{125}I-human GH (hGH),a hormone possessing both growth-promoting and lactogenic properties.

MATERIALS AND METHODS

Membrane preparation

Male and female New Zealand rabbits, 4-90 days of age, were killed by decapitation between 09.00 and 11.00 h and their brains removed and dissected as previously described (2). The hypothalamus, cerebellum, cerebral cortex, pons-medulla and a specimen of liver were homogenized at 4°C in 20 volumes of 0.3 M sucrose using a Polytron PT-10. The homogenate was fractionated by differential centrifugation to yield 600 x g, 15,000 x g and 100,000 x g pellets, according to the

method described by Posner et al. (15). Membranes from
3-4 brain regions were pooled for each experiment.

Binding assay

The binding assay was performed with slight modification as described by Shiu et al. (17) with 100,000
x g pellet, which is referred to as the main membrane
preparation containing lactogenic receptors. The membrane pellet was resuspended in ice-cold 25 mM Tris-
HCl, 10 mM $MgCl_2$, pH 7.4, for protein measurement (12)
and for binding assay. ^{125}I-labeled hGH (spec. act.
76-113 µCi/µg), iodinated using a modification of the
Hunter and Greenwood method (10)was purchased from
New England Nuclear (Boston, Ma, U.S.A.). The integrity of the labeled hormone was verified on membranes
from early lactating rabbit mammary gland and from
female rat liver. In the binding assay, approximately
60,000 cpm of labeled hormone were added to each tube,
containing 0.2 mg of membrane protein in a final vol
of 0.5 ml assay buffer (25 mM Tris-HCl, 10 mM $MgCl_2$,
0.1% bovine serum albumin, pH 7.4).

After 16 h of incubation at 20°C, bound and free
^{125}I-hGH were separated by low-speed centrifugation for
30 min at 4°C. The supernatant was decanted and the
membrane pellet was counted for radioactivity in a
Packard auto-gamma counter. The specific binding was
calculated as the differences between binding in the
absence and the presence of excess (2 µg/ml) of unlabeled hGH, expressed as percent of the total counts
added to the incubation medium.

Scatchard analyses (16) of the hGH binding to
hypothalamus, pons-medulla and liver membranes were also performed by transformation of binding data from
the competition studies with increasing concentrations
of unlabeled hGH, mixed with a fixed amount of tracer.
The dissociation constant (K_d) and binding capacity (n)
were determined for unlabeled hormone concentrations
between 1.6 and 60 ng/ml. Scatchard plots of binding
data of hGH to hypothalamus and pons-medulla membranes
were analyzed by assuming two independent noncoopera-
tive classes of binding sites, using the limiting
slopes technique of Hunston (9). Degradation studies of
labeled tracer for possible hormone damage during iodi-

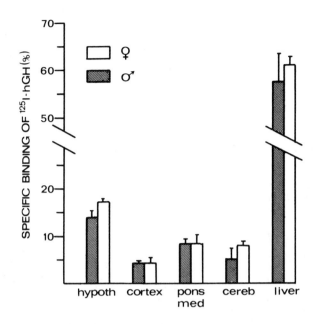

FIG. 1 - Specific binding of ^{125}I-hGH to membranes from liver and from different regions of the rabbit brain. Values are means of 3-5 experiments.

nation or incubation with membrane preparation were performed, but no corrections have been made for Scatchard analysis, owing to the low degrading activity.

The binding specificity of ^{125}I-hGH was tested with the following unlabeled hormones: ovine PRL (NIAMDD-oPRL-14), rat GH (NIAMDD-1-4), rat LH (NIAMDD-1), rat FSH (NIAMDD-RP-1), human GH (NIAMDD-RP-1) and porcine insulin (Schwarz/Mann).

In order to gain insight into the mechanism of hGH binding to its hypothalamic receptor, membranes from male rabbit hypothalamus were incubated in the presence of increasing concentrations of concanavalin A (Con A, Pharmacia, Uppsala). The reaction was carried out with either ^{125}I-hGH or ^{125}I-ovine prolactin (oPRL) The binding was determined as previously described. To reverse the inhibition induced by Con A the competitive sugar α-methyl-D-mannopyranoside (Sigma Chemicals, U.S.A., 50 mM) was added to the reaction mixture after 3 h. oPRL was iodinated (spec. activ. 40 μCi/μg) using the method of Bolton and Hunter (1).

All results are expressed as group arithmetic means and standard deviation of the means. Statistical comparisons between group means were carried out using the Student's t-test.

RESULTS

As reported in Fig. 1, among the different brain

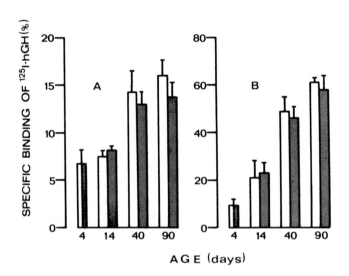

FIG. 2 - Specific binding of ^{125}I-hGH to membranes from hypothalamus (A) and from liver (B) of male (hatched bars) and female (open bars) rabbits at different stages of development. Values are means of 3-4 experiments.

areas examined, the hypothalamus of both male and fe-male rabbits shows the highest specific binding of labeled hGH with values that are about one-fourth of the binding found in the liver. In the other brain regions the specific binding of hGH is very low, except for the pons-medulla where it is about one-half of the binding in the hypothalamus.

The specific binding of labeled hGH to hypothala-mic membranes was quite low in 4-day rabbits of both sexes. A slight increase in binding occurred in 14-day

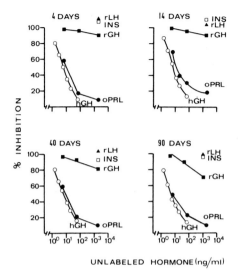

FIG. 3 - Competitive inhibition of the specific binding of ^{125}I-hGH to hypothalamic membranes from male rabbits at different stages of development by increasing concentrations of unlabeled hormones.

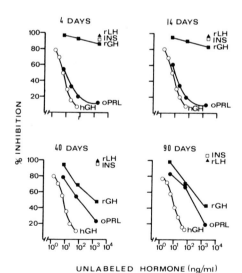

FIG. 4 - Competitive inhibition of the specific binding of ^{125}I-hGH to liver membranes from male rabbits at different stages of development by increasing concentrations of unlabeled hormones.

animals, and a further increase in 40-day animals. The
same pattern was observed in the specific binding to
liver membranes of the same animals (Fig. 2). No
significant difference between male and female rabbits
of various ages was found.the specific binding of hGH
to hypothalamic membranes varied from 31 to 55% of
total counts bound.
    Fig. 3 shows the specificity of binding of ^{125}I-
hGH to hypothalamic membranes from male rabbits at
different stages of development. Addition of increasing
amounts of unlabeled hGH resulted in a substantial
decrease in binding of labeled tracer.
A similar inhibition was observed for oPRL, but not for
rat GH or rat LH, or for porcine insulin.
    Similar results were obtained with liver membranes

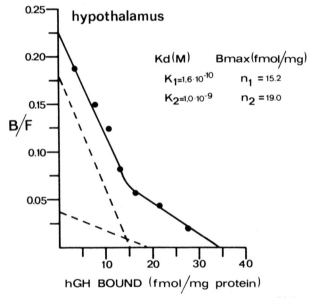

FIG. 5 - Scatchard plot of the binding of ^{125}I-hGH to
rabbit hypothalamic membranes.

from 4-day and 14-day rabbits. With liver membranes
from 40-day and 90-day rabbits addition of rat GH was
able to induce an evident decrease in binding of ^{125}I-
hGH, whereas oPRL showed a reduced inhibitory activity
(Fig. 4).
    Scatchard analysis of the binding of hGH to hy-
pothalamus and pons-medulla revealed the presence of

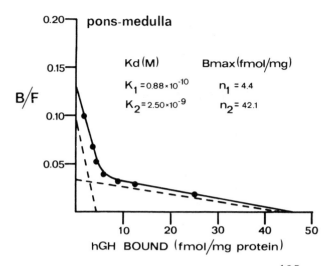

FIG. 6 - Scatchard plot of the binding of ^{125}I-hGH to rabbit pons-medulla membranes.

two independent classes of binding sites, differing in affinity by 6.3- to 28.4-fold (Fig. 5 and 6).

The Scatchard analysis of hypothalamic membranes from rabbit at different stages of development revealed a marked progressive increase with age of hGH binding capacities. No substantial difference was found in dissociation constant value in 14-day animals in comparison to adult rabbits, whereas the hypothalamus of 4-day rabbits showed a single class of high-affinity binding sites (Fig. 7).

Fig. 8 shows the effect of Con A on hGH and oPRL binding to hypothalamic membranes. Although Con A inhibited specific prolactin binding by about 60%, only 25% inhibition of specific hGH binding was observed. When α-methyl-D-mannopyranoside was added to the reaction mixture to release bound Con A, hormone binding increased, but did not return to control levels.

DISCUSSION

Brain lactogen binding sites have been identified thus far only in the rat by radioautographic methods *in vivo* using ^{125}I-hGH (19), whereas Dorn et al. (4) with immunohistochemical methods was not able to demonstrate the presence of GH binding sites in human brain

material. On the other hand, Lechan et al. (11) have
described the presence of neurons in the rat brain that
contain a substance bearing immunological similarity

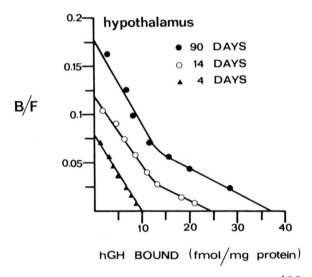

FIG. 7 - Scatchard plots of the binding of ^{125}I-hGH
to hypothalamic membranes from rabbit at different
stages of development.

to hGH, and Hansen and Hansen (6) immunocytochemically
demonstrated somatotropin-like and prolactin-like
activity in the brain of the fish Calamoichthys calaba-
ricus.

Recently, we have demonstrated the presence of
specific prolactin binding sites in membranes obtained
from rabbit hypothalamus (2). These sites showed structural specificity, high affinity, saturability and
optimum pH, and their number has been shown to vary
during ontogenesis (13) and during physiological hyper-
prolactinaemic states (lactation) and after administration of ovine prolactin or prolactin releasers and
inhibitors (3). The present results confirm our previous data on the presence in the rabbit hypothalamus of

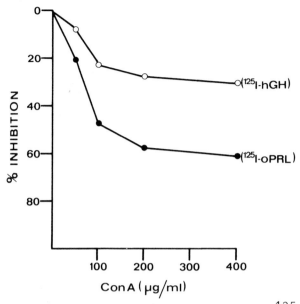

FIG. 8 - Effect of Con A on the binding of ^{125}I-hGH and ^{125}I-oPRL to hypothalamic membranes.

specific binding sites able to recognize polypeptide hormones endowed with lactogenic activity.

The binding of ^{125}I-hGH to membranes from rabbit hypothalamus shows kinetic properties typical of hormone-receptor interactions: high affinity, saturability and specificity. Significant changes in specific binding of hGH in the hypothalamus and liver as a function of the stage of development were observed. The development of hypothalamic specific binding sites for hGH occurred between 4 and 40 days of age both in male and female rabbits.

The presence of two independent classes of hGH binding site in membranes from hypothalamus and pons-medulla is in accordance with the results obtained by Herington et al. (7) in the rat liver and by Hughes(8) in the rabbit liver. It is interesting to note that membranes from 4-day animals presented only one class of binding site (with higher affinity)suggesting an earlier development of these receptors.

As far as hormonal specificity is concerned during development, it remains unchanged in the hypothalamus, whereas the liver of 40-day and 90-day rabbits was shown to have a second hGH binding site with the specificity of a non-lactogenic growth hormone binding site, in accordance with the results of other workers (5,15).

From the results obtained with Con A it is clear that although both hGH and oPRL do bind to the same molecular site, their binding properties show differ-.ent sensitivities to membrane alterations due to the action of Con A.

In conclusion,our finding demonstrating the existence of binding sites for hGH in the rabbit hypothalamus could suggest that the central nervous system is an important site of action for GH, probably related with a mechanism of autoregulation.

ACKNOWLEDGEMENTS

We thank C. Ghè for his skilful technical assistance and the NIADDK and Dr. A.F. Parlow for providing unlabeled hormone. Partial support was obtained by Consiglio Nazionale delle Ricerche, Italy(CT 81.00217).

REFERENCES

1. BOLTON, A.E. and HUNTER, W.M.(1973): Biochem. J.,
   133: 529-539.
2. DI CARLO, R. and MUCCIOLI, G.(1981): Life Sci.,
   28: 2229-2307.
3. DI CARLO, R. and MUCCIOLI, G.(1981): Brain Res.,
   230: 445-450.
4. DORN, V.A., BERNSTEIN, H.G., AHRENDT, E. and
   ZIEGLER, M. (1982): Acta histochem., 70: 150-152.
5. FIX, J.A., LEPPERT, P. and MOORE, W.V. (1981):
   Horm. Metab. Res., 13: 508-515.
6. HANSEN, B.L. and HANSEN, G.N. (1982): Cell Tissue
   Res.,222: 615-627.
7. HERINGTON, A.C., VEITH, N. and BURGER, H.G. (1976):
   Biochem. J., 158: 61-69.
8. HUGHES, J.P. (1979): Endocrinology, 105: 414-420.
9. HUNSTON, D.L. (1975): Anal. Biochem., 63: 99-109.
10. HUNTER, W.M. and GREENWOOD, F.C. (1962): Nature,
    194: 495-496.

11. LECHAN, R.M., NESTLER, J.L. and MOLITCH M.E.(1981): Endocrinology, 109: 1950-1962
12. LOWRY, O.H., ROSEBROUGH, N.J., FARR, A.L. and RANDALL, R.J. (1951): J.Biol.Chem.,193: 265-275.
13. MUCCIOLI, G., BELLUSSI, G., LANDO,D. and DI CARLO R. (1982): Develop. Brain Res., 4: 244-247.
14. MULLER, E. and PECILE, A. (1966): Proc. Soc. Exp. Biol., 122: 1289-1291.
15. POSNER, B.I., KELLY, P.A., SHIU, R.P.C. and FRIESEN, H.G. (1974): Endocrinology, 95: 521-531.
16. SCATCHARD, G. (1949): Ann. N.Y. Acad. Sci., 51: 660-672.
17. SHIU, R.P.C., KELLY, P.A. and FRIESEN, H.G.(1973): Science, 180: 968-970.
18. TANNENBAUM, G.S. (1980): Endocrinology, 107: 2117-2120.
19. VAN HOUTEN, M., POSNER, B.I. and WELSH, R.J.(1980): Exp. Brain Res., 38: 455-461.
20. VOOGT, J.L., CLEMENS, J.A., NEGRO-VILAR A., WELSCH, C. and MEITES, J. (1971): Endocrinology, 88: 1363-1367.

CNS Receptors—From Molecular
Pharmacology to Behavior, edited by
P. Mandel and F. V. Defeudis.
Raven Press, New York © 1983.

High Affinity Binding Site for γ-Hydroxybutyric Acid in Rat Brain

M. Maitre, J. F. Rumigny, J. Benavides, J. J. Bourguignon,
C. G. Wermuth, C. Cash, and P. Mandel

*Centre de Neurochimie du CNRS and INSERM U 44, Université Louis Pasteur,
67084 Strasbourg Cedex, France*

γ-Hydroxybutyric acid (GHB) was first synthesized in order to
obtain an analogue of GABA (10). But, administered to animals,
this compound was found to induce a behavioural depression, often
called "anaesthesia" (9), which is paralleled by an EEG pattern of
petit mal epilepsy (21). Besides these neurophysiological effects,
exogenous GHB induces a decrease in brain glucose consumption (24)
and in the level and turnover rate of acetylcholine (20), serotonin (22) and especially dopamine (15,26) in various regions of
the rat brain. The fact that GHB exists naturally in the brain at
concentrations ranging from $2.10^{-6}M$ to about $3.10^{-5}M$ is some evidence that GHB may play a functional role in this organ (16,22).
Since GHB has been identified as a reductive catabolite of GABA,
a specific succinic semialdehyde reductase has been isolated and
characterized (17). This enzyme reduces only succinic semialdehyde
and some structurally related compounds (e.g. 2 methyl succinic
semialdehyde or 2 phenyl succinic semialdehyde). Unlike other al-
dehyde reductases, this enzyme is not inhibited by barbiturates or
some branched-chain fatty acids such as valproic acid (17). Under
physiological conditions *in vitro*, this SSA reductase is specifically involved in the synthesis of [^{3}H] GHB from [^{3}H] GABA (19).
Immunocytochemical studies have demonstrated the presence of this
enzyme specifically in neurons and in some dendrites and axonal
terminals (27). Thus, it was interesting to investigate the possible existence of a specific GHB receptor in the rat brain, near
the sites of GHB synthesis, which could mediate the actions
of endogenous GHB and the multiple effects of administered GHB.
The existence of these receptors implicates the presence of high
affinity binding sites. The existence and characterization of
such binding sites is the subject of the present report.

METHODS

[2,3 ^{3}H] GHB potassium salt (specific activity 40 Ci/nmol) was obtained from the CEA (France). Radiochemical purity was checked by thin-layer chromatography in 3 different solvent systems. Crude membranes from rat brain were prepared by homogenisation with a polytron of a crude mitochondrial fraction (P_2 fraction) in ice-cold deionized water. Membranes were centrifuged at 50,000 g for 20 min, and stored at -20°C for one night. For binding assays, membrane suspensions were thawed, washed twice more with 20 vol of ice-cold deionized water and resuspended in the incubation medium. Buffers used for binding assays consisted of either PIPES (1,4-piperazine-diethanesulfonic acid) or potassium phosphate ($KH_2 PO_4$ / $K_2H PO_4$). In both cases, the salt concentration was 50 mM and the pH 6.5 at 0°C. The two buffers used gave essentially the same results. Different ions (Ca^{++}, Mg^{++}, Cl^-) were tested on the binding but no significant variations were observed.

Binding experiments were carried out in small tubes each containing 100 μl of membrane suspension (about 1 mg protein), 300 μl of buffer containing [^{3}H] GHB at the desired concentration and 200 μl of buffer with or without the test substance. After incubation for 30 min at 0°C, the tubes were centrifuged at 55,000 g for 20 min in a Beckman R 25 Rotor. The supernatant was aspirated and the pellet rapidly washed twice with 800 μl ice-cold incubation buffer. Pellets were then resuspended in 250 μl water by vortexing and the tritium label was determined by liquid scintillation spectrometry in 10 ml of Rotiszint 22 (Roth, West Germany).

RESULTS

The specific [^{3}H] GHB binding was linear in the range of protein concentrations used (between 0.5 and 2 mg/600 μl incubation medium). Moreover, specific binding reached equilibrium at 0°C after 10 min incubation. However, an incubation time of 30 min at 0°C was usually adopted. Thin-layer chromatographic analysis of the bound [^{3}H] GHB displaceable by 5 mM non-radioactive GHB showed that at least 98% of the radioactivity was [^{3}H] GHB.

Under these experimental conditions, specific [^{3}H] GHB binding to crude membranes was saturable with increasing concentrations of [^{3}H] GHB (Figure 1). In contrast, non-specific binding was not saturable, but increased linearly with [^{3}H] GHB over the concentration range tested. At low concentrations (under 40 nM [^{3}H] GHB), two plateaux in the specific binding curve could be detected, possibly indicating that two binding systems of high affinity and low capacity are saturated before the appearance of a third system with a larger capacity.

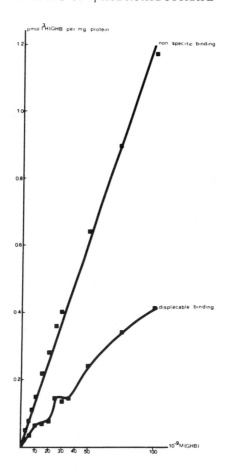

FIG. 1. Saturation curve of GHB binding to
a rat brain membrane fraction. Non-specific
binding is linear (3 separate experiments).

Effect of pH

Specific [^{3}H] binding is strongly pH-dependent. Maximal binding was observed at pH 5.5 (Figure 2) and a very large decrease
at neutral pH was observed. However, significant binding occurs at
pH 6.5. This optimum pH of 5.5 cannot be due to lactonization of
GHB as this binding is not displaceable by gamma-butyrolactone.
Moreover, ^{1}H - NMR spectroscopy performed on GHB incubated in the
binding buffer at pH 5.5 and 0°C shows that the lactonic form of
GHB is not present in significant quantity. Therefore, the pH
optimum of 5.5 for GHB binding suggests that protonation of the
ligand (PKa = 4.7) and/or of the binding site is a condition necessary for the most active conformation.

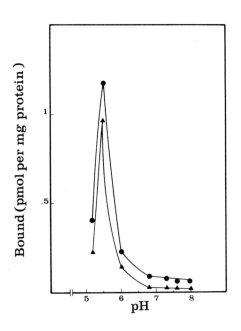

FIG. 2.   pH-dependence of [^{3}H] GHB binding
(25 nM) to rat brain membranes.
Upper curve : binding displaceable by
              5 mM GHB
Lower curve : binding displaceable by
              10 μM GHB

Kinetic Parameters of GHB Binding

[^{3}H] GHB concentrations were increased from 25 nM to 300 nM (specific activity 4 Ci/mmol); specific binding (displaceable by
5 mM non-radioactive GHB) was plotted by the Scatchard method.
The results are in favor of 2 populations of binding sites (or
possibly the existence of negative cooperativity) (Figure 3).
Computer analysis of the data using the mathematical treatment
of Feldman (7) (two binding sites/one ligand) indicated that the
high affinity binding has a Kd_1 of 95 nM and a $Bmax_1$ of 0.56 pmol/
mg protein and the lower affinity site a Kd_2 of 16 μM and $Bmax_2$
of 46 pmol/mg protein.
The characteristics of the high affinity binding site (Kd =
95 nM) are similar in magnitude to those for established neuro-

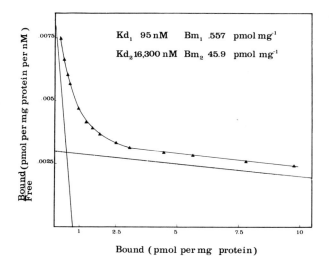

FIG. 3. Analysis by Scatchard plot of [^{3}H] GHB binding to rat brain membranes (3 separate experiments). GHB concentrations starting at 25 nM.

TABLE 1

[^{3}H] GHB displacement by some analogues and other compounds

Compound	% inhibition of GHB binding at 10 μM
GHB	52 ± 2
γ-butyrolactone	n.s.
2-methyl GHB	24 ± 0.7
2-phenyl GHB	n.s.
3-methyl GHB	59 ± 0.7
3-ethyl GHB	43 ± 8
3-n-propyl GHB	5 ± 1
3-isopropyl GHB	n.s.
3-hydroxy GHB	19 ± 4
3-phenyl GHB	n.s.
3-benzyl GHB	n.s.
2,3-dimethyl GHB	n.s.
4-methyl GHB	45 ± 4
3-hydroxypropionic acid	n.s.
5-hydroxyvaleric acid	43 ± 4
2-hydroxyethane sulfonic acid	7 ± 0.4
3-hydroxypropane sulfonic acid	n.s.
4-hydroxybutane sulfonic acid	n.s.
cis 4-hydroxycrotonic acid (cis-HCA)	n.s.
3-methyl (HCA)	n.s.
3-isopropyl (HCA)	n.s.
trans 4-hydroxycrotonic acid (trans-HCA)	59 ± 0.5
3-methyl trans-HCA	n.s.
O-hydroxymethylbenzoic acid	n.s.
GABA,(±) baclofen, isoguvacine	n.s.
dopamine	n.s.
picrotoxine	n.s.
ethosuccinimide, trimethadione	n.s.

For this study the membranes were added to the incubating buffer containing 25 nM [^{3}H] GHB and 10 μM of the tested substance. Results are expressed as the percentage inhibition of the binding displacable by 5 mM GHB (mean ± SD of 3 separate experiments performed in quadruplicate which varied less than 5%). n.s. : no significant inhibition.

transmitters, such as GABA (12) and serotonin (13). This site
appears to be specific for GHB (see Table 1) as GABA, baclofen,
isoguvacine, muscimol, bicuculline and picrotoxin had no significant effects on GHB binding at a concentration of 10 µM. At
this same concentration, some compounds structurally related to
GHB had better capacity than GHB itself to displace specific
binding. This is especially the case for trans-4 hydroxycrotonic
acid. These results are a possible indication that the binding
site requires GHB or its analogues in an open structure and semi-
extended conformation.

   This GHB binding system is clearly distinct from the GHB transport process which occurs optimally at pH 7.4 and is strongly dependent on the presence of a Na^+- gradient (1).

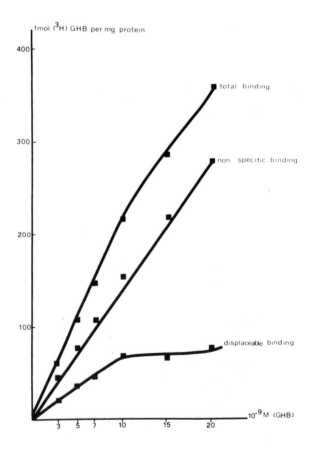

FIG. 4.   Saturation curve of GHB binding
to a rat brain membrane fraction at low
concentrations of GHB (below 25 nM).

Existence of a High Affinity,
Positive Cooperative System for GHB

At lower concentrations of [³H] GHB (< 25 nM), rat brain membranes exhibit a third apparently specific GHB binding system.
In this range of GHB concentration (2-20 nM) the specific binding
is also saturable (Figure 4). However, in this case, using a [³H]
GHB concentration of 2 nM (specific activity 40 Ci/mmol), displacement of bound [³H] GHB by increasing concentrations of non-
radioactive GHB produced a rather unusual result (Figure 5). At
a low concentration of GHB (< 10^{-8}M), the specific binding of
[³H] GHB increases until 150% of the control value obtained with
2 nM [³H] GHB. Higher concentrations of GHB (> 10^{-8}M) displaced
the specific radiolabelling. This phenomenon is typical of a

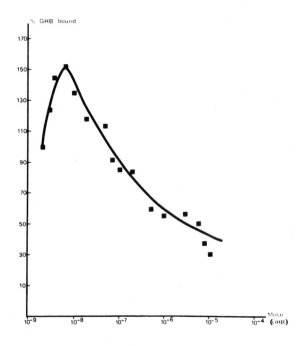

FIG. 5. Displacement of bound [³H] GHB (2 nM)
by increasing concentrations of non-radioactive GHB. The bound GHB increases at low
concentrations of non-radioactive GHB (below
10^{-8}M).

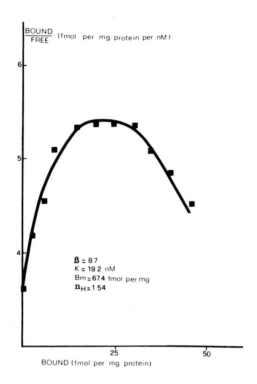

FIG. 6.   Analysis by Scatchard plot of
[³H] GHB binding to rat brain membranes
(4 separate experiments). GHB Concentrations between 1 and 15 nM.

positive cooperative process at low concentration of GHB. Using
[³H] GHB concentrations ranging from 10^{-9}M to 12.10^{-9}M, binding
results were plotted by the Scatchard method. The curve obtained
(Figure 6) is concave downwards with a well pronounced maximum.
This type of curve is characteristic of a system showing positive
cooperativity. According to the mathematical treatment using the
data by Thakur et al. (24) in their "statistical mechanical
model", a non-linear regression line (Gauss-Newton-fitting) can
be obtained which indicates a single class of site with 9-fold
positive cooperativity (β = 8.75 $\pm$ 2.8). Maximum binding capacity
is about 70 femtomol/mg protein ($\bar{B}$max = 67.4 $\pm$ 3.5 femtomol/mg
protein) with an affinity constant of 20 nM ($\bar{K}$d = 19.2 $\pm$ 1.8 nM).
From the position of the maximum in the Scatchard plot, the Hill
coefficient can be estimated to 1.54. The characteristics of this
positive cooperativity binding sites are not modified by the pres-

ence of 1 μM of GABA, muscimol or baclofen.

Although this high affinity binding site for GHB appears to be specific, it is not the only cooperative system that has been described in the brain for putative neurotransmitters. In particular, glycine-binding exhibits similar characteristics (3,28).

TABLE 2. Subcellular distribution of GHB binding sites (1)

Fraction	displaceable by 10 μM GHB RB	displaceable by 5 mM GHB RB	% protein recovered
Nuclear	0.44	0.52	7.6
Microsomal	1.28	1.23	20.4
Myelin (A)	0.71	0.80	7.1
Nerve endings (B)	1.40	1.83	5.2
Nerve endings (C)	4.54	4.25	8.7
Nerve endings + mitochondria (D)	1.11	1.12	11.0
Mitochondria (E)	0.95	0.97	6.1
Cytosol	N.D.	N.D.	33.5

RB : relative binding :

$$\frac{\text{% binding displaceable by x μM non-radioactive GHB}}{\text{% protein recovered}}$$

(1) Average of three experiments
N.D. : binding not determined.

[3H] GHB High Affinity Binding Sites Are Located In Neurons

Distribution of γ-hydroxybutyrate binding sites in subcellular fractions

Subcellular fractionation of rat brain was carried out according to the method of DeRobertis et al. (4). Membranes were prepared from the different fractions by the method previously described. Binding assays were performed using 25.10^{-9}M [3H] GHB. In Table 2, results are expressed as relative binding (RB) in the different fractions. The richest compartment was membranes derived from fraction C of the sucrose gradient, which has been described by DeRobertis et al. to contain essentially nerve endings. Nuclear, myelin and mitochondrial fractions are almost devoid of GHB binding sites. In the richest fraction of GHB binding sites (fraction C), GHB binding was saturable and the affinity constant of this binding, plotted by the Scatchard method, gave essentially the same results as for crude membranes. The existence of the high affinity, positive cooperative binding site was not tested. However, for the two other sites described for total crude membranes, the binding capacity was enriched 9-fold for the high affinity site and about 5-fold for the low affinity site ($Bmax_1$

changing from 0.55 pmole/mg to 5.1 pmole/mg and $Bmax_2$ changing
from 46 pmol/mg to 231 pmole/mg). All these data are in favor of
a distribution of the GHB binding sites almost exclusively at the
synaptic level.

Distribution of γ-hydroxybutyrate sites in isolated neurons and glial cell cultures

Pure neuronal primary cultures from chick embryo brain were
obtained according to the method of Pettmann et al. (14). Cultures of pure glial cells were obtained by the method of Booher
and Sensenbrenner (2). Neuronal (6 days old) and glial cells (14
days old) were rinsed, homogenised in water using a Polytron and
centrifuged at 50,000 g for 20 min. The pellet was washed once
more with water and resuspended in the incubation buffer used for
the binding experiment. In chicken embryo neuronal cultures, [³H]
GHB binding is present at a level of 50 fmoles/mg protein, whereas
in glial cultures, no binding was apparent (mean of 3 experiments
which vary less than 15%).

The existence of GHB binding sites on neuronal membranes and
especially on membranes of synaptic origin, the neuronal localization of GHB synthesis (26), and the existence of high affinity
uptake by plasma membrane vesicles from synaptic origin (1)
supports a neurotransmitter role for GHB in brain.

Distribution of GHB Binding Sites in Various Rat Brain Regions and During Ontogenesis

Rat brain regions were dissected according to the method of
Glowinski and Iversen (8). GHB binding was measured as previously
described using 25 nM [³H] GHB. Results are summarized in Table 3.

TABLE 3

Regional distribution of [³H] GHB binding

Region	[³H] GHB binding 10^{-15} mole mg^{-1}	different from whole brain
Whole brain	220 ± 52	
Olfactory bulbs	567 ± 85	$p < .005$
Frontal cortex	248 ± 25	$p > .05$
Striatum	296 ± 14	$p < .05$
Hippocampus	465 ± 27	$p < .001$
Thalamus	89 ± 16	$p < .01$
Hypothalamus	107 ± 32	$p < .02$
Cerebellum	15 ± 3	$p < .001$
Pons Medulla	n.d.	
Spinal cord	24 ± 5	$p < .001$

GHB binding was measured as described under Materials and
Methods using 25 nM [³H] GHB (+ 5 mM GHB for estimating
background). Results are mean ± SD (3 separate experiments
performed in quadruplicate which varied less than 5%).
n.d. : no binding detected under our assay conditions.

TABLE 4

[^{3}H] GHB binding in 6-day-old and adult rat brain

	Displacable by 5 mM GHB	Displacable by 10 µM GHB
Adult	353 ± 70	183 ± 37
6 days after birth	145 ± 26 *	51 ± 9 *

GHB binding([^{3}H] GHB binding, 10^{-15} mole per mg protein) was measured as described under Materials and Methods using 25 nM [^{3}H] GHB. Results are mean ± SD (3 separate experiments performed in quadruplicate which varied less then 5%).
* : significantly different from adult (p < .005)

Heterogeneity of GHB binding site distribution appears to be appreciable although the experiment was performed on hand-dissected brain regions. It should be noted that high densities of GHB binding sites are present in the anterior part of the CNS, while in the caudal part (cerebellum, pons-medulla, spinal cord), the density is very low. During development, (between 6 days after birth and adult) the densities of GHB binding sites increases about twofold in total brain (Table 4). Apparently there is no strict correlation between specific binding site distribution and the distribution of the biosynthetic enzyme of GHB (18) (specific succinic semialdehyde reductase – SSR2). For example, cerebellum and pons-medulla, which exhibit a relatively high SSR2 activity, have only a low receptor density. It has been reported that during the same period, the density of GHB receptor increases almost twofold. An explanation of these discrepancies might involve consideration of several pools of GHB. Changes in the sizes of these pools may occur during development. If GHB is a neurotransmitter, one might expect a better correlation between receptors and terminal area densities. In fact, a lack of correlation between receptor densities for a neurotransmitter and the endogenous content of its synthesizing enzyme does occur, as has already been described for serotonin (11) and GABA (6).

ACKNOWLEDGEMENTS

This work was supported by CNRS, ATP "Pharmacologie des récepteurs des neuromédiateurs".

REFERENCES

1. Benavides, J., Rumigny, J.F., Bourguignon, J.F., Wermuth, C.G., Mandel, P. and Maitre, M. (1982): J. Neurochem., 38:1570-1575.
2. Booher, J. and Sensenbrenner, M. (1972): Neurobiology, 2:97-105.
3. DeFeudis, F.V., Fando, J. and Orensanz Muñoz, L.M. (1977): Experientia, 33:1068-1070.
4. DeRobertis, E., Pellegrino De Iraldi, A., Rodriguez de Lores Arnaiz, G. and Salganicoff, L. (1962): J. Neurochem., 9: 23-35.
5. Doherty, J.D., Hattox, S., Ando, N., Snead, O.C. and Roth, R. H. (1976): Fedn. Proc. Fedn. Am. Socs. Exp. Biol., 35:270.
6. Enna: S.J. (1979): In: GABA-Biochemistry and CNS Functions, edited by P. Mandel and F.V. DeFeudis, pp. 323-337. Plenum Press, New York.
7. Feldman, H.A. (1972): Anal. Biochem., 48:317-338.
8. Glowinski, J. and Iversen, L.L. (1966): J. Neurochem., 13: 655-669.
9. Laborit, H. (1973): Progr. Neurobiol., 1:255-263.
10. Laborit, H., Jouany, J.M., Gerard, J. and Fabiani, F. (1960): Press Méd., 68:1867-1869.
11. Nelson, D.L., Herbert, A., Bourgoin, S., Glowinski, J. and Hamon, M. (1978): Molec. Pharmacol., 14:983-995.
12. Olsen, R.W. (1981): J. Neurochem., 37:1-13.
13. Peroutka, S.J. and Snyder, S.H. (1979): Mol. Pharmacol., 16: 687-699.
14. Pettmann, B., Louis, J.C. and Sensenbrenner, M. (1979): Nature, 281:378-380.
15. Roth, R.H., Walters, J.R. and Aghajanian, G.K. (1973): In : Frontiers in catecholamine research, edited by E. Usdin and S.H. Snyder, pp. 567-574. Pergamon Press, Oxford.
16. Roth, R.H. and Giarman, N.J. (1970): Biochem. Pharmacol., 19: 1087-1093.
17. Rumigny, J.F., Maitre, M., Cash, C. and Mandel, P. (1980): FEBS Lett., 117:111-116.
18. Rumigny, J.F., Cash, C., Mandel, P. and Maitre, M. (1982): Neurochem. Res., 7:555-561.
19. Rumigny, J.F., Cash, C., Mandel, P., Vincendon, G. and Maitre, M. (1981): FEBS Lett., 134:96-98.
20. Sethy, V.H., Roth, R.H., Walters, J.R., Marini, J. and Van Woert, M.M. (1976): Naunyn-Schmiedeberg's Arch. Pharmac., 295:9-14.
21. Snead, O.C., Yu, R.K. and Huttenlocker, P.R. (1976): Neurology, 26:51-56.
22. Snead, O.C. and Morley, B.J. (1981): Develop. Brain Res., 1:579-589.
23. Spano, P.P. and Przegalsniski, E. (1973): Pharmac. Res. Commun., 5:55-69.

24. Taberner, P.V., Rick, J.T. and Kerkut, G.A. (1972): *J. Neuro-chem.*, 19:245-254.
25. Thakur, A.K., Jaffe, M.L. and Rodbard, D. (1980): *Anal. Bio-chem.*, 107:279-295.
26. Walters, J.R., Aghajanian, G.K. and Roth, R.H. (1972): *Bio-chem. Pharmac.*, 21:2111-2121.
27. Weissmann-Nanopoulos, D., Rumigny, J.F., Mandel, P., Vincendon, G. and Maitre, M. (1982): *Neurochem. Intern.* (in press).
28. Werman, R. (1978): In : *GABA-Biochemistry and CNS Functions*, edited by P. Mandel and F.V. DeFeudis, pp. 287-303. Plenum Press, New York.

CNS Receptors—From Molecular
Pharmacology to Behavior, edited by
P. Mandel and F. V. Defeudis.
Raven Press, New York © 1983.

Quantitative Receptor Autoradiography: Application to the Study of Multiple Serotonin Receptors in Rat Cortex

J. M. Palacios

Preclinical Research, Sandoz Ltd., CH-4002 Basel, Switzerland

In recent years methods have been developed that allow the localization of receptors for drugs and neurotransmitters at the light- and electron-microscopic levels, using the technique of autoradiography (1). Two important developments in this field have been the availability of an in vitro method for the labeling of receptors for autoradiography (2) and the adaptation of this technique, thanks to the use of a ^{3}H-sensitive film, for quantitative microdensitometric determination of receptor densities (3-5).

Because of the use of in vitro conditions for labeling of receptors, allowing for the utilization of drugs with different affinities for specific receptor subtypes, and because of its high anatomical resolution, the quantitative autoradiography of receptors is a method especially well suited for the study of multiple receptors for a neurotransmitter (6).

In this paper I shall describe methods for the computer-assisted microdensitometric measurement of receptor concentrations and the application of this technology to the study of the laminar distribution of serotonin-1 (5HT-1) and serotonin-2 (5HT-2) (7-8) receptors in the rat cortex.

QUANTITATIVE RECEPTOR AUTORADIOGRAPHY

Labeling of receptors for autoradiography

The brains from adult male rats (Wistar, 250 g body weight) were used in all experiments described in this paper. Ten-micron slide-mounted sections were prepared as previously described (2). Serotonin receptors were labeled with ^{3}H-LSD as described by Meibach et al., (9) and Young and Kuhar (10). Serotonin-2 receptors were also labeled with ^{3}H-spiperone as described by Palacios et al., (11).

The different components of the binding of these ligands were analyzed by using drugs with different affinities for serotonin and dopamine receptors. Serotonin, spiperone, ketanserin and cinanserin were used in the study of 5HT receptors. Sulpiride and ADTN (2-amino-6,7-dihydroxy-1,2,3,4-tetrahydronaphthalene) were used to block dopamine receptors.

Generation and Standardization of Autoradiograms

Autoradiograms were generated by apposing the labeled tissue sections against a ^{3}H-sensitive film (^{3}H-ultrofilm, LKB, Sweden). Exposure time was one and two months. Standards containing different amounts of a ^{3}H-labeled, non-volatile substance were exposed along with the labeled sections. These standards were prepared with brain paste as described by Unnerstall et al. (12,13). Because of the different self-absorption for β-particles by white and gray matter (14), two different sets of standards were prepared by using regions of the brain enriched in gray or white matter. Figure 1 shows a plot of the densitometric readings of these two sets of standards, and demonstrates a more than 3-fold greater self-absorption for beta-particles by the white matter compared with the gray matter. Use of standards containing only white matter or mixtures of white and gray matter will result in overestimation of the receptor concentrations in gray matter areas. In this study gray matter standards were used in all experiments.

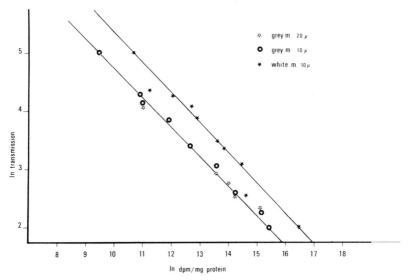

Fig. 1. Double logarithmic plot of transmission versus concentration of radioactivity in the standards,
in dpm/mg of protein. Gray matter standards, cut
at 10 or 20 μm thickness, produced the same standard
curves. White matter standards produced a parallel
standard curve, but displaced to the right, indicating that for the same amount of radioactivity these
standards have a more than 3-fold lower optical
density.

Computer-assisted quantification of the autoradiograms

Autoradiograms were analyzed using a computerized image-ana-
lysis system developed in our laboratories (Schweizer et al.).
A television camera coupled to a microscope is used to digita-
lize the autoradiographic image into a 256x256 matrix of digital
numbers. The areas of interest are outlined in the image displayed in a television monitor using a light-sensitive pen. The
mean density of the area is calculated by a microprocessor that
is programed to transform it into a receptor density. For this
the quantification process is initiated by the reading of the
standard curve. This generates a factor for the transformation
of optical density into radioactivity concentration in dpm/mg
of protein. Taking into account the specific activity of the
ligand used in the experiment, the optical densities are converted to receptor concentrations, in fmol/mg of protein.

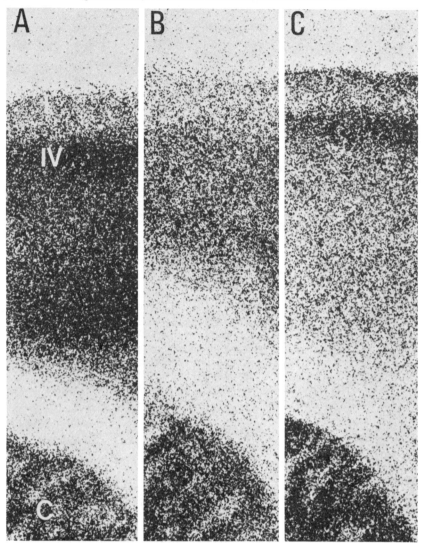

Fig. 2. Autoradiographic localization of ^{3}H-LSD
binding sites in the rat cortex. A is a photomi-
crograph of the autoradiogram from a tissue section incubated with 5nM ^{3}H-LSD. Note a high density of autoradiographic grains in lamina IV (IV),
in the layers below this one and in the nucleus
caudate-putamen (C). B shows a section, consecutive to that in A, incubated with 0.1 μM ketanserin
to block 5HT-2 receptors. Note the reduction of
autoradiographic grains, particularly in laminae
I (I) and IV. The section shown in C was incubated
with 30 nM serotonin to block 5HT-1 receptors.
A considerable decrease in the binding of ^{3}H-LSD
to the deepest cortical layers can be observed.

LAMINAR DISTRIBUTION OF SEROTONIN-1
AND SEROTONIN-2 RECEPTORS IN THE RAT CORTEX

As an example of the application of quantitative autoradiographic methods to the study of multiple neurotransmitter receptors, I shall describe the localization of 5HT-receptors in the rat frontal cortex.

Tritiated LSD and ^{3}H-spiperone were used as ligands for these receptors. Binding of ^{3}H-LSD was observed in all areas and layers of the rat cortex, but varied in the different areas and laminae.

Figure 2A shows the distribution of ^{3}H-LSD binding sites in the frontal cortex of the rat. Binding was elevated in laminae IV, V and VI, while the density of autoradiographic grains was somewhat lower in laminae I, II and III.

A section consecutive to the one shown in Fig. 2A, incubated with ^{3}H-LSD in the presence of 0.1 µM ketanserin, a specific blocker of 5HT-2 receptors (15), is shown in Fig. 2B. Binding of ^{3}H-LSD was decreased in all layers of the cortex but particularly in the laminae I, II, III and IV. Co-incubation of ^{3}H-LSD with 30 nM serotonin, a concentration that will block preferentially binding to 5HT-1 receptors, resulted in the inhibition of ^{3}H-LSD binding to sites localized mainly in the deep laminae V and VI.

It is apparent that 5HT-1 and 5HT-2 receptors have a differential distribution in the frontal cortex; 5HT-1 receptors are concentrated in laminae V and VI and 5HT-2 receptors in laminae I through IV.

These results were confirmed by using ^{3}H-spiperone, a neuroleptic that binds to 5HT-2 receptors in the cerebral cortex (7,8,11). Fig. 3A shows the localization of ^{3}H-spiperone binding sites in the rat cerebral cortex and demonstrates an enrichment of sites in the laminae I and IV and lower densities in the other laminae. The addition of 1 µM concentration of the neuroleptic sulpiride, that specifically blocks dopamine receptors (8), to the incubation medium resulted in a complete blockade of the binding of ^{3}H-spipe-

rone to the nucleus caudate-putamen (Fig. 3B), without affecting
the binding in the cortex. On the other hand, 0.1 µM ketanserin
completely inhibited the binding of ^{3}H-spiperone to cortical sites
without affecting binding to the sites in the caudate-putamen.
These results demonstrate again the presence of 5HT-2 receptor
sites in the more external cortical layers. Similar results were
obtained in these and previous experiments (11) using other displacing agents such as ADTN, cinanserin and 5HT.

A further confirmation of the laminar distribution of 5HT-re-
ceptors in the rat cortex has been provided by the autoradiographic localization of [3]H-5HT binding sites. Rainbow et al., (3)
have shown that the binding sites for [3]H-5HT, under conditions in
which 5HT-1 receptors are preferentially labeled, are concentrated in the deepest cortical laminae IV through VI.

Finally, in order to obtain a quantitative estimation of the
distribution of 5HT receptors in the rat cortex, complete displacement curves were constructed using consecutive saggital sections
and increasing concentrations of different displacers, such as
5HT, ketanserin, cinanserin and spiperone. As an example, Fig. 4
shows the results obtained using ^{3}H LSD as ligand and 5HT as displacer. When the mean receptor density of a cross section of the
cortex ("Total cortex", Fig. 4A) was measured, it was observed
that 5HT displaced ^{3}H-LSD binding in a biphasic manner. Fifty
to 60% of the binding sites were sensitive to low 5HT concentrations (IC_{50} approximately 2-3 nM) while the remaining ^{3}H-LSD
sites required higher 5HT concentrations (IC_{50} around 0.3-1 µM)
to be blocked.

The quantitative analysis of the separate laminae (Fig. 4B) confirmed the qualitative results discussed above. Biphasic displacement curves were found in all the cortical layers, with the exception of lamina I that appears to contain mainly 5HT-2 receptors. Lamina IV was also rich in 5HT-2 receptors although about
30% of the sites were of the 5HT-1 type. Laminae V and VI were
enriched in 5HT-1 sites, although 5HT-2 sites were also present
in variable proportion (40 and 25% of the total, respectively).

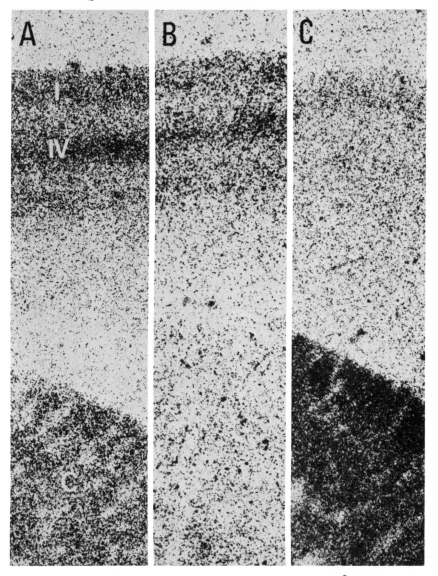

Fig. 3. Autoradiographic localization of ^{3}H-spi-
perone binding sites in the rat cortex. A shows
the binding of 0.4 nM ^{3}H-spiperone to cortical
layers (I and IV) and to sites in the nucleus
caudate-putamen (C). The effects of co-incubation with 1 μM sulpiride are shown in B. Note
the inhibition of the binding of ^{3}H-spiperone
to sites in the caudate, without effects on the
cortical binding. C shows the effects of ketanserin (0.1 μM) on the binding of ^{3}H-spiperone.
The cortical sites were blocked while the sites
in the caudate were not affected.

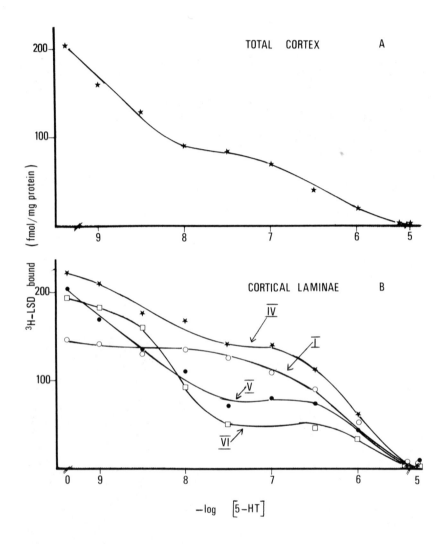

Fig. 4. Displacement curves of 5 nM ³H-LSD binding to the rat cortex by 5-HT as determined microdensitometrically. In A the mean density of the cortex was measured. B shows the displacement curves for individual laminae (I, IV, V and VI). Points are the means of 9 measurements, three for each of three animals. The standard deviation was always less than 5% of the mean value.

In conclusion, by using quantitative, computer-assisted, auto-radiographic techniques it was possible to demonstrate the differential laminar distribution of 5HT receptor subtypes in the rat cortex. The pharmacological characteristics and the relative proportions of these receptors were also analyzed with high anatomical resolution.

Because of the different afferent and efferent connections of the cortical laminae one could suggest that activation or blockade of one or the other 5-HT receptor subtype will influence brain function in a differential way.

REFERENCES

1. Kuhar, M.J. (1981): Trends in Neurosci., 4: 60-64.
2. Young, W.S., III and Kuhar, M.J. (1979): Brain Res. 179: 255-270.
3. Rainbow, T.C., Bleisch, W.V., Biegon, A. and McEwen, B.S. (1982): J. Neurosci. Methods 5: 127-138.
4. Penney, J.B., Pan, H.S., Young, A.B., Frey, K.A. and Dauth, G.W. (1981): Science 214: 1036-1038.
5. Palacios, J.M., Niehoff, D.L. and Kuhar, M.J. (1981): Neurosci. Letters 25: 101-105.
6. Snyder, S.H. and Goodman, R.R. (1980): J. Neurochem. 38: 153-175.
7. Peroutka, S.J. and Snyder, S.H. (1979): Mol. Pharmacol. 16: 687-699.
8. List, S. and Seeman, P. (1981): Proc. Natl. Acad. Sci., USA 78: 2620-2624.
9. Meibach, R.C., Maayani, S. and Green, J.P. (1980): Eur. J. Pharmacol. 67: 371-382.
10. Young, W.S., III and Kuhar, M.J. (1980): Eur. J. Pharmacol. 62: 237-239.
11. Palacios, J.M., Niehoff, D.L. and Kuhar, M.J. (1981): Brain Res. 213: 277-289.
12. Unnerstall, J.R., Kuhar, M.J., Niehoff, D.L. and Palacios, J.M. (1981): J. Pharmacol. Exp. Ther. 218: 797-804.
13. Unnerstall, J.R., Niehoff, D.L., Kuhar, M.J. and Palacios, J.M. (1982): J. Neurosci. Methods, 6: 59-73.
14. Alexander, G.M., Schwartzman, R.J., Bell, R.D., Yu, J. and Renthal, A. (1981): Brain Res. 223: 59-67.
15. Leysen, J.E., Awouters, F., Kennis, L., Laduron, P.M., Vandenberk, J. and Janssen, P.A.J. (1981): Life Sci. 28: 1015-1022.

CNS Receptors—From Molecular
Pharmacology to Behavior, edited by
P. Mandel and F. V. DeFeudis.
Raven Press, New York © 1983.

Biochemical and Physiological Characterization of Adenosine Receptors in Rat Brain

M. Reddington, K. S. Lee, P. Schubert, and G. W. Kreutzberg

*Nerve Cell Biology Group, Max Planck Institute for Psychiatry,
8 Munich 40, Federal Republic of Germany*

The classical concept of neurotransmission consists
of the presynaptic release of a neurotransmitter that
directly depolarises or hyperpolarises the postsynaptic
membrane, increasing or decreasing the probability of
discharge and thus defining the basic excitatory or inhibitory nature of a synapse. This idea has been extended in recent years to include so-called 'neuromodulators', i.e. substances which are capable of
modifying the release or action of a primary neurotransmitter. Among the substances fulfilling such a
neuromodulatory role, the purine, adenosine, is
currently receiving considerable attention(3,12,18,25).
Adenosine has been shown to interact with the effects
of biogenic amines on brain adenylate cyclase either
in a stimulatory, synergistic manner (2,15) or as an
inhibitor of ß-adrenergic agonist-stimulated cyclic
AMP accumulation (23). Further, it is a potent
attenuator of nerve cell activity in both peripheral
and central neurons (3,5,12,16). In this respect it
is of particular interest that the behavioural effects
of methylxanthines (e.g. caffeine), which are known to
be adenosine receptor antagonists, might be mediated
via a reversal of the depressive action of endogenous
adenosine.

In vitro brain slice preparations have proved to be
invaluable for studying the basic physiological and
pharmacological parameters relating to purinergic
neuromodulation (5,10). The rat hippocampal slice,
for instance, allows both extra- and intracellular

analyses of the effects of adenosine on nerve cell
activity. The depressive action of adenosine on
evoked populations EPSPs in the CA1 region of this
preparation is illustrated in Fig. 1. Electrophysiological analyses of these evoked responses indicate
that the depressive action of adenosine occurs
primarily at the synaptic level rather than by
changing the activity of afferent fibres (16). This
is consistent with studies with peripheral nerves
where adenosine has been shown to inhibit transmitter
release at both cholinergic and adrenergic synapses(3).
By analogy, this suggests a possible presynaptic site
of adenosine action also in hippocampal neurons.
However, from intracellular studies in rat hippocampal
slices there is some indication also of a postsynaptic
component of the response to adenosine (21).
  The depressive action of adenosine on synaptic transmission and its effects on cyclic AMP accumulation in
brain slices and cell cultures are mediated via extracellular receptors (2,4,5,23). Recently, progress has
been made in the biochemical characterisation of
adenosine receptors using radioligand binding methods
(1,20,26,27). In this chapter we present studies
based on both electrophysiological and biochemical
approaches to the receptors mediating the synaptic
effects of adenosine.

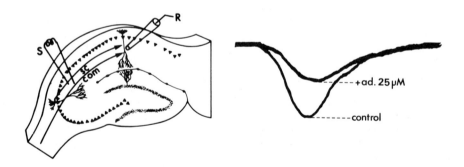

FIG: 1. Depressive action of adenosine on evoked
EPSPs in a rat hippocampal slice preparation. The
positions of the stimulating (s) and recording (r)
electrodes are shown in the schematic diagram on
the left. Evoked EPSPs were depressed on superfusion of the slices with adenosine (right).

CLASSIFICATION OF ADENOSINE RECEPTORS

Investigations of the interaction of adenosine and adenosine derivatives with adenylate cyclase have provided the basis for the classification of adenosine receptors. Extracellular adenosine receptors have been subdivided into two classes depending on several pharmacological criteria and on whether adenylate cyclase is inhibited or stimulated (Table 1). These receptor types have been variously designated as R_i and R_a (9) or as A_1 and A_2 (23). Since the latter system of nomenclature is now gaining wider acceptance it will be used exclusively in this chapter.

TABLE 1. Classification of adenosine receptors

A_1 type	A_2 type
High stereospecificity for isomers of phenyl-isopropyladenosine (PIA) (L-PIA≫ D-PIA)	Low stereospecificity (L-PIA≈D.PIA)
N^6-substituted derivatives e.g. PIA or cyclohexyl-adenosine (CHA) more effective than adenosine	PIA or CHA almost as effective as adenosine
L-PIA more effective than N-ethylcarboxamido-adenosine (NECA)	NECA more effective than PIA
Inhibits adenylate cyclase	Stimulates adenylate cyclase

In addition to its actions via extracellular receptors, adenosine can also inhibit adenylate cyclase via an intracellular site, termed the P-site (8). This site differs from the extracellular sites in its structural specificity. In general, adenosine derivatives modified in the ribose moiety retain P-site activity whereas their affinities for extracellular sites are reduced.

THE RECEPTOR MEDIATING THE DEPRESSIVE ACTION OF ADENOSINE ON HIPPOCAMPAL SYNAPTIC TRANSMISSION

The availability of several of the adenosine derivatives used to distinguish between receptors of the A_1 and A_2 subtypes has made possible the identification of the class of receptor which mediates the

depressive action of adenosine on synaptic transmission in the rat hippocampal slice preparation.
Dose-response curves for the effects of various
nucleosides on hippocampal evoked EPSPs showed the
criteria for an A_1- rather than an A_2-receptor to be
fulfilled (see Table 1). In particular, the relative
effectiveness of adenosine analogues was as follows:
L-phenylisopropyladenosine (L-PIA)» D-PIA, cyclo-
hexyladenosine (CHA) > L-PIA > adenosine and L-PIA >
N-ethylcarboxamidoadenosine (NECA)(Figs.2,4; ref.14).
The receptor type mediating the synaptic action of
adenosine and its derivatives is therefore similar
to that mediating an attenuation rather than a stimulation of adenylate cyclase. These data support
previous reports that the structural requirements of
nucleoside derivatives for the depression of hippocampal evoked potentials differ from those for the
stimulation of cyclic AMP accumulation (13,22). It
remains to be shown, however, whether the action of
adenosine on synaptic transmission is mediated via a
reduction in adenylate cyclase activity or if the
A_1-receptor is in this case coupled to another, as
yet uncharacterised, effector system.

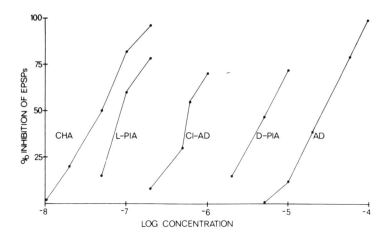

FIG. 2. Dose-reponse curves for the depression of
hippocampal evoked EPSPs by adenosine derivatives.
For methodological details see ref. 14. Abbreviations
for the derivatives are as in Table 2.

CHARACTERISATION OF ADENOSINE RECEPTORS
IN RAT BRAIN USING LIGAND BINDING TECHNIQUES

The recent availability of radioactively-labeled
nucleoside derivatives of high specific activity has

made possible a more direct approach to the study of adenosine receptors using ligand binding methods. High affinity binding sites with the characteristics of A_1-receptors have been demonstrated with ³H-CHA (1), ³H-PIA (20) and ³H-chloroadenosine (³H-Cl.AD)(26,27). Similar approaches to the A_2-receptor have been less successful due to methodological difficulties arising from the lower affinity of this receptor for nucleoside derivatives. Some indication for the presence of a binding site with properties similar to an A_2-adenosine receptor has been reported in guinea pig brain using the labeled antagonist ³H-diethylphenylxanthine (³H-DPX)(1). More recently, a site of relatively low affinity, possibly related to an A_2-receptor, which binds ³H-adenosine, ³H-CHA and ³H-NECA was shown to be present in a plasma membrane preparation from rat liver (19).

³H-CHA Binding to Rat Brain Membranes

In our studies we have employed ³H-CHA to characterise nucleoside binding sites in rat brain. A saturation curve for the binding of ³H-CHA to a crude membrane fraction from rat cerebral cortex is shown in Fig. 3a. Scatchard analysis of the data gave a curvilinear plot indicating the presence of multiple binding

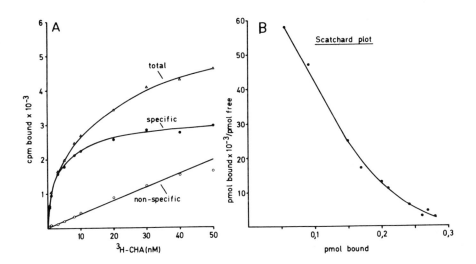

FIG. 3. Binding of ³H-CHA to a crude membrane fraction from rat cerebral cortex. Membranes (0.5 mg/ml) were incubated for 90 min. at 25° with ³H-CHA as described in ref. 14. A) Saturation curve. B) Scatchard plot.

sites or of negative cooperativity (Fig. 3b). On the
assumption of two independent binding sites, apparent
K_d values of 2.8 nM and ca. 20 nM were obtained. The
relative affinities of several substances for the high
affinity ^{3}H-CHA binding site are shown in Table 2. As
described for membranes from guinea pig and bovine
brain (1), the relative affinities of nucleoside derivatives are consistent with the properties of an A_1-
adenosine receptor. The relative abilities of CHA,
L-PIA, D-PIA and Cl.AD to inhibit ^{3}H-CHA binding are
remarkably similar to their relative effects on hippocampal evoked potentials (see Fig.4; ref.14). Further,
[3]H-CHA binding was inhibited by the methylxanthines,
caffeine, theophylline and 8-phenyltheophylline with a
rank order corresponding to their action as adenosine
receptor antagonists. On the other hand, the P-site
agonist, adenine 9,ß-D-arabinofuranoside, and several
blockers of the membrane-bound adenosine transporter
were without effects commensurate with their abilities
to interact with the P-site or adenosine carrier,

TABLE 2.   Pharmacology of high affinity ^{3}H-CHA
           binding sites in rat cerebral cortex

	K_i (nM) [a]
Nucleosides.	
Cyclohexyladenosine (CHA)	2.8
L-phenylisopropylad.(L-PIA)	3.5
2-chloroadenosine (Cl.AD)	10.5
N-ethylcarboxamidoad.(NECA)	15.0
D-PIA	150
adenine-9-ß-D-arabino-furanoside	100,000
Antagonists.	
8-phenyltheophylline	310
theophylline	10,400
caffeine	100,000
Adenosine uptake inhibitors.	
6-(nitrobenzyl)thioinosine	11,500
6-(2-OH-5-nitrobenzyl)-thioguanosine	38,500
6-(2-OH-5-nitrobenzyl)-thioinosine	100,000

[a]Calculated from displacement curves using the
relationship: $K_i = IC_{50}/(1+C/K_d)$, where C is the
concentration of ^{3}H-CHA (1 nM) and K_d is taken
from a Scatchard analysis using only labeled
ligand (2.8 nM).

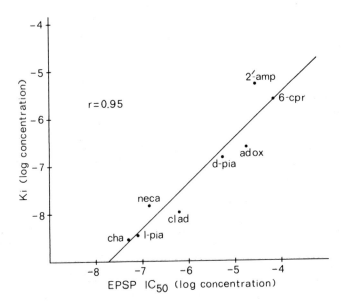

FIG. 4. Correlation between the abilities of various adenosine derivatives to depress evoked EPSPs in a hippocampal slice preparation and to inhibit the binding of ^{3}H-CHA to membranes from rat brain; adox: adenosine oxide, 6-cpr: 6-chloropurine riboside; other abbreviations as in TABLE 2.

respectively. These data strongly suggest that the high affinity ^{3}H-CHA binding site in rat brain represents an A_1-receptor of the type which mediates the depressive action of adenosine on synaptic transmission. Studies on ^{3}H-CHA binding sites might therefore be expected to lead to important insights into the extent and properties of purinergic neuromodulation in the CNS.

Subcellular Distribution of ^{3}H-CHA Binding Sites

Subcellular fractionation of rat cerebral cortex showed ^{3}H-CHA binding to be highest in a synaptosomal fraction, specific binding being enriched sixfold compared with an unfractionated membrane preparation (Table 3). The observed differences in ^{3}H-CHA binding activity appear to reflect differences in the number of binding sites rather than in affinity: curved Scatchard plots yielding apparent K_d values similar to those in crude, unfractionated membranes as in Fig. 3 were obtained with both synaptosomal and microsomal fractions (data not shown). These data are

TABLE 3. Subcellular distribtuion of ^{3}H-CHA binding
          sites in rat cerebral cortex

Fraction	Enrichment[a]
Total membranes[b]	1
nuclear fraction	1.08
microsomes	2.31
myelin	1.03
synaptosomes	6.47
mitochondria	1.50

[a]refers to cpm bound per mg protein in a given
fraction compared to the total membrane fraction.
[b]100,000 g, 1 hour pellet.

consistent with a presynaptic localisation of A_1-
adenosine receptors in the CNS, as expected by analogy
with the observed inhibition of neurotransmitter release from peripheral nerves (3). However, care must
be taken in the interpretation of data from subcellular
fractionation experiments since synaptosomal fractions
also contain membrane fragments from other sources.
This must be borne in mind especially when dealing with
A_1-adenosine receptors since they have been reported
to be present in primary cultures from foetal rat
brain which are enriched in astrocytes (23).

Regional Distribution of ^{3}H-CHA Binding Sites in Rat Brain

[3]H-CHA binding sites are widely distributed in the
mammalian CNS being particularly enriched in the hippocampus (7,11). Their distribution in the hippocampus
as revealed by autoradiography of labeled brain sections, is quite heterogeneous (Fig. 5). In general,
cell body regions exhibit sparse labeling while dendritic zones are positive for ^{3}H-CHA binding. Dense
labeling is observed in: 1) CA1 apical and basal dendritic zones, 2) granule cell dendritic zone, and
3) CA3 basal dendritic zone. Less ^{3}H-CHA binding is
observed in the apical dendritic region of CA3
than the basal part. Assuming that this labeling is
associated with synaptic structures this would imply
a different degree of purinergic modulation of synapses forming contacts with different regions of the
CA3 pyramidal cells.

The high density of labeling in CA1 corresponds to
the presence of considerable activity of 5'-nucleo-
tidase, the enzyme responsible for the extracellular
formation of adenosine from 5'-AMP, whereas the basal
dendrites of CA3, which bind ^{3}H-CHA, are relatively

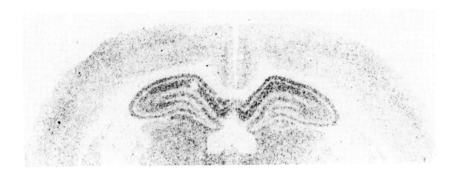

FIG. 5. Autoradiograph of ^{3}H-CHA binding to rat brain.
Cryostat sections were incubated for 90 min at 25°
with 5 nM ^{3}H-CHA and exposed as in (7).

poor in the enzyme (17). The functional significance
of differences in the relationship between adenosine
formation and receptor concentration remains to be
explored.

A_1-RECEPTOR CONCENTRATION AS A DETERMINANT OF THE
STRENGTH OF ADENOSINE-MEDIATED NEUROMODULATION

The heterogeneous distribution of A_1-adenosine receptors in rat brain raises the question as to the
functional significance of differences in receptor
density. The theoretical implications of differences
in receptor number have been considered by Williams
and Lefkowitz (24) in a discussion of the regulation
of ß-adrenergic receptors. In the case of receptors
tightly bound to an effector system (such that occu-
pation of each receptor site evokes a response) an
increase in the number of receptors would lead to an
increase in the maximal response without a change in
apparent affinity (i.e. EC_{50} or IC_{50}). Alternatively,
if 'spare' receptors are present, i.e. if only a small
number of receptors must be occupied to evoke a maximal
response, increasing the number of receptors would lead
to a shift in the dose-response relationship to the
left (i.e. an increase in apparent affinity) without
any change in maximal response.
We were able to approach this problem in a relatively
homogeneous cell population by comparing the concentration of A_1-adenosine receptors in the CA1 region of
the rat hippocampus with the effects of adenosine on
evoked EPSPs in the same region. This was made possible by the intriguing observation that membranes
prepared from the dorsal aspect of the hippocampus

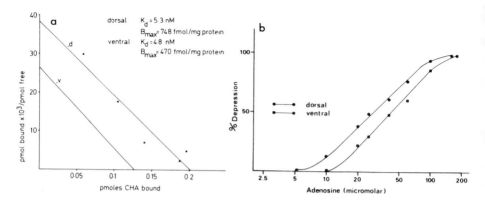

FIG. 6.   (A) Scatchard plot of ³H-CHA binding to crude
membranes from dorsal (d) and ventral (v)hippocampus.
The similarity in slopes and the differences in inter-
cept with the abscissa indicate a difference in number
of binding sites rather than in affinity. For convenience, the data were analysed as a straight line plot
as opposed to a curvilinear plot as shown in FIG. 3.
(B) Dose-response curves for the depression of evoked
EPSPs by adenosine in slices from the dorsal (d) or
ventral (v) hippocampus. Stimuli were applied as
shown in FIG. 1.

bound more ³H-CHA than did those from the ventral
part (6). This was due to a difference in the number
of binding sites rather than in affinity (Fig. 6a) and
was also observed in membranes from the CA1 area of
these hippocampal regions.
    Analysis of dose-reponse curves for adenosine in the
CA1 region of slices from the dorsal and ventral hippocampus suggests the presence of spare A₁-adenosine
receptors. First, the fact that in both regions
adenosine at high enough concentrations will completely abolish evoked EPSPs indicates the presence of
A₁-receptors on the majority of activated neurons.
The difference in receptor number in these regions can
therefore be taken to indicate that neurons in the
CA1 region of the dorsal hippocampus carry more A₁-receptors than their more ventral counterparts. A consequence of this higher receptor concentration is a
shift to the left of the dose-response curve for the
action of adenosine on evoked EPSPs in this region
compared to the ventral slices (Fig. 6b). A given
concentration of adenosine thus evoked a greater response in the CA1 neurons of the dorsal than in the
ventral hippocampus. The maximum response, however,
is the same in both regions. These data suggest the
presence of spare A₁-adenosine receptors on hippocampal

neurons and indicate that the concentration of A_1-receptors in a neuronal population is an important determinant of the strength of adenosine action. Differences in the distribution, or changes in the concentration of A_1-receptors would therefore have important consequences for the strength of purinergic neuromodulation.

CONCLUSION

The purine, adenosine, exerts a powerful depressive action on synaptic transmission in neurons of the rat hippocampus. This effect is mediated by a receptor of the A_1 subclass, which would inhibit rather than stimulate adenylate cyclase. The depression of evoked potentials by adenosine is therefore not mediated by a simple second messenger scheme involving an increase in adenylate cyclase activity. On the other hand, it remains to be established whether a decrease in cyclic AMP synthesis mediates this effect, or if the A_1-receptor is in this case coupled to a different effector system.
The A_1-adenosine receptor has been further characterised in rat brain using ligand binding techniques. High affinity binding sites for the potent A_1-receptor agonist, ^3H-CHA, show a specific distribution in the CNS. It could be shown in a relatively homogeneous neuronal population in the hippocampus that the number of adenosine receptors is an important factor determining the strength of adenosine action. The availability of both biochemical and in vitro electrophysiological techniques for approaching the effects of adenosine on central neurons provides an imporant tool for the further investigation of purinergic neuromodulation.

REFERENCES

1. Bruns, R.F., Daly, J.W. and Snyder, S.H. (1980):
   Proc. Natl. Acad. Sci. USA. 77:5547-5551.
2. Daly, J.W. (1977): 'Cyclic Nucleotides in the
   Nervous System'. Plenum Press, New York.
3. Fredholm, B.B. and Hedqvist, P. (1980): Biochem.
   Pharmacol., 29:1635-1643.
4. Huang, M. and Daly, J.W. (1974): Life Sci., 14:
   489-503.
5. Kuroda, Y., Saito, M. and Kobayashi, K. (1976):
   Brain Res., 109:196-201.
6. Lee, K.S., Reddington, M., Schubert, P. and
   Kreutzberg, G.W. (1982): Brain Res. (in press).
7. Lewis, M.E., Patel, J., Edley, S.M. and Marangos,
   P.J. (1981): Eur. J. Pharmacol., 73:109-110.

8. Londos,C. and Wolff, J. (1977): Proc. Natl. Acad. Sci.USA, 74:5482-5486.
9. Londos,C., Cooper, D.M.F. and Wolff, J. (1980): Proc. Natl. Acad. Sci. USA, 77:2551-2554.
10. Lynch, G. and Schubert, P. (1980) Ann. Rev. Neurosci., 3:1-22.
11. Murray, T.F. and Cheney, D.L. (1982): Neuropharmacology, 21:575-580.
12. Phillis, J.W. and Wu, P.H. (1981): Prog. Neurobiol. 16:187-239.
13. Reddington, M. and Schubert, P. (1979): Neurosci. Lett., 14:37-42.
14. Reddington, M., Lee, K.S. and Schubert, P. (1982) Neurosci. Lett., 28:275-279.
15. Sattin, A. and Rall, T.W. (1970): Mol. Pharmacol., 6:13-23.
16. Schubert, P. and Mitzdorf, U. (1979): Brain Res., 172:186-190.
17. Schubert, P., Komp, W. and Kreutzberg, G.W. (1979): Brain Res., 168:419-424.
18. Schubert, P., Lee, K.S., Reddington, M. and Kreutzberg, G.W. (1982): In 'Molecular, Cellular and Behavioral Neurobiology of the Hippocampus', edited by W. Seifert (in press) Academic Press, London.
19. Schütz, W., Tuisl, E. and Kraupp, O. (1982): N.-S. Arch. Pharmacol., 319:34-39.
20. Schwabe, U. and Trost, T. (1980): N.-S. Arch. Pharmacol., 313:179-187.
21. Siggins, G.R. and Schubert, P. (1981): Neurosci. Lett., 23:55-60.
22. Smellie, F.W., Daly, J.W., Dunwiddie, T.V. and Hoffer, B.J. (1979): Life Sci., 25:1739-1748.
23. Van Calker, D., Müller, M. and Hamprecht, B. (1979) J. Neurochem., 33:999-1005.
24. Williams, L. and Lefkowitz, R.J. (1978): 'Receptor Binding Studies in Adrenergic Pharmacology', Raven Press, New York.
25. Williams, M. (1982): In 'Handbook of Neurochemistry Vol. 6', edited by N. Marks and R. Rodnight (in press). Plenum Press, New York.
26. Williams, M. and Risley, E.A. (1980): Proc. Natl. Acad. Sci. USA, 77:6892-6896.
27. Wu, P.H., Phillis, J.W., Balls, K. and Rinaldi, B. (1980): Can. J. Pharmacol., 58:576-579.

CNS Receptors—From Molecular
Pharmacology to Behavior, edited by
P. Mandel and F. V. DeFeudis.
Raven Press, New York © 1983.

Specific Binding of Radiolabelled Antidepressants to Brain Astroglial Cells

Patricia M. Whitaker and Jerry J. Warsh

Clarke Institute of Psychiatry, Toronto, Canada

In the past two decades, it has become generally accepted that functional alterations of central neurotransmitter systems, such as serotonin or noradrenaline, may contribute to the appearance of depressive disorders (1,7,36). Consequently, much of the research on depression has been directed towards identifying these specific neurochemical changes, often by studying the mechanism of action of the psychotropic drugs used to treat the disorder. A commonly studied group of drugs, therefore, are the tricyclic antidepressants, such as imipramine, a number of which are available in a radiolabelled form of high enough specific activity to be used in direct binding assays. Similarily, the atypical antidepressant mianserin is also available for use in binding assays.

Most of the research on neurotransmitter function in affective disorders has focused on the neuronal systems themselves and extraneuronal influences have been virtually ignored. Recently, however, a number of reports have appeared suggesting that astrocytic glial cells may have a major role in modulating neurotransmission and may thus be a target of antidepressant action.

For example, astroglial cells have been shown to have a high capacity active transport system for GABA (17), noradrenaline (14, 28), dopamine (28) and serotonin (14, 33). The removal of transmitter from post-synaptic sites effectively eliminates continued neurotransmission. The clearance of neurotransmitter from the synapse by glial uptake, therefore, may be a major means by which these cells modulate neurotransmission. If one of the means by which antidepressants exert their therapeutic effect is by inhibition of uptake processes, as has been suggested (8,20), then the site of action of these drugs may actually be on glial cells rather than, or in addition to, neuronal cells.

In addition to neurotransmitter uptake inhibition, antidepressants may also exert their effects by interactions with specific receptor sites. These drugs may have an acute effect on serotonergic (31), alpha-adrenergic (35), histaminergic (34) and muscarinic cholinergic (10, 32) receptors. After chronic treatment with antidepressants, their effects are also evident on serotonergic (21, 29), beta-adrenergic (5) and possibly dopaminergic (2, 22) receptors. Astroglial cells possess a number of these specific receptor sites for neurotransmitters. These include beta-adrenergic receptors (3, 25), dopaminergic receptors (15, 16) muscarinic cholinergic receptors (12) and serotonergic receptors (9, 18). The beta-adrenergic (11, 25) and possibly also the serotonergic (9) receptors are linked to adenylate cyclase. One recent report has shown that the beta-adrenergic linked cyclase is down-regulated in astroglial cells after prolonged exposure to antidepressants (19).

In consequence of these findings, we began studying the possible role of brain astroglial cells as the site of action of antidepressants, by observing the interactions of radiolabelled antidepressants with the rat clonal astroglial cell line C_6. We report here principally our findings with ^{3}H-imipramine and also some preliminary results with ^{3}H-mianserin, both of which bind in a saturable high affinity manner to glial cells.

METHODS

Culturing of C_6 glial cells

Cells were grown in plastic tissue culture flasks (Falcon, 75 cm^2 surface area) in 25 ml of F_{10} growth media supplemented with 15% heat-inactivated horse serum and 2.5% heat-inactivated fetal calf serum and containing 200 units/ml penicillin-G and 200 mcg/ml of streptomycin. The flasks were incubated in a humidified atmosphere of 5% CO_2 and 95% air at 37° C. The medium was changed every three days.

For subculturing, monolayer colonies were washed and briefly incubated with 0.1% Viokase (Gibco) in phosphate-buffered saline (140 mM NaCl, 3 mM KCl, 0.15 mM KH_2PO_4, 8 mM Na_2HPO_4, pH=7.1). The cells were then resuspended in growth media and diluted one to ten into fresh culturing flasks.

The astrocytic nature of the colonies was checked periodically by an indirect immunocytochemical procedure using an antibody to glial fibrillatory acidic protein.

Direct binding assays using ^{3}H-imipramine

Glial cells were prepared for use in the assays by rinsing twice
with buffer (120 mM NaCl, 5 mM KCl, 50 MM Tris, pH=7.4) and then
harvested by scraping with a rubber policeman. The cells were
resuspended in buffer at a final concentraion of 2.5-3.0 million
cells/0.2 ml and sonicated for 10 seconds.

^{3}H-imipramine binding to glial cells was assayed in triplicate
at five different concentrations of radioligand ranging from 0.6
to 6.0 nM. For competition studies a radioligand concentration
of 0.75 nM was used. Desipramine at a final concentration of
1,000 nM was used to define specific binding.

The following aliquots were incubated at 0-4° C   for 90 min :
0.1 ml ^{3}H-imipramine, 0.1 ml   buffer or buffer containing
desipramine or (for the competition studies) competing drugs, and
0.2 ml   cell suspension. Following incubation 0.2 ml   from
each test tube was diluted into 4.0 ml   of buffer and filtered
under vacuum through Whatman GF/B filters. Filters were washed
three times with 4.0 ml   of buffer each time before being placed
in liquid scintillation vials with 10 ml   Aquasol (New England
Nuclear) for counting.

Drugs for these studies were kindly donated by Astra Lakemedel
Ab (zimelidine, norzimelidine), Rhone-Poulenc Pharma Inc.
(mepyramine), Ciba-Geigy (chlorimipramine, imipramine,
desipramine) and Lilly Research Laboratories (fluoxetine).

Direct binding assays using ^{3}H-mianserin. The preparation of
glial cells was the same as that described for ^{3}H-imipramine
binding but the buffer was 50 mM Tris alone.

Binding of ^{3}H-mianserin was determined at ten different ligand
concentrations ranging from 0.1 to 10 nM. Specific binding was
defined by 500 nM unlabeled mianserin. The following aliquots
were incubated for 30 min   at room temperature: 0.2 ml
radioligand, 0.2 ml   buffer or buffer containing unlabelled
mianserin, and 0.2 ml   cell suspension. After incubation, 3.5
ml of buffer were introduced into each tube and the entire
contents filtered under vacuum through Whatman GF/B filters. The
tubes were rinsed with a further 3.5 ml   of buffer and the
contents again filtered. The filters were placed into liquid
scintillation counting vials with 10 ml   Aquasol and the
radioactivity counted.

^{3}H-serotonin uptake into C$_6$ glial cells. Cells were prepared as
described above but Hank's balanced salt solution was used for
rinsing and resuspending at a final concentration of 12.5 to 15
million cells/ml.

For measuring uptake the following aliquots were incubated at

$37^\circ C$ (for total uptake) or $0^\circ C$ (for nonspecific uptake) for 8 min : 0.2 ml cell suspension, 0.1 ml of ^{3}H-serotonin (final concentration ranging from 250 to 2,000 nM), and 1.7 ml Hank's balanced salt solution. Active uptake was stopped by placing the tubes into ice . Cells were pelleted by centrifugation (21,000 g for 15 min) at $4^\circ C$. The supernatant was aspirated and the cells were resuspended in 1.0 ml distilled water and frozen ($-20^\circ C$) overnight. Cells were then thawed and a 0.5-ml aliquot placed in a liquid scintillation vial with 10.0 ml Aquasol for counting radioactivity.

RESULTS

Scatchard analysis (30) of astroglial sites labelled with ^{3}H-imipramine revealed apparently only one type of saturable high affinity non-interacting site with a K_D of 1.72 nM and a B_{max} of 202 fmoles/mg protein. Analysis of ^{3}H-mianserin binding revealed one type of site which was saturable and had a K_D of 3.9 nM and a B_{max} of 116 fmoles/mg protein.

Competition curves of various tricyclic antidepressants and other drugs on ^{3}H-imipramine labelled sites were steep with radioligand binding totally inhibited over a one-hundredfold range of competing ligand concentrations. This type of competition curve further suggests that the radioligand labels only one type of site (38) (Fig. 1.). The IC_{50} values (concentration of a drug which reduces radioligand binding by 50%) of a series of drugs are given in Table 1.

Results of ^{3}H-serotonin uptake into C_6 cells are given in Fig. 2.

Table 1. The IC_{50} Values of Drugs Competing for Sites on Astroglial Cells Labelled by ^{3}H- Imipramine

Drug	IC_{50} (nM)
Antidepressants	
Amitriptyline	76
Chlorimipramine	80
Nortriptyline	100
Desipramine	116
Serotonin Uptake Inhibitors	
Fluoxetine	78
Zimelidine	194
Norzimelidine	408
Others	
Chlorpromazine	74
Mepyramine	102

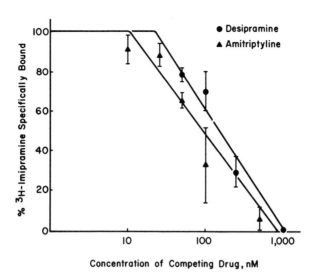

FIG.1 Competition curves of two tricyclic antidepressants for sites labelled by ^{3}H-imipramine in C_6
astroglial cells. Each point represents the mean of at
least three determinations done in triplicate.

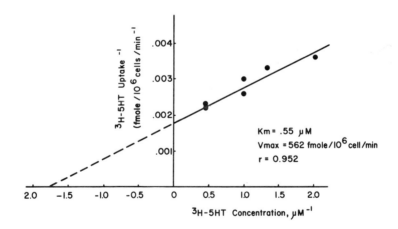

FIG.2 ^{3}H-serotonin uptake by C_6 astroglial cells. Each
point represents a single determination done in
triplicate.

DISCUSSION

A major difficulty in any study investigating the functions of astroglial cells is the problem of obtaining a source of pure cells which have the metabolic and morphological properties of the cell in vivo. Bulk isolation procedures from fresh brain result in a poor yield of cells. Furthermore, the non-physiological nature of the methods used may lead to destruction of some types of receptors (12). This may explain the results of an earlier study investigating ^{3}H-imipramine binding in glial fractions which failed to show any binding (6). Perhaps the most normal astrocyte population to study are those grown as primary cultures; however the exact nature and purity of the resulting cells may vary from lab to lab. The C_6 cell line, although derived originally from a chemically-induced tumour, is considered a good model of astrocytes in vivo (4). Furthermore, the cell line is readily available, allowing investigators in different laboratories to compare results.

On the basis of binding studies following lesions of serotonergic pathways, several recent investigations have suggested that the ^{3}H-imipramine binding site is associated with, or identical to, the pre-synaptic serotonin uptake site (24,27). Although it is possible that a certain amount of ^{3}H-imipramine binding in brain does occur pre-synaptically, the criteria of decreased binding after lesioning for showing pre-synaptic occurrence may not be entirely valid. There are at least two other explanations for the loss of sites after lesions. Binding sites occurring post-synaptically may also degenerate following removal of the innervating neuron (13). Another possibility is that the binding sites occur to a large extent on astroglial cells. Following a lesion, astrocytes surrounding an affected synapse undergo extensive morphological changes becoming capable of considerable phagocytic activity. It is possible that during these reactive changes some normally occurring membrane properties, such as binding sites for ^{3}H-imipramine, are lost.

An additional finding which argues against ^{3}H-imipramine labelling exclusively pre-synaptic uptake sites, is the work of Laduron et. al. (23). These workers showed that after subcellular fractionation of rat cortex, the fractions richest in ^{3}H-imipramine binding do not correlate with the fractions highest in serotonin uptake.

It is possible that ^{3}H-imipramine labels a variety of sites on astroglial cells. Although shallow competition curves are usually observed when multiple sites are being labelled, this is not always the case, especially if the competing ligand does not have a high degree of selectivity for sites being labelled (38).

One site labelled by ^{3}H-imipramine may be a serotonin transporting site. To test this hypothesis, we have quantified serotonin uptake into our cell line and we are currently investigating the inhibitory effects of tricyclic antidepressants and specific serotonin uptake inhibitors on this uptake. However, there are other sites which our data suggests may also be labelled. The relatively high potency of compounds such as mepyramine and chlorpromazine, substances not known to inhibit serotonin uptake, is suggestive of histamine receptor involvement. Although to date there are no reports of histamine receptors associated with astroglial cells, it is known that in whole brain antidepressants do interact with a histamine receptor (35). Furthermore, the labelling of sites on glial cells by ^{3}H-mianserin could indicate the presence of histamine receptors, as this ligand is known to label these receptors (37). We are therefore beginning work aimed at assessing the possible occurrence of histamine receptors on C_6 cells. As other studies have shown the possible involvement of alpha-adrenergic, serotonergic and muscarinic cholinergic receptors in antidepressant drug action, we will expand our studies to include a search for these receptor types as well.

CONCLUSION

The neuromodulatory capability of brain astroglial cells has long been overlooked as a possible means by which psychotropic drugs exert their effects. The presence of high affinity binding sites for at least two different antidepressants on C_6 cells indicate the role these cells may play in antidepressant drug action in general. Further studies using the C_6 cell line, as well as primary cultures and bulk isolated cells, are being undertaken in order to assess the physiological significance of these sites.

ACKNOWLEDGEMENTS

The skilled technical assistance of Carley Vint and Rosemary Morin is gratefully acknowledged. The manuscript was prepared with the secretarial assistance of Mrs. Susan McNally. This work is supported by a grant from the Medical Research Council of Canada.

REFERENCES

1. Adolphe, A.B., Dorsey, E.R. and Napoliello, M.J. (1977): Dis. Nerv. System, 38(10):841-846.

2. Antelman, S.M. and Chiodo, L.A. (1981): Biol. Psychiatry, 16(8):717-727.
3. Barovsky, K. and Brooker, G. (1980): J. Cyclic Nucleotide Res., 6(4):297-307.
4. Benda, P., Lightbody, J., Sato, G., Levine, L. and Sweet, W. (1968): Science, 161:370-371.
5. Bergstrom, D.A. and Kellar, K.J. (1979): J. Pharmacol. Exp. Ther., 209:256-261.
6. Briley, M.S., Fillion, G., Beaudoin, D., Fillion, M.P. and Langer, S.Z. (1980): Eur. J. Pharmacol. 64:191-194.
7. Bunney, W.E. (1975): Psychopharmacol. Comm., 1:596-609.
8. Carlsson, A., Jonason, J., Lindqvist, M. and Fuxe, K. (1969): Brain Res., 12:456-460.
9. Fillion, G., Beaudoin, D., Rouselle, J.C. and Jacob, J. (1980): Brain. Res.:361-374.
10. Fjalland, B., Christensen, A.V. and Hyttel, J. (1977): Naunyn-Schmiedberg's Arch. Pharmacol., 301:5-9.
11. Gilman, A.G. and Nirenberg, M. (1971): Proc. Natl. Acad. Sci., 68:2165-2168.
12. Guainieri, M., Krell, L.S., McKhann, G.M., Pasternak, G.W. and Yamamura, H.I. (1975): Brain Res., 93:337-342.
13. Hattori,T. and Fibiger, H.C. (1982): Brain Res., 238:245-250.
14. Henn, F.A. and Hamberger, A. (1971): Proc. Natl. Acad. Sci., 69(11):2686-2690.
15. Henn, F.A., Anderson, D.J. and Sellstrom,A. (1977): Nature, 266:637-638.
16. Henn, F.A. and Henn, S.W. (1980): Prog. Neurobiol., 15:1-17.
17. Hertz, L., Schousboe, A., Boechler, N., Mukerji, S. and Fedoroff, S. (1978): Neurochem. Res., 3:1-14.
18. Hertz, L., Baldwin, F. and Schousboe, A. (1979): Can. J. Physiol. Pharmacol., 57:223-226.
19. Hertz, L., Mukerji, S. and Richardson, J.S. (1981): Eur. J. Pharmacol., 72:267-268.
20. Iversen, L.L. (1965): J. Pharm. Pharmacol., 17:62-64.
21. Kellar, K.J., Cascio, C.S., Butler, J.A. and Kurtzke, R.N. (1981): Eur. J. Pharmacol., 69:515-518.
22. Koide, T. and Matsushita, H. (1981): Life. Sci., 28: 1139-1145.
23. Laduron, P.M., Robbyns, M. and Schotte, A. (1982): Eur. J. Pharmacol., 78:491-493.
24. Langer, S.Z., Moret, C., Raisman, R.,Dubocovich, M.L. and Briley, M. (1980): Science, 210:1133-1135.
25. Lucas, M. and Bockaert, J. (1977): Mol. Pharmacol., 13: 314-329.
26. Maas, J.W. (1975): Arch. Gen. Psychiatr., 32:1357-1361.
27. Paul., S.M., Rehavi, M., Rice, K.C., Ittah, Y. and Skolnick, P. (1981): Life Sci., 28:2753-2760.
28. Pelton, E.W., Kimelberg, H.K., Shipherd, S.V. and Bourke, R.S. (1981): Life. Sci., 28:1655-1663.
29. Savage, D.D.,. Mendels, J. and Frazer, A. (1980): Neuropharmacology, 19:1063-1070.
30. Scatchard, G. (1949): Ann. N. Y. Acad. Sci., 51:660-672.

31. Seeman, P., Westman, K., Coscina, D. and Warsh, J.J. (1980): Eur. J. Pharmacol., 66:179-191.
32. Snyder, S.H. and Yamamura, H.I. (1977): Arch. Gen. Psych., 34: 236-239.
33. Suddith, R.L., Hutchinson, H.T. and Haber, B. (1978): Life Sci., 22:2179-2188.
34. Taylor, J.E. and Richelson, E. (1980): Eur. J. Pharmacol., 67:41-46.
35. U'Prichard, D.C., Greenberg, D.A., Sheehan, P.P. and Snyder, S.H. (1978): Science, 199:197-198.
36. Van Praag, H.M. (1980): Compr. Psychiat., 21(1):30-54.
37. Whitaker, P.M. and Cross, A.J. (1980): Biochem. Pharmacol., 29:2709-2712.
38. Whitaker, P.M., Kish, S.J., and Madras, B.K. (1982): Rev. in Pure and Applied Pharmacol. Sci., manuscript submitted.
39. Zaborszky, L., Leranth, C. and Palkovits, M. (1978): Brain Res. Bull., 4:99-117.

Subject Index

Subject Index

NOTE: British and American spellings are used in the text. For consistency, this index uses American spellings only.